Fundamentals of
KINESIOLOGY
Second Edition

Mississippi State University

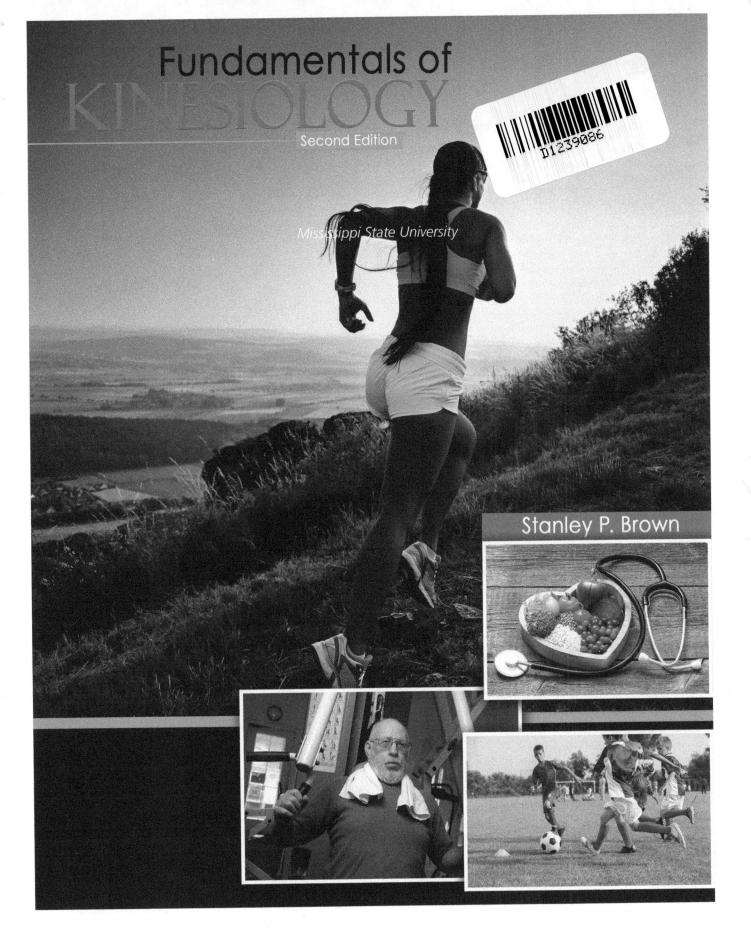

Stanley P. Brown

Kendall Hunt
p u b l i s h i n g   c o m p a n y

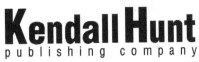

Cover image © Shutterstock, Inc.

Kendall Hunt
publishing company

www.kendallhunt.com
Send all inquiries to:
4050 Westmark Drive
Dubuque, IA 52004-1840

Copyright © 2013, 2016 by Kendall Hunt Publishing Company

ISBN 978-1-4652-9768-6

Printed in the United States of America

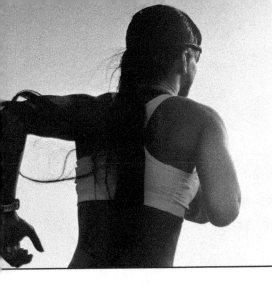

CONTENTS

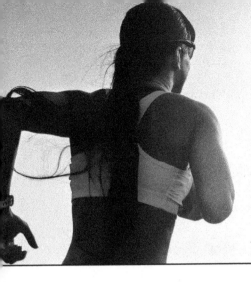

ACKNOWLEDGMENT

CHAPTER 1:

Stanley P. Brown, Ph.D.
Professor of Clinical Exercise Physiology
Department of Kinesiology
Mississippi State University

Gregg Twietmeyer, Ph.D.
Assistant Professor of Sport Studies
Department of Kinesiology
Mississippi State University

CHAPTER 2:

Synthia Sydnor, Ph.D.
Associate Professor of Kinesiology
Department of Kinesiology and Community Health
University of Illinois at Urbana-Champaign

CHAPTER 3:

Stamatis Agiovlasitis, Ph.D.
Associate Professor of Clinical Exercise Physiology
and Disability
Department of Kinesiology
Mississippi State University

CHAPTER 4:

Stanley P. Brown, Ph.D.
Professor of Clinical Exercise Physiology
Head, Department of Kinesiology
Mississippi State University

CHAPTER 5:

Matthew A. Masucci, Ph.D.
Associate Professor of Interdisciplinary Sport Studies
Chair, Department of Kinesiology
San José State University

CHAPTER 6:

Adam Love, Ph.D.
Assistant Professor of Socio-Cultural
Studies in Recreation and Sport
Management
Department of Kinesiology, Recreation,
and Sport Studies
University of Tennessee

Lars Dzikus, Ph.D.
Associate Professor of Sport Studies
Department of Kinesiology, Recreation,
and Sport Studies
University of Tennessee

CHAPTER 7:

Adam Love, Ph.D.
Professor of Socio-Cultural Studies in Recreation
and Sport Management
Department of Kinesiology, Recreation,
and Sport Studies
University of Tennessee

Brian Gearity, Ph.D.
Clinical Assistant Professor
Director of Master's of Art
in Sport Coaching
Graduate School of Professional
Psychology
University of Denver

CHAPTER 8:

Stanley P. Brown, Ph.D.
Professor of Clinical Exercise Physiology
Head, Department of Kinesiology
Mississippi State University

CHAPTER 9:

Andreas Kavazis, Ph.D.
Associate Professor
Director, Muscle Biochemistry Laboratory
School of Kinesiology
Auburn University

CHAPTER 10:

Megan Elizabeth Holmes, Ph.D.
Assistant Professor of Exercise Epidemiology
Department of Kinesiology
Mississippi State University

CHAPTER 11:

John Lamberth, Ph.D.
Associate Professor of Anatomical Kinesiology
Department of Kinesiology
Mississippi State University

Adam C. Knight, Ph.D.
Associate Professor of Biomechanics
Department of Kinesiology
Mississippi State University

CHAPTER 12:

Adam C. Knight, Ph.D.
Associate Professor of Biomechanics
Department of Kinesiology
Mississippi State University

CHAPTER 13:

Heather E. Webb, Ph.D., ATC, LAT
Associate Professor of Exercise and Sport Science
Department of Kinesiology
Texas A&M University, Corpus Christie

CHAPTER 14:

Leah E. Robinson, Ph.D.
Associate Professor of Kinesiology
School of Kinesiology
Research Associate Professor, Center for
Human Growth and Development
University of Michigan

Kara K. Palmer, M.Ed.
School of Kinesiology
University of Michigan

CHAPTER 15:

Kathleen T. Foley, PhD, OTR/L
Associate Professor

School of Occupational Therapy
Brenau University

Patricia L. Perez, PT, DScPT, OCS
Assistant Professor
Department of Physical Therapy
University of Alabama at Birmingham

CHAPTER 16:

George L. Hoyt, III, Ph.D.
Professor of Kinesiology
Chair, Department of Kinesiology
Methodist University

Stanley P. Brown, Ph.D.
Professor of Clinical Exercise
Physiology
Head, Department of Kinesiology
Mississippi State University

CHAPTER 17:

Pei-Chun Hsieh, Ph.D., CTRS
Assistant Professor
Department of Rehabilitation Sciences
Temple University

CHAPTER 18:

James M. Rankin, Ph.D., AT, ATC
Associate Professor of Athletic Training
Department of Kinesiology
University of Toledo

CHAPTER 19:

Katherine J. Coffey, PED
Associate Clinical Professor of Kinesiology
Department of Kinesiology
Texas Women's University

CHAPTER 20:

B. Christine Green, Ph.D.
Professor of Recreation, Sport & Tourism
Director, Sport+Development Laboratory
Department of Recreation, Sport
and Tourism
University of Illinois at Urbana-Champaign

Laurence Chalip, Ph.D.
Professor of Recreation, Sport
and Tourism
Department of Recreation, Sport
and Tourism
University of Illinois at Urbana-Champaign

CHAPTER 21:

Donald L. Rockey, Jr. Ph.D.
Associate Professor of Recreation and Sport Studies
Department of Kinesiology, Recreation
and Sport Studies
Coastal Carolina University

CHAPTER 22:

Stanley P. Brown, Ph.D.
Professor of Clinical Exercise Physiology
Head, Department of Kinesiology

Benjamin Wax, Ph.D.
Associate Professor of Kinesiology
Division of Education
Mississippi State University – Meridian Campus

Matthew McAllister, Ph.D.
Assistant Professor of Exercise Physiology
Department of Kinesiology
Mississippi State University

CHAPTER 23:

Guy Hornsby, Ph.D.
Assistant Professor of Exercise Science
Department of Health and Physical Education
Glenville State College

Margaret E. Stone, M.S.
Director, Center of Excellence for Sport Science and
Coach Education Director, Olympic Training Site
East Tennessee State University

Michael H. Stone, Ph.D.
Associate Professor of Exercise Science
Department of Exercise and Sport Science
East Tennessee State University

CHAPTER 24:

Stanley P. Brown, Ph.D.
Professor of Clinical Exercise Physiology
Head, Department of Kinesiology
Mississippi State University

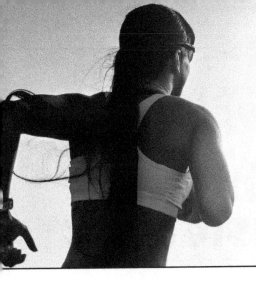

The ability to move is as basic to human nature as the ability to think and reason. Given the historic importance of mobility to survival, and in more contemporary times to health, it is no wonder that what we call *kinesiology*, the science of movement, developed into a distinct academic field. The study of physical activity, exercise, and sport is at its apex; not since the ancient Greeks has the *sound mind in a sound body* concept taken on such prominence.

Part One of *Fundamentals of Kinesiology* explores how the academic discipline came to be (Chapter 1) and the importance of studying movement using cultural studies as a model (Chapter 2). We then examine the impact of disability on society (Chapter 3) and survey relevant professional issues important to the field of kinesiology (Chapter 4).

The adage, "With time comes change," rings true with respect to the old field of physical education. Within one generation sweeping changes occurred to create the fastest growing discipline in higher education today. The opportunities that await students of kinesiology upon graduation have greatly expanded since the days when physical education defined the extent and scope of the field. This book presents a comprehensive treatment of these opportunities.

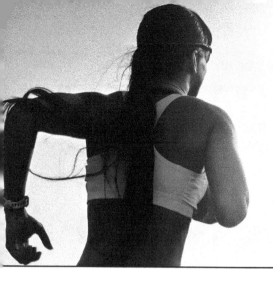

Chapter 1

INTRODUCTION TO KINESIOLOGY

OUTLINE

OBJECTIVES

1. Describe the relationship among kinesiology, exercise science, sport studies, and physical education.
2. Explain the meaning of interdisciplinary, crossdisciplinary, transdisciplinary, and multidisciplinary.
3. Describe the contributions of scientists during the development of the foundations of the exercise sciences.
4. Identify the events that precipitated the emergence of kinesiology as a transdisciplinary field.
5. Identify and discuss the roles of individuals and cultures that have made important contributions to the history of kinesiology.

Kine comes from two Greek words—kinesis (movement) and kinein (to move).

The ability to move is basic to our nature, affecting all human endeavors. In its richest sense, *kinesis* or motion is at the very heart of our being. As Twietmeyer has argued, "motion is a fundamental aspect of human nature, encompassing all that human beings are and do" (19). Therefore, it is not surprising that throughout history, various cultures have explored human movement, often ascribing deep significance to it. We perceive the world around us through our senses and with an inquisitive mind; however, more than anything else inherent to our being, it is the ability to move that allows us to interact with a constantly changing environment and the threats and challenges of the world around us.

Early humans had to teach and learn physical skills to survive. This, "physical education," if you will, has been considered by some to be the first rudimentary attempts at instruction in the psychomotor realm of learning. It had numerous purposes. For example, some physical activities were taught for survival and may have included things such as boating, fishing, fowling, and hunting, usually for the purpose of seeking food, clothing, and shelter. However, there were other reasons for teaching physical skills. Acrobatics, board games, chance games, guessing games, and various sporting pursuits were used for entertainment purposes. Military training required instruction in archery, boxing, sword play, chariot racing, gladiatorial events, jumping contests, running, equestrian activities, and wrestling. Access to many of these activities was usually determined by citizenship, social status, and wealth, and may even have been tied to rites of passage rituals for advancement to adulthood.

Most life activities require the ability to move. Today, the types of activities may be vastly different, but movement, whether engaged in for work, leisure, or other forms of human pursuit is still essential. When that ability is removed, something truly precious has been lost and people in such a state suffer as a result. This point can be seen empirically in our own experience whether by reflecting on a past injury or on the cessation of one's participation in a sport or recreation activity. An injury, for example, which results in a lack of mobility, always makes one appreciate the "rudimentary" skills one has temporarily lost (such as walking, jumping, or throwing). Moreover, in the most fundamental sense, to cease moving "is not simply to become sedentary, but to cease being human. It is death" (19). Movement, therefore, is a central aspect of human experience. To be human is to move, though not everyone can do so with equal ability due to genetic predisposition, physical trauma, or illness. With scientific discovery progressing at an exponential rate, it is no wonder that the science of movement, what has come to be known as *Kinesiology*, has developed as an academic discipline.

Kinesiology has a rich history, primarily traced through its precursor, physical education. The term, kinesiology, is only a little more than 100 years old having first been used in 1894 as the basis of the title of a textbook exploring educational gymnastics. Through most of the intervening century, the word was associated with an academic course of various titles. It was not until 1967 that the world's first Department of Kinesiology was launched at the University of Waterloo in Canada. Since then, academic departments centered on physical education and/or exercise science have changed their title to kinesiology in ever-increasing numbers. The next section explores why this may be the best model to adopt.

THE ACADEMIC SETTING

The last half of this chapter is devoted to discovering the roots of kinesiology as an academic field. First, however, the chapter explores how kinesiology fits within the framework of higher education. It is important for students to grasp how the study of movement intersects with a broad spectrum of the sciences and the humanities, fields of study that typically comprise university curricula and that serve kinesiology as parent disciplines.

In the early 1960s, the field of *Physical Education* was challenged to become a well-respected discipline within higher education. James Bryant Conant, the former President of Harvard University and U.S. ambassador, published a series of works in the late 1950s and early 1960s critical of American public education.

The third installment entitled, *The Education of American Teachers*, was especially hard on graduate physical education (4). The following is a key excerpt from the book:

> I am far from impressed by what I have heard and read about graduate work in the field of physical education. If I wished to portray the education of teachers in the worst terms, I should quote from the descriptions of some graduate courses in physical education. To my mind, a university should cancel graduate programs in this area. If the physical education teacher wishes to enter into a research career in the field of physiology of exercise and related subjects, he should use the graduate years to build on his natural science background a knowledge of the physiological sciences that will enable him to stand on an equal footing with the undergraduate major in these sciences.

Many have understood the last sentence to be a tacit insult that equates graduate work in physical education with undergraduate work in the sciences. Therefore, the "common view" of Conant's impact on the field has been that he was highly critical of the discipline. On this reading, Conant's indictment of physical education sent shock waves through physical education faculty ranks, but it should not have surprised anyone. Prior to the 1960s, physical education graduate curricula had little, if any, science course work required of students. The field of physical education at the doctoral level had evolved from earlier in the 20th century into generalist preparation (broad study as opposed to specialization in a narrow field). Graduates were prepared to teach a wide variety of courses. The result of this type of graduate education was that physical education faculty were ill prepared to produce relevant research, which requires more in-depth preparation (specialist training) of the type found more typically in the sciences and other units of the academy.

Therefore, according to proponents of the "common view," the result of Conant's criticism of teacher education and his remarks that graduate physical education be eliminated was a serious and immediate examination of existing physical education curricula (9). Franklin Henry, a pioneer in motor behavior and a respected leader in physical education in the middle of the 20th century, led an introspective movement that resulted in strengthening curricular requirements and producing specialists in the emerging exercise sciences. The result was that people entering higher education as university faculty were better prepared to be productive researchers. This move toward disciplinarity and more specialization worked well as evidenced by the larger body of research literature published by physical education faculty members beginning in the time period of the mid- to late 1960s.

There is, however, an "alternative view" of Conant's impact, which, in our estimation, more fully explains his influence on the history of kinesiology. The main difference between the "common view" and the "alternative view" is the degree to which change should be ascribed to Conant. On the common view, Conant is a key catalyst to change. In the "alternative view," he is understood as one in a long line of influences on a field without a settled philosophy. On this view, "Conant's work is not seminal to kinesiology but rather fits into a broader history; a history of contention and debate over the meaning, purpose, and value of the field" (20).

Defenders of this view point to several facts that they argue moderate Conant's impact and contextualize it within a larger and longer philosophic debate about the meaning and purpose of physical education/kinesiology. First, Conant's book was not focused on physical education. His comments amount to 5 pages in a 200-page book. To whatever degree there was a reaction to Conant among physical educators, it was clearly disproportionate to the criticism. This means that other factors must have been at work. Second, not everything Conant says about physical education is negative. For example, Conant called physical education and coaching "two important functions" (4). One would not expect an unremitting critic of physical education to say such things. Finally, defenders of the "alternative view" have argued that the over-reaction of the field to the criticism reflects the tenuous nature of the field's own self-understanding and that this can be seen in the historical record. From this perspective, Conant was only one in a long line of important voices attempting to influence the philosophy of kinesiology.

"In fact, calls to 'liberalize' or humanize the field, as well as calls to 'intellectualize' the field by making it more scientific, both preceded and followed Conant's critique—just as such disparate calls continue today. To properly understand the transformation of physical education into kinesiology historians must look both beyond and before the work of James Bryant Conant" (20).

It is beyond to purview of this chapter to settle this debate. Fortunately, for our purposes, it suffices to merely introduce the debate as a way to convince readers that the nature and purpose of kinesiology are matters of contention. Budding kinesiologists should think about these issues, because the answer to such questions makes a difference. *You* will shape the future of the field.

Whatever one makes of Conant's challenge to the field of physical education as well as Henry's subsequent response, it is clear that since the 1960s, a paradigm shift has occurred. Many different areas of study emerged from physical education. One important question for the future of kinesiology is this: how can kinesiology continue to grow and evolve without losing its vital connection to physical education? This has taken on renewed urgency as many programs in physical education have been dropped around the United States.

No matter which interpretation of Conant's impact is more accurate, things have changed. Over the intervening decades, departments of physical education in colleges and universities, riding a wave of specialization, experienced changes that led to even more focus on the science content in their curricula. With this came a gradual realization that the term physical education was somehow deficient in communicating the new scope and focus of these departments. While many different labels have been used for those academic units studying exercise, sport, physical activity, and movement, the argument is made in this text that *Kinesiology* is the term best suited to carry the mantle of the academic discipline into the future.

Why then is kinesiology the best name for the field? While it is beyond the scope of this book to start a new front on this old debate, it is sufficient to state here that the term kinesiology is succinct and matches up well with other mainstream disciplines that use the suffix "ology" as part of the descriptive word signifying a field of study.

Logos is a Greek word that simply means knowledge. It forms the root of the "ology" suffix, which means—*the study of*. Thus, biology is the study of life, sociology is the study of human society, and anthropology is the study of humanity. Likewise, kinesiology is the study of movement in broad terms with a focus on physical activity, exercise, and sport.

One new field, *Exercise Science*, has subsequently become an integral part of kinesiology. Another newly established field, *Sport Studies*, has had a much more recent ascendency as an independent field of study. There are also several professional fields connected to kinesiology by a common body of knowledge. Kinesiology's disciplinary and professional subfields use their own tools of investigation to expand the knowledge base, but in doing so often rely on the techniques of other disciplines, thus giving them a strong multidisciplinary approach.

DISCIPLINARITY

Figure 1.1 presents kinesiology and its connections to related *cross-* and *multi*-disciplinary units. Common to all the disciplines and professions linked to kinesiology is the idea of movement. It can be argued that these fields have largely become or are on the way to becoming more autonomous, thus giving kinesiology the mantle of *parent discipline* and transforming it into a *trans*-disciplinary field of study. The subunits of kinesiology, therefore, work on many levels at once, each necessarily connected to kinesiology through parent disciplines from which they draw research tools to expand their unique body of knowledge.

Figure 1.2 illustrates the idea of disciplinarity, an important concept in higher education. When we speak of a discipline, we speak not merely of a body of knowledge, but also of a set of practices by which that knowledge is acquired, confirmed, implemented, preserved, and reproduced. Universities institutionalize knowledge through disciplines. Disciplines do this differently by varying the ways they structure themselves, establish

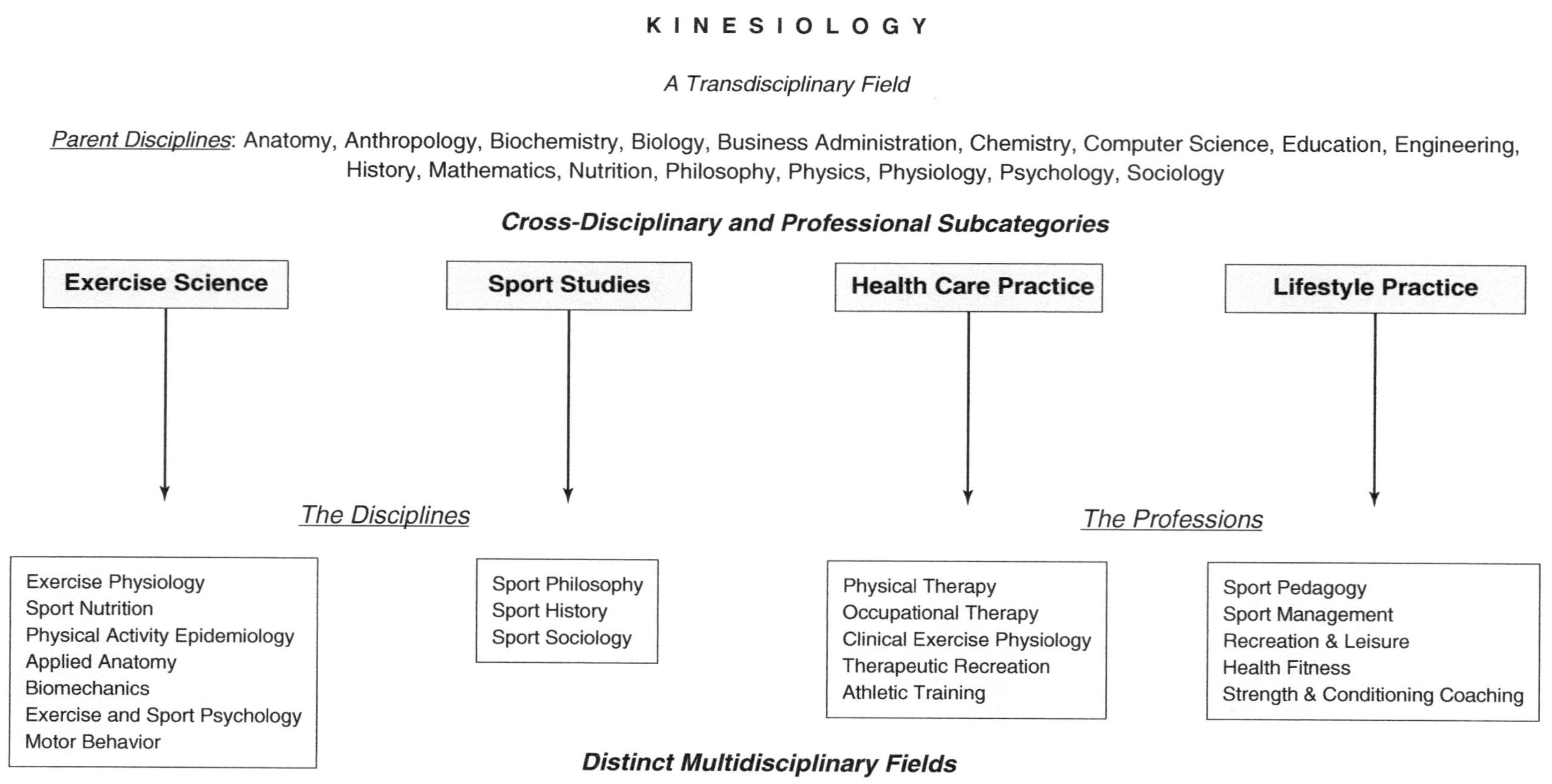

KINESIOLOGY

A Transdisciplinary Field

Parent Disciplines: Anatomy, Anthropology, Biochemistry, Biology, Business Administration, Chemistry, Computer Science, Education, Engineering, History, Mathematics, Nutrition, Philosophy, Physics, Physiology, Psychology, Sociology

Cross-Disciplinary and Professional Subcategories

Exercise Science	Sport Studies	Health Care Practice	Lifestyle Practice

The Disciplines

The Professions

Exercise Physiology
Sport Nutrition
Physical Activity Epidemiology
Applied Anatomy
Biomechanics
Exercise and Sport Psychology
Motor Behavior

Sport Philosophy
Sport History
Sport Sociology

Physical Therapy
Occupational Therapy
Clinical Exercise Physiology
Therapeutic Recreation
Athletic Training

Sport Pedagogy
Sport Management
Recreation & Leisure
Health Fitness
Strength & Conditioning Coaching

Distinct Multidisciplinary Fields

Figure 1.1. *Kinesiology, the study of movement, physical activity, exercise and sport, broadly serves to bring cohesion to those disciplines and professions that have a unique connection via a common body of knowledge. As shown, kinesiology draws on many parent disciplines in expanding its knowledge base through scientific research. Kinesiology is a transdisciplinary field of study associated with a number of crossdisciplinary fields that in turn are connected (some loosely, some strongly) with the various disciplines and professions of kinesiology.*

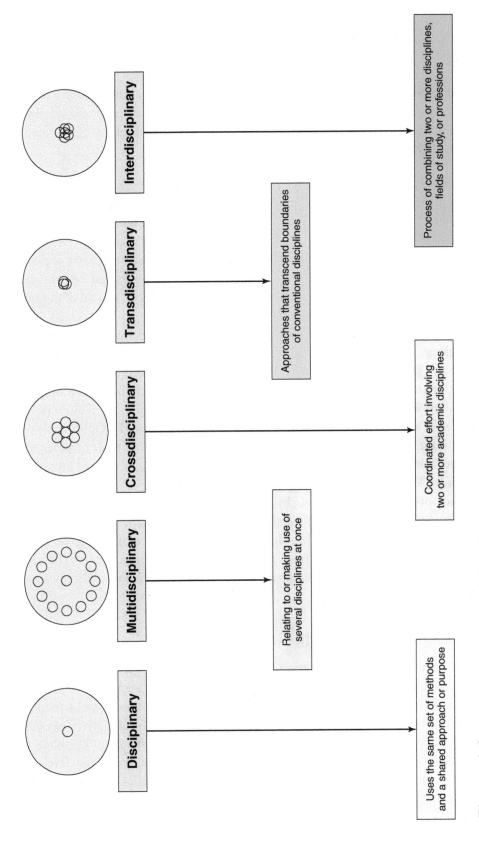

Figure 1.2.   *Looking beyond a single discipline*

identities, maintain boundaries, regulate and reward practitioners, manage consensus and dissent, and communicate. Disciplines also differ in the internal coherence of their methodology and subject matter. Quoting Franklin Henry (10):

> An academic discipline is an organized body of knowledge collectively embraced in a formal course of learning. The acquisition of such knowledge is assumed to be an adequate and worthy objective as such, without any demonstration or requirement of practical application. The content is theoretical and scholarly as distinguished from technical and professional.

Academic disciplines, therefore, have the following components: (1) body of knowledge, (2) conceptual framework, and (3) methods of inquiry involving exact processes and procedures. Typically, most disciplines are discrete, that is, the topic is limited to a particular subject matter. For example, mathematics, biology, and chemistry are distinct fields of learning with their own formalized body of knowledge.

As shown in Figure 1.1, there are several disciplines that coalesce around movement as the body of knowledge to form the transdisciplinary field of kinesiology. Each of these disciplines may be considered multidisciplinary in their approach to science. Exercise physiology, for example, relies on several of the parent disciplines at once: physics, biology, biochemistry, and physiology.

Multidisciplinarity in this context has to do with making use of several disparate disciplines simultaneously to expand the knowledge base. Exercise science and sport studies (referring to Figure 1.1) "cross" disciplinary lines by seeking to give cohesiveness to their respective disciplines. Kinesiology itself would be considered "trans" disciplinary, or transcending the boundaries of conventional disciplines (including its parent disciplines) to form an even wider cohesiveness. In time, kinesiology may achieve true interdisciplinarity, which may best be described as a result of opportunism in knowledge production (17). Opportunism in this context means that researchers in kinesiology are apt to readily acquire the research tools of other disciplines when necessary to test specific hypotheses. The benefit to this "borrowing" of others' tools of investigation is an even greater expansion of the knowledge base.

Broadly, the study of movement, exercise, physical activity, and sport is what distinguishes the crossdisciplinary fields of *Exercise Science* and *Sport Studies* and the professions oriented to these fields from the parent academic disciplines that support them. In studying movement, these crossdisciplinary fields use specific principles from the parent disciplines and through rigorous scientific inquiry attempt to describe and develop causal relationships that expand our understanding. This process has led to a virtual explosion of the knowledge base within kinesiology.

Exercise Science and Sport Studies

The term exercise science refers to the application of science to the phenomenon of exercise. This text treats exercise as being inclusive of all human movement, including random or infrequent movement, work, habitual activity, training done for fitness or health, dance, sport, leisure activities of all sorts, and activities of daily living. Any movement that can be imagined can be studied using one or more of the disciplines of exercise science.

The phrase application of science in the above definition is somewhat vague. There are many branches of science that can be applied to exercise science. Psychological applications led to the development of motor behavior (Chapter 14) and exercise and sport psychology (Chapter 13). Physics was used in exploring mechanics of movement (biomechanics—Chapter 12). Biology and chemistry were the foundations of exercise physiology (Chapter 8).

Multidisciplinary research among the disciplines of exercise science is becoming increasingly common, and it is clear that the supporting sciences for these different disciplines are not unique in their applications. For example, physics is used in explaining the dynamics of cardiovascular function in exercise physiology, biomechanics borrows from neuromuscular function on occasion, and motor behavior specialists have adapted dynamical systems theory from physics to measure galvanic skin response and heart rates.

The recent evolution of *Sport Studies* as a crossdisciplinary field has led to new opportunities for kinesiology students. *Sport Studies* has three major disciplinary tie-ins: philosophy, history, and sociology. Each of these has multidisciplinary connections that help expand and enrich our understanding of movement better than what can be done solely within one discrete field of study.

The multidisciplinary approach can be illustrated this way. For example, physical activity epidemiologists study how exercise and physical activity affect disease incidence in populations. This rather new discipline within *Exercise Science* can benefit from an understanding of the sociological characteristic of the population of individuals being studied. In this case, understanding sociology (the study of human society) may help research scientists study disease patterns related to physical inactivity in a population more effectively. This is an example of a "multi" disciplinary approach within two "cross" disciplinary fields of kinesiology—*Exercise Science* and *Sport Studie*s.

THE HISTORY OF KINESIOLOGY

Table 1.1 places the disciplines and professions of kinesiology in the approximate time frame of their emergence, lists important early contributors to each field, and gives the major events that established each area. As mentioned at the start of the chapter, teaching others physical skills has always been an important activity to human. It was necessary for survival, and throughout history, it was necessary if the community was to be perpetuated. Other physical skills were also taught, and in that respect, education within the realm of the physical had very early beginnings, but which culture systemized this form of learning?

Table 1.1. The disciplines and professions of kinesiology, their academic foundation, and important contributors

Discipline/ Profession	~Date	Key Contributors	Key Events and Important Work
KINESIOLOGY DISCIPLINES			
Exercise Physiology	1927s–1950s	Thomas Cureton David B. Dill S. M. Horvath	Harvard Fatigue Laboratory, exercise physiology labs founded, Journal of Applied Physiology established, ACSM founded
Sports Nutrition	1980s	Melvin Williams David Lamb	Studies investigating contribution of nutrition to athletic performance, nutrition and human performance texts published
Physical Activity Epidemiology	1990s	Steve Blair Ralph Paffenbarger	Studies establishing physical inactivity as a disease risk factor
Biomechanics	1980s	John Basmajian, Peter Cavanaugh, David Winter, James Hay	Orthotics, diabetic foot ailments, posture and balance, locomotion, electromyography, movement analysis with sport applications
Exercise and Sport Psychology	1960s	Rainer Martens Robert Singer Daniel Landers	Incorporation of NASPSPA, applied research using scientific psychology as a model

(Continued)

Discipline/ Profession	~Date	Key Contributors	Key Events and Important Work
Motor Behavior	1960s	Franklin Henry Anna Espenschade G. Lawrence Rarick	Memory drum theory, publication of major textbooks on motor development
Sport History	1970s	Marvin Eyler Guy Lewis	Completion of seminal dissertations
Sport Sociology	1970s	Gerald Kenyon George Sage	Treatises on the sociology of sport, major textbooks
Sport Philosophy	1960s–1970s	Elwood Davis Earle Zeigler	Important graduate programs, first meeting of the Philosophic Society for the Study of Sport
KINESIOLOGY PROFESSIONS			
Physical Therapy	1810s–1920s	Per Henrik Ling Mary McMillan	Royal Central Institute of Gymnastics founded in Sweden, British nurses form the Chartered Society of Physiotherapy, 1894 polio epidemic, the first higher education facilities teach physical therapy
Occupational Therapy	1790s–1910s	Phillipe Pinel Susan Tracy William Rush Dunton	Moral treatment and occupation, an approach to treating people with mental illness, National Society for the Promotion of Occupational Therapy formed
Clinical Exercise Physiology	1970s	Roy Shephard John Holloszy	Exercise training as a rehabilitative agent for several patient populations
Therapeutic Recreation	1940s–1950s	Elliott Avedon	Hospital recreation section of the American Recreation Society formed
Athletic Training	1950s	Robert Behnke William E. Newell	Accreditation, education program
Sport Pedagogy	1960s	Francklin Henry Nathaniel Gage	Henry's article on physical education as an academic discipline, Gage's *Handbook of Research on Teaching*
Sport Management	1960s	James Mason	Education program established at Ohio University
Recreation and Leisure	1960s	Charles Brightbill	Formation of the National Recreation and Park Association in the United States
Health Fitness	1970s	Karl Stoedefalke John Faulkner	ACSM certification programs established, ACSM's Guidelines for Exercise Testing and Prescription published
Strength and Conditioning Coaching	1950s–1960s	Martin Broussard Francis Drury	Studies on strength and conditioning training with application to coaching

Educating the physical has at different time periods been overvalued, merely tolerated, or completely denounced. Whatever ideals of human excellence held sway in a given time period and culture usually dictated the opinions educational leaders favored regarding this form of education. At least four lines of thought have existed through history: the Greek (aesthetic), the monkish (ascetic), the military (knightly), and the modern (scientific).

Greece

The Greeks were the earliest Western culture to systematically organize learning for physical pursuits beyond those necessary to acquire the basic necessities of life. That is, physical education was part of a formal course of learning. All men had to learn warring skills, but to the Greeks the pursuit of leisure was equally important. For example, Greek culture established some of the earliest recorded athletic events. They also developed the gymnasium (the word literally means a place for naked exercise) where males disrobed to pursue sport, exercise, and intellectual curiosity (philosophical debates). It is to the Greeks, therefore, that we usually look for the origins of physical education, but in truth, if our previous assertions regarding the centrality of motion to human being are accurate, there probably is no singular beginning.

Nevertheless, there is much in ancient Greece worth admiring and perhaps even emulating. The Greek philosophy of education took the body seriously and considered that no lasting value can accrue from its neglect. Much of their philosophy, literature, music, and especially art reflected the love of the physical and an appreciation of the human form. Yet, as a close examination of any culture reveals there were paradoxes, contradictions, and countercurrents as well. Consider the three following examples:

1. Even as Plato and Aristotle could both insist on the importance of physical education, Plato also insisted that death frees the soul from the body "because the body confuses the soul, and does not allow it to acquire truth and wisdom whenever it is associated with it" (15). At the very least, this complicates our understanding of Plato as a friend of physical education. Moreover, Plato and Aristotle were both Athenians and we must be careful to avoid haphazardly applying Athenian values to all of the Greeks.
2. Although the Greeks admired physical beauty for its own sake, they also ruthlessly pursued victory by any means, including in events that sullied and disfigured the human form. The *pankration*, for example, was essentially an ancient, no holds barred, version of MMA (Mixed-Martial Arts).
3. Even as women were clearly treated as second-class citizens in ancient Greek sport—they could not, for example, even attend the ancient Olympic Games—there is emerging and intriguing evidence that women (especially girls) were significantly involved in and interested in sport. Let us examine each point in turn.

Arguably, the backdrop for the eventual systematization of physical training was an idea unique to the Greeks—the best man was one sound in *mind and body*. Plato, in his work, *Timaeus*, says it best:

> Everything that is good is fair, and the fair is not without proportion. Now, we perceive lesser symmetries and comprehend them, but about the highest and greatest we have no understanding, for there is no symmetry greater than that of the soul to the body. This, however, we do not perceive, nor do we allow ourselves to reflect that when a weaker or lesser frame is the vehicle of a great and mighty soul, or conversely, when a little soul is incased in a large body, then the whole animal is not fair, for it is defective in the most important of all symmetries; but the *fair mind in the fair body* (emphasis mine) will be the fairest and loveliest of all sights to him who has the seeing eye (16).

Embodied in this statement is the concept of the *Greek Ideal*. Education served as the vehicle through which this concept was inculcated into the psyche of the people. Through education, the Greeks set out to produce a higher order of men. The term *Paideia* referred to this systematic rearing toward self-improvement as a way to develop the ideal member of the *Polis* (city-state). The goal of education in the Greek city-states was to prepare the child for adult activities as a model (body and mind) citizen. The ideal citizen of Athens was to be a person educated in the arts of both peace and war, making necessary schools for education of the mind and exercise fields for education of the body. Moderation was key. In Sparta, the ideal male citizen was to be a warrior, while the ideal female citizen was to be strong enough to be a wife and mother (and thereby survive the rigors of childbirth). As sport historian Don Kyle puts it, the Spartans were interested in "girl power for manpower" (13).

It is worth noting that Aristotle found this Spartan form of pedagogy wanting because it allegedly lacked the Athenian ideal of moderation.

> "In our own day some of those states which have the greatest reputation for looking after their youth aim at producing an athletes' condition, to the detriment of both the appearance and growth of the children's bodies; while the Spartans, who have avoided that error, nevertheless by severity of exercise render them like wild animals, under the impression that it is particularly conducive to courage. But, as has been often pointed out, the care of the young must not be directed to producing one virtue only, nor this one more than the rest"(1).

In sum, despite contradictions and inconsistencies in both theory and execution, the Greek ideal followed Homer, who insisted in the *Illiad* that a citizen must be "a speaker of words and a doer of deeds." The whole person was to be educated.

Turning our attention to the Greek desire for victory, it is clear that the key idea for understanding Greek athletics and physical education is *arête*, which means something akin to virtue or excellence. What must be emphasized here is that *arête*—whether understood as virtue or excellence—was a concrete rather than abstract concern for the Greeks. That is, they wanted to unambiguously see excellence "in the moment." It is for this reason that victory was so important. To win, to be better than all others in that time and place, was to visibly demonstrate *arête*. It is for this reason that the Greeks were willing to pursue brutal and dangerous sports such as boxing and pankration. It is also for this reason that the Greek athletic circuit has no judged or team events. In such circumstances, winning and therefore *arête* would have been ambiguous.

What then did the Greek athletic circuit consist of? There were four major festivals and myriad lesser festivals. The major festivals held in Olympia, Delphi, Corinth, and Nemea were *stephanitic* or "crown" games. Each festival was religious in character and dedicated to one of the gods of the Greek pantheon. The Olympic Games, for example, were dedicated to Zeus, whose temple at Olympia was one of the seven ancient wonders of the world. While the Olympic Games and Nemean Games were named for their locations, the Games in Corinth were called the Isthmian Games due to Corinth's geographic feature of being on the isthmus between the Peloponnesus and the Greek mainland, whereas the Games in Delphi were called the Pythian Games after the name of the priestess at Delphi's famous Oracle.

Although the Olympic Games were the oldest and most prestigious, all of the *stephanitic* games were important. So important in fact that, contrary to conventional wisdom, the Greeks were not amateurs and had no concept of amateurism. They competed to win, and winners were rewarded handsomely by their home city-states. As historian David C. Young points out, "It is true that the officials at the Olympic games [sic] gave the victorious a crown of olives, nothing more. That is because the athletes' own home cities would reward them with lavish prizes" (21). Any doubt in this regard should be eliminated by the fact that the lesser Greek festivals are known as *chrematitic* or "money" games because of the explicit cash awards that were given to the victors at these games. Athletic competition was basically a way for warrior-athletes to prove to the gods and their fellows that they embodied *arête*, that then and there they were superior to all other competitors. Winning in the games was at once an athletic achievement and a form of obeisance, honoring the gods by proving one's allegiance to the Greek Ideal.

Finally, let us consider the role of women in sport in ancient Greece. The paradox of women's athletics is perhaps best exemplified by Cyniska, the Spartan princess, who was the first woman to win at the ancient

Olympic Games. You are likely asking yourself how she could win when she wasn't allowed to attend the games. The answer is simple. The victors in the chariot races were the owners of the horses rather than the charioteers. As such, Cyniska could win in absentia. How ought such a victory be interpreted? On the one hand, she won. On the other hand, she could only do so in absentia. On the one hand, the evidence suggests that she was proud of her victory as this inscription shows:

> "Kings of Sparta were my fathers and brothers, and I, Cynisca, winning the race with my chariot of swift-footed horses, erected this statue. I assert that I am the only woman in all Greece who won his crown" (12).

On the other hand, there is good evidence that her brother encouraged her to enter as a way to embarrass a political rival, by showing that, "entering chariots at Olympia was about money, not skill," so much so that even a woman could do it (12). Was Cyniska's victory a step forward for women's athletics or simple confirmation of their second class status? Perhaps it was both.

Similarly, other evidence of women's participation in ancient Greece is suggestive of both greater participation than one would expect and also of the relative neglect of women's athletics. Young women, for example, competed every four years in a separate festival at Olympia dedicated to Hera, the wife of Zeus. There is also limited evidence of young women competing at the Pythian, Nemean, and Isthmian Games. It is not clear, based on such limited evidence, how common such participation was or even whether the women competed in their own division. Finally, there is suggestive evidence in Athens for female athletics. There is a *palaistra* (wrestling school) on the grounds of the Sanctuary of Artemis. As archeologist Stephen Miller points out, "This must have been a wrestling school for girls and women since the Sanctuary of Brauronian Artemis was a strictly female cult..." (14).

As with the previous examples, what these facts mean for the nature and practice of women's athletics in ancient Greece is not entirely clear. The sources are too sparse. Does the limited evidence suggest that women were not very involved in sport or does the limited evidence merely mean that their involvement garnered little attention? Should we focus on the lack of recognition the dearth of sources suggests or would we be better off emphasizing that women were far more involved in ancient Greek athletics than most suppose? Finally, it is worth noting that the neglect of women's athletics (and the impact of this neglect on the historical record) is still with us today. Again, Miller is instructive, "If two thousand years from now [current] newspapers are the only athletic records that survive, what will historians conclude about the relative importance of women's athletics today" (14)?

Rome

Although we cannot go into great detail, no history of physical education and kinesiology would be complete without at least a brief survey of Rome. For our purposes, we must limit ourselves to a few brief points. The Roman focus was neither as religious nor as competitive as the Greeks. For Rome, sport was about spectacle. This can be seen most prominently in the three great *Ludi Romani* (Roman games): the *circus*, the *naumachia*, and the *munera*. The circus consisted of chariot races on a mile-long track between four teams of different colors (e.g. red and blue) each of which had passionate factions of fans. The *Circus Maximus* in Rome could hold 150,000 spectators (8). The *naumachia* were staged naval battles. The floor of the Roman Colosseum could be flooded via aqueduct for such events. Finally, the most famous of Roman sports, the *munera*, or blood sports, consisted of gladiatorial combat as well as elaborate animal hunts. The Flavian amphitheater, or Roman Colosseum, was the most famous site of the *munera* but hardly the only site. The Colosseum was a technical marvel, which included seating for 50,000, elaborate trap doors in the floor for stage effects such as animal releases, and a huge awning to protect spectators from the Sun.

What, in summary, can be said of the Greeks and the Romans? Physical training constituted a central component of life for citizens of Greek city-states. The goal was an education for mind *and* body to unite the *man of action* with the *man of wisdom* to produce a well-integrated person. The Romans, in turn, introduced spectacle, technology, and medicine into sport and physical activity. Their engineering prowess and thirst for distraction and entertainment foreshadow modernity in important ways. Similarly, Galen's work with Roman gladiators, as we shall see, is of foundational importance for the field of sports medicine. Arguably, however, the Greek Ideal (however imperfect) is the most important influence on the fields of physical education and later still, kinesiology. This influence is significant, since it is kinesiology with its Greek root meaning centering on movement and the study of exercise, physical activity, and sport that best exemplifies today's ideal: the education of the "whole person."

Middle Ages

It is often argued that this idea was subsequently lost as the Christian Church became predominate in Europe in the periods of time after the fall of Rome in A.D. 476 known sequentially as the Middle Ages. Christians at the time (and now) were (are) said to be "anti-body" and "anti-pleasure" because of their fear of "carnal" sin and their focus on an other-worldly salvation. At best, such assertions are misleading, and at worst, they are outright false. It cannot be denied that isolated cases can be found to support such claims. Yet, this is not unique. As we have seen, the Greek ideal was neither uniformly consistent nor uniformly followed. Moreover, whether one considers the Bible, the great historical theologians, or the basic doctrines of Christianity, one sees that, "Although some Christians might claim that the human body is evil, it is an un-Christian belief" (18).

As you consider three brief examples, remember that the truth or falsity of Christianity is not the issue. The issue is rather the definition and implications of the central claims of the faith. The truth of the argument being made is independent of whether or not Christianity itself is true.

First, consider that according to the Book of Genesis, human beings are the pinnacle of creation and that God says that creation (which includes the human body) is "very good" (Genesis 1:31). Second, consider this quote regarding the source of man's sin from St. Augustine (arguably the most influential post apostolic theologian in the history of the Church). In the *City of God*, Augustine wrote, "Moreover, it was not the corruptible flesh that made the soul sinful; on the contrary, it was the sinful soul that made the flesh corruptible" (2). It was a focus on self—a corrupt will—not embodiment, which caused man's fall. Sin is a function of rebellion, not physicality. Finally, consider the importance of embodiment in the central doctrines of Christianity such as the incarnation or resurrection. The incarnation is the belief that God became man, that "the Word [Jesus Christ] became flesh and dwelt among us" (John 1:14). The doctrine of resurrection is the claim that the physical death and resurrection of Jesus is the basis for the hope of eternal life (1st Corinthians 15: 16–18). Given the centrality of embodiment to the Bible and to Christian theology and tradition, it is clear that no consistent account of Christianity claimed that the human body is evil. Of course, that doesn't mean no one ever tried.

However, the common claim that the Middle Ages period of Western history was not kind to the Greek ideal, which sought equality of education for the mind, and the body should be moderated if not overturned. Here, as with the Greeks and what follows, we see an echo of the contemporary debate over Conant. History (and cultures) is complex and almost never uniform. As a result our depictions of history are often caricatures, whereas our convictions about history are often clouded by our own biases. That is, we only pay attention to those aspects of the past that confirm or justify our own worldview. None of this is to argue that real answers to historical questions cannot be found, but rather to insist on the importance of engaging historical questions in pursuit of truth, since the truth is often well below the surface of things. If all we ever engage is the surface of things, the truth will rarely be found. History, even in kinesiology, needs to be studied carefully.

Renaissance and Enlightenment

The Renaissance period is another good example of this complexity. Fourteenth-century Italy saw a renewed emphasis on Greek learning. Renaissance humanists, like the Greeks, wanted education to develop man's intellectual, spiritual, and physical powers for the enrichment of life. Their humanistic curriculum included history and physical games and exercises in addition to the Middle Ages' emphasis on the seven liberal arts. Physical development was, therefore, encouraged. Later in the renaissance period, however, physical development, so important to the early humanist ideal of the well-rounded man, was removed to be replaced once again by harsh, repressive discipline.

Throughout this period, too, the militaristic ideal existed side-by-side with the ascetic, especially in England (but also elsewhere on continental Europe) where it was important to the nobility of the time. The idea was an exaggeration to the other extreme; where the ascetic overly stressed the soul (the mind) to the exclusion of the body, the nobility stressed the body for warfare to the exclusion of the mind. During the 18th and 19th centuries, there was a rising tide of nationalism throughout Europe. It is against this backdrop that physical education developed and expanded.

In many ways, *The Greek Ideal*, the idea of a sound mind in a sound body with equal attention to both, became the modern model for physical education. Nevertheless, here, too, we will see rejections and contradictions of this model. With the rise of science in the enlightenment, the idea was to advance knowledge through the scientific method. New perspectives on nature and man's place within it were introduced. As breakthroughs in the sciences of biology, chemistry, and physiology occurred, there was a rise also in "scientific" medicine that helped facilitate the modern era of physical education. The practice of medicine became more grounded in science than in myth as the scientific revolution caught on. As a result, the general well-being of the populace gradually increased.

This era is replete with the ideas of individuals as to the best way to systematize the training of the human body. Throughout the latter part of the 18th century, word of the benefits of exercise became increasingly well known in Europe and in America.

Greek Revivalism had also been spreading throughout Europe for decades, and in 1807, the first classical statues to be exhibited in Great Britain were put on display (Figure 1.3). The statues depicting elegant and muscularly symmetrical bodies, a picture of the *Greek Ideal*, were a huge success. The average citizen viewing these perhaps could not help but find that his or her own body was somewhat lacking in comparison.

Figure 1.3. Hercules holds up the apples he stole from the Hesperides in the eleventh of his twelve labors. Could the well-chiseled musculature have caused 18th-century males to turn to exercise?

Jean Jacues Rouseau's book *Émile*, published in 1762, sets forth a hypothetical plan for the naturalistic education of youth, including education of the body. It was a highly politicized statement against the state of education of the day and was partly responsible for his expulsion from France. The book started an education revolution of sorts based on Rouseau's vision of the *natural man* in whom the mind and body acted synergistically. Johann Basedow founded a school in Dessau, Germany, the *Philanthropinium*, based on Rouseau's educational principles. The school's curriculum included three hours of daily physical education and recreation.

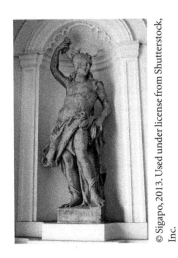

Figure 1.3. *Hercules holds up the apples he stole from the Hesperides in the eleventh of his twelve labors. Could the well-chiseled musculature have caused 18th-century males to turn to exercise?*

© Sigapo, 2013. Used under license from Shutterstock, Inc.

Johan Simon became the first full-time physical educator in Basedow's school and included in the curriculum what he called "Greek Gymnastics" (running, leaping, wrestling, and throwing). The repertoire of exercises increased over time to include manual labor and military drills. Other individuals developed their own schools, and this movement became known as *Philanthropic Education*. Notable among these were Christian Salzmann who hired as his physical educator, Johann Guts-Muths. Guts-Muths, via his popular works on exercise, would go on to be very influential in the early physical education movement.

Three early innovators who followed in this vein were Friedrich Jahn (of Germany), Per Ling (of Sweden), and Franz Nachtegall (of Denmark). Jahn developed the *Turnverein* movement, which were associations centered around gymnastics. Their goal was to strengthen the youth of Germany. The central component of Jahn's system was the *Turnplatz*, an outdoor exercise area with equipment for jumping, vaulting, balancing, and climbing. The exercisers (gymnasts) were known as *Turners*. Jahn emphasized nationalism and the building of strong bodies for German defense in the face of foreign aggression. In this regard, physical education was a means, not an end. The hope of German freedom lay in the development of strong, sturdy, fearless youth. Physical education had only one value. The charm, joy, drama, and meaning found in play had no role in the Turner movement. Here, arguably, is one of the contradictions of the *Greek Ideal* in modernity. Human beings—both men and women—are more than mere bodies. Yet, to treat the body as a tool of health is to neglect the needs of the whole person (and thereby the most attractive element of the *Greek Ideal*). Health is necessary, but not sufficient for a good life. Nevertheless, his system spread to the United States in the 19th century when German immigrants developed *Turnvereins* in the new world. Although the Turner movement did not survive for long in the United States, the impulse to reduce physical education (and kinesiology) to a "means to health" is alive and well.

Why did the Turner movement fail in the United States? To put it perhaps too bluntly and certainly too briefly, Turner exercises were boring and sports were fun. Modern sports were an Anglo-American innovation that spread around the world via the British Empire and American missionary and trading activity (7). Unlike what had been the dominate influence on the continent, the nationalistic fervor to build strong bodies for national defense never took hold in Great Britain, a dominate world power at the time. The British Isle never faced territorial threat the way other countries had, therefore, instead of physical education for strength and defense, they stressed sport and games to develop character. The English philosopher John Locke advocated a sound mind/sound body concept paralleling the *Greek Ideal*. This influenced the *British Amateur Sport Ideal*—playing the game for the game's sake—an idea similar in some ways to the ancient Greek's love of athleticism and competition. Thus, British sports and recreational pastimes divided by class lines took hold. Here the idea of *Muscular Christianity* became dominate in the Victorian era centered on a vigorous masculinity emphasizing spiritual and moral character achieved principally through team sports. The greatest innovator in Great Britain at the time was Archibald Maclaren who also emphasized physical activity for health and treating physical training as a science.

Exercise as Medicine

Galen (A.D. 129–210), a Roman (of Greek ethnicity) physician, surgeon, philosopher, and the most prominent medical researcher of antiquity, considered it a physician's duty to use exercise to promote health and prevent disease. To that end, he emphasized what physicians in antiquity called *Regimen*, the centrality of exercise and diet as key factors in the maintenance of health.

Galen was heavily influenced by two Greek physicians of several centuries prior: Herodicus (a physician and athlete) and Hippocrates (the father of preventive medicine). Herodicus (5th century B.C.) is the first person to combine sports with medicine. He considered bad health to be the result of imbalance between diet and physical activity, recommending strict diet and regular exercise training. He applied this treatment method to his patients and is, therefore, usually considered to be the father of sports medicine. Hippocrates (460–370 B.C.) wrote three books on regimen, noting that, "Eating alone will not keep a man well; he must also take exercise."

Following in their ideological footsteps, Galen coined the term *scientific hygiene*, an area of study that in his day was close in meaning to our understanding of the science of exercise physiology. He followed the Hippocratic School of Medicine that believed in logical science grounded in observation and experimentation instead of superstition. He built his medical theory upon the *naturals* (of or with nature—physiology), the *non-naturals* (things not innate—health), and the *contra-naturals* (against nature—pathology). He viewed hygiene (named after the goddess of health, Hygieia) and the uses and abuses of what he referred to as the *six things non-natural* to be central in his theory. As opposed to the innate qualities that disposed one to good or bad health, what we might call today genetic predisposition, there were six factors external to the body over which a person had some control: (1) air and environment, (2) food (diet) and drink, (3) sleep and wake, (4) motion (exercise) and rest, (5) retention and evacuation, and (6) the passions of the mind (emotions). Held in balance and used in moderation, these factors could lead to health, but if abused in either extreme (too much or too little) could lead to disease (3). An example of this balance can be seen in a warning found in his treatise, *Art of Medicine*:

> When, for example, the body is in need of motion, exercise is healthy and rest morbid; when it is in need of a break, rest is healthy and exercise morbid. Exercise should cease as soon as the body begins to suffer.

One of Galen's works on the "art of health" was a treatise titled, *On Hygiene*. In it he provides an excellent understanding of the difference between exercise and the regular bodily movement:

> It does not seem that all movement is exercise, but only when it is vigorous. . . The criterion of vigorousness is change of respiration; those movements which do not alter the respiration are not called exercise. But if anyone is compelled by any movement to breathe more of less faster, that movement becomes exercise for him.

Galen was also interested in what would much later become the science of biomechanics. He produced the equivalent of a medical textbook entitled, *On the Function of the Parts*, in which he elucidated the differences between sensory and motor nerves and between agonist and antagonist muscles.

Galen thought that regimen (exercise and diet) produced good health, but he was adamant about a balanced approach. Where exercise was concerned, Galen seems not to have had a high regard for athletics. He did not approve of the excesses in which athletes routinely engaged and indicated that these would lead to later misery in life as chronic overexertion during years of athletic pursuit would eventually prove detrimental to health years later.

This view of the rigors of athletic competition had a lasting influence on Western medicine, and Galen's thoughts on medical practice in general went unchallenged through the Middle Ages and Renaissance periods. As the enlightenment took hold and the progress of science gradually brought medicine into the modern era, dubious practices began to end in favor of those that had a stronger emphasis in science. At this time, advances in chemistry and physiology provided a stronger basis for the practice of medicine. The old idea of exercise as medicine as advocated by Galen and his Greek predecessors was gaining popularity again.

Galen's negative view of athletics had a strong effect on physicians and influenced the budding field of scientific medicine in the 19th century. It was not without some basis in fact because it had always been the case that athletes tended to acquire debilitating injuries as a result of competition. Moreover, Galen had years of experience treating the injuries of Roman gladiators, which could obviously be severe.

The Advent of Physical Education

Despite the partial truth of Galen's reservations regarding ancient sport, there were many physicians who participated in sport and in the mid- to late 19th century. They would coin a new term, *physical education*, as indicative of the task of teaching children the "laws of health." In effect, then, the beginnings of the field of physical education were grounded in the *non-natural* tradition of Galen (3).

Physicians played a role in the new field of study from the beginning. In the 1885 founding of the Association for the Advancement of Physical Education (AAPE), there were 11 physicians of the 49 individuals present at the meeting. At the turn of the 20th–century, physicians comprised nearly 15% of the 600 member organization. The membership of the American Association for the Advancement of Physical Education (AAAPE) two years later (the word American was added in 1886) would not be substantially different in makeup from that of the American Physiological Society founded in 1887.

Physical education and the field of medicine had an early connection through close philosophical ties to the *non-natural* tradition of preventive medicine. Physical education in the 19th century focused on health instruction and bodily development. Many early pioneers in physical education came from medical backgrounds and were interested in scientific applications related to health. A typical example of the type of work done by both pedagogically trained physical educators and those who were trained physicians was the anthropometric measurements (body dimension measures such as height, weight, and girth) popular just before and after the end of the 19th century. When World Wars I and II led to research on physical fitness as related to military performance, relatively little of the sophisticated research was done by physical educators. The same was true of perceptual motor research stimulated by demands of aviator training in World War II. These wars also required the use of ergonomics in design of military equipment and involved applications of principles of biomechanics by engineers rather than by physical educators. Instead, most physical educators in the first two or three decades of the 20th century were largely concerned with K-12 curriculum development.

Physical education at the beginning of the 20th century shifted from its roots in the *non-natural* tradition to an emphasis on sports following the British model that asserted that moral benefits outweighed any health value. In this way, formalized physical education in schools and professional programs in colleges and universities gradually became associated more with sports skills and less with health outcomes. As the close association with sports grew, coaches became more and more important in physical education programs, which tended then to further increase the overreliance on competitive athletics that had come about. This idea eventually became inculcated in the minds of the public. Competitive sports could suffice and substitute for Galen's idea of exercise, something that Galen would have denied. This moved exercise away from everyday life. In the "practice" of physical education, sports and games became dominate. Galen's *Laws of Health* as they had become known in the 19th century also became less prominent as a necessary part of medicine in the 20th century as the focus of medical practice turned to disease, pharmacology, surgery, and care of the sick (3). It is only within the last 40 years with the advent of the exercise sciences that Galen's ideas have had an ascendency once again.

The 19th Century and the Rise of Exercise Physiology

Attention has been given to health, fitness, anatomy, and physiology by physicians and other scholars at least as far back as the Golden Age of Greece. However, not until the latter part of the 19th century was the foundation for what would become the discipline of exercise physiology being laid. Among numerous journal articles and books dealing with various aspects of physiology published during that period, two books by Flint dealt specifically with aspects of exercise physiology. Shortly thereafter, the first exercise physiology course was taught by George Wells Fitz, M.D., in the short-lived (1892–1900) Department of Anatomy, Physiology, and Physical Training at Harvard University. The course was part of a science-based physical education curriculum and included experimental investigation and 6 hours per week of laboratory study. Its prerequisites included a course in general physiology (or its equivalent) at the medical school.

The 1919 text *Physiology of Muscular Exercise* by Bainbridge was updated by Arlie Bock and Bruce Dill in 1928. Dill commented:

> We think now of 1925 as a remote period in exercise physiology, but I was astonished recently to count over 400 references in our 1928 edition of Bainbridge.

About that same time, A.V. Hill's important work *Muscular Movement in Man* was published followed by Schneider's and McCurdy and Larson's physical education-based texts on exercise physiology in the 1930s. *Research Quarterly* contained a few articles related to exercise physiology in the 1930s, and physical educators Arthur Steinhaus and F.A. Hellebrandt contributed important exercise physiology reviews in prestigious physiology journals during this foundational period.

Laboratories devoted to exercise physiology in the context of physical education were set up in two institutions in which YMCA fitness directors were trained. Arthur Steinhaus at George Williams College in 1923 and James McCurdy at Springfield College in 1927 directed these early ventures. In later years, Peter Karpovich would be extremely productive in further research and development at Springfield, Massachusetts.

L.J. Henderson's brainchild, the Harvard Fatigue Laboratory, was established in 1927 and flourished until its closure in 1947. David Bruce Dill was director during that period, entering as a chemist and exiting as one of the world's outstanding figures in exercise physiology. The impact of the Harvard Fatigue Laboratory and Bruce Dill can hardly be overestimated. The Laboratory contributed importantly during World War II in two ways: (1) research was done that directly related to military personnel performance and (2) several scientists left the laboratory to work in other research centers that were involved in military-related research (5, 6). Following a precipitous loss of federal funding after World War II, a reluctant decision was made to close the fatigue laboratory. Dill relates:

> . . . I do not consider it to have been an irreparable loss to physiology. Successful organisms have a way of reaching maturity, declining, and dying, but not without perpetuating their kind.

"Graduates" of the Harvard Fatigue Laboratory established their own laboratories across the country and around the world, and continued the work of exercise physiology in their own spheres of influence. Those scientists who were the first- or second-generation exercise physiologists after the closure of the Harvard Fatigue Laboratory were instrumental in developing the first generation of well-trained exercise physiologists from physical education backgrounds.

Among a group of 11 individuals responsible for founding the ACSM in 1954 were physical educators Karpovich, Larson, and Steinhaus. The other founders, representatives of medicine and physiology, understood the importance of physical education's relationship to "sports medicine." Interestingly, the term sports medicine, as used at the founding of the ACSM, is synonymous with exercise science in today's understanding. Sports medicine today carries the connotation of athletic training, one of the professions associated with kinesiology. In the early stages, ACSM's focus was on athletics, injuries, fitness, and physiology. Only in years to come did diversification cover the range of exercise sciences, with a strong emphasis on exercise physiology. In ACSM's founding year, the 10th international congress on sports medicine was held in Luxembourg, the first meeting having been in Amsterdam in 1928. ACSM, therefore, met a long-overdue need in America.

While most scholarly early work in exercise physiology was still being done by scientists outside the realm of physical education, there was increasing recognition of the importance of exercise physiology in undergraduate and graduate physical education programs. Two additional textbooks were published in the early 1960s by R.E. Johnson and Ernst Jokl. Johnson's was an edited volume that saw frequent use as a graduate reference, but there was no text really suitable for graduate study at this time. Not a coincidence, this was the period during which Conant recommended cancelling graduate physical education. Conant's challenge produced a rapid response and exercise physiology grew into a discipline within the field of physical education. However, physical education as we know it today bears little resemblance to what existed at the time of Conant's report, evolving into a profession while the field of study we now call kinesiology emerged as its disciplinary counterpart.

The result of Conant's challenge was a widespread move toward requiring graduate students with a major or emphasis in exercise physiology to take graduate courses (and undergraduate prerequisites when appropriate) in departments of physiology, anatomy, and chemistry. Three obvious effects were: (1) with increased rigor, doctoral programs changed from 2–3 years in residence to 4–5 years, (2) graduates were able to compete on a more equal footing, publishing in sophisticated refereed journals and earning the respect of scientists outside of physical education, and (3) for the first time, a group of individuals were clearly defined as exercise physiologists. No longer was exercise physiology the exclusive domain of individuals trained in physiology, biochemistry, or medicine who just happened to have an interest in exercise. Exercise physiology had come of age.

Several increasingly sophisticated texts on exercise physiology, some clearly suitable for graduate study, were published in the 1960s and 1970s. The first edition of Åstrand and Rodahl's text found wide acceptance by graduate faculties. ACSM first published *Medicine and Science in Sports* in 1969. Although the journal's intended sports medicine audience was wide-ranging and interdisciplinary, a strong exercise physiology emphasis evolved.

ACSM's *Medicine and Science in Sports*, becoming *Medicine and Science in Sports and Exercise* in 1980 was an important new forum for exercise physiology papers. ACSM's manual on standardization of professional preparation for individuals interested in exercise leadership at several levels, along with guidelines for testing and prescription has been an important contribution to institutions that have responded to the need for training at the undergraduate and graduate levels of individuals seeking careers in corporate fitness, clinical exercise physiology settings, or related areas.

These new employment opportunities, emerging in significant number in the early 1970s and increasing into the 1990s and into the new century, breathed new life into many university physical education programs that had experienced decreasing interest in their traditional teacher education undergraduate and master's level graduate degrees.

Contributions from abroad have been especially important for the history of exercise physiology. Per-Olof Åstrand's textbooks make him perhaps one of the most influential. We quote him now to close the chapter. In a paper published in 1992, he asked this question, "Why has a subdiscipline entitled exercise physiology developed?"

In the second decade of the 21st century, that question should now be turned to address the broader disciple. We rephrase the question now—Why has Kinesiology developed? It is clear that as "old school" physical education was challenged to become a respected academic discipline, a refocusing took place in which science and research became central. Using the research tools of its parent disciplines, kinesiology emerged as the disciplinary counterpart with physical education in turn evolving into a profession focused on teacher preparation. Kinesiology today harkens strongly to Galen's *non-natural* tradition, a tradition that through the most of the 20th-century physical education had abandoned.

SUMMARY

The study of movement, physical activity, exercise, and sport is a vital and necessary academic pursuit given human's reliance on movement, a basic attribute necessary to remain healthy and vibrant. History also clearly indicates the universal appeal of physical activity and sport to all human beings. There is no known human culture in which it did not or does not exist. History is replete with the roots, controversies, debates, successes, and failures of what has come to be known as kinesiology. Ancient physicians knew of the importance of *regimen*, of which exercise was a key ingredient for health. Through the centuries, though, this knowledge was often obscured as the human body was devalued in favor of the education of the mind. In the enlightenment as the practice of modern medicine grew, Galen's principles gave the fledgling discipline of physical education the central core on which to establish itself. This, however, arguably was lost in favor of teaching students sports and games. This, of course, was not wholly without reason. As we saw, austere efforts such as the Turner movement based on sober duty simply did not appeal to most human beings. Instead they were drawn to play and delight. Which means, even at a clinical level, games may be better medicine than exercise. Medicine is only effective when people take it (11).

Can play and health be balanced? Are delight and duty compatible? To remain a vital part of 20th-century academic life, faculty of the 1960s and1970s pushed the discipline back toward science and health, arguably at the expense of play and delight. It out of this contested and evolving history that what we know of today as kinesiology has emerged. Who are we as kinesiologists? Whom do we serve as kinesiologists? What are our primary values, that is, what should kinesiology be about? History, philosophy, and experience (practice) all *inform* these questions, but you, as the future leaders of kinesiology, must be prepared to *answer* them. They will not answer themselves

REFERENCES

1. Aristotle. *Politics*. Translated by T. Sinclair and T. J. Saunders. New York: Penguin Books, 1981.

2. Augustine St. *The City of God*. Translated by G. G. Walsh, D. B. Zema, G. Monahan, and D. J. Honan. New York: Bantam Doubleday, 1958.

3. Berryman, J. W. "Motion and Rest: Galen on Exercise and Health." *Lancet* 380 (2012): 210–211.

4. Conant, J. B. *The Education of American Teachers*. New York: McGraw-Hill, 1963.

5. Dill, D. B. "The Harvard Fatigue Laboratory: Its Development, Contributions, and Demise." *Circulation Research (Supplement I)* 20–21 (1967): I-161–I-170.

6. Folk, G. E. "The Harvard Fatigue Laboratory: Contributions to World War II." *Advances in Physiological Education* 34 (2010): 119–127.

7. Guttmann, A. *Games and Empires: Modern Sports and Cultural Imperialism*. New York: Columbia University Press, 1994.

8. Guttmann, A. *Sports: The First Five Millennia*. Amherst and Boston: University of Massachusetts Press, 2004.

9. Henry, F. M. "Physical Education—An Academic Discipline." In *Proceedings of the Annual Meeting of the National College Physical Education Association for Men* (pp. 6–9). Washington, D.C.: AAHPER, 1964.

10. Henry, F. M. "The Academic Discipline of Physical Education." *Quest* 29 (1978): 13–29.

11. Hochstetler, D. R. "Another Look at 'Exercise Is Medicine.'" *The Journal of Physical Education, Recreation & Dance* 85 (2014): 7–8.

12. Kyle, D. G. "The Only Woman in All Greece: Kyniska, Agesilaus, Alcibiades and Olympia." *Journal of Sport History* (2003): 183–203.

13. Kyle, D. G. *Sport and Spectacle in the Ancient World* (2nd ed.). Malden: Wiley-Blackwell, 2015.

14. Miller, S. *Ancient Greek Athletics*. New York: Yale University Press, 2004.

15. Plato. *Five Dialogues*. Translated by G. Grube. Indianapolis: Hackett Publishing, 2002.

16. Plato. Timaeus. Translated by B. Jowett. Kindle Edition, 2012.

17. Post, Robert C. "Debating Disciplinarity." *Faculty Scholarship Series* (2009). Paper 164. http://digitalcommons.law.yale.edu/fss_papers/164.

18. Twietmeyer, G. "A Theology of Inferiority: Is Christianity the Source of Kinesiology's Second-Class Status in the Academy?" *Quest* 60 (2008): 452–466.

19. Twietmeyer, G. "Kinesis and the Nature of the Human Person." *Quest* 62 (2010): 135–154.

20. Twietmeyer, G. "What Is Kinesiology? Historical & Philosophical Insights." *Quest* 64 (2012): 4–23.

21. Young, D. C. *The Olympics Myth of Greek Amateur Athletics*. Chicago: Ares Publishers, 1984.

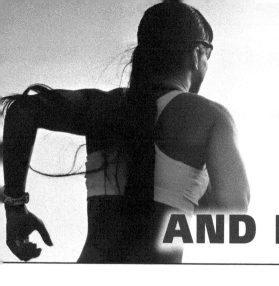

Chapter 2

EXERCISE, SPORT, AND PHYSICAL CULTURE

OUTLINE

OBJECTIVES

1. Overview tenets, purpose, and value of the humanities, specifically cultural-interpretive studies related to exercise, sport, and physical culture.

2. Introduce selected (canonical and recent) cultural studies' key terms, concepts, scholars, and works associated with the study of physical culture.

3. Sample criticism of the history and sociology of science regarding exercise, sport, and physical culture-related fields of study.

4. Inspire readers to think about how cultural analysis and the humanities can be uniquely used in their lives to effect social justice.

In a world of ever-new discoveries, inventions, scandals, and triumphs, what are the specific knowledges, ideas, and themes associated with cultural (interpretive, qualitative, humanistic) studies related to physical activity, exercise, and sport that will have enduring resonance—timeless value—to students and graduates of kinesiology, whatever their changing interests and long-term career directions? What are the issues coming onto the scene now that will help us anticipate upcoming directions in our fields of study and future careers? This chapter details foundational themes and theories of cultural interpretive studies and the humanities, all of which taken together offer a valuable, critical lens through which to view and live in the world, possibly transforming it for the better. The chapter also sketches some of the ideas of foundational (canonical) thinkers of cultural studies who are influential to the fields collectively located within the discipline of kinesiology. Fresh approaches to assess and understand exercise, sport, and physical culture experiences in new, changing times are likewise presented.

CULTURAL STUDIES

Overall, the field of cultural studies is concerned with understanding culture. Culture is anything and everything that humans endlessly create, perform, and live in. This may include, but is not limited to, ideas, beliefs, art, language, industry, everyday rituals, sport, and play. Those working in the humanities and cultural studies create nuanced definitions of things in order to reflect the knotty elaborateness of human life. Charles Fruehling Springwood studies sport and race, and understands culture as:

> . . . a semantic terrain, a space both historical and spatial, where the practices of signification and representation are enacted—where people represent themselves and their histories to themselves and others. As an unfolding process . . . culture is always politically situated, conflictural, and potentially empowering . . . such a slippery notion of culture allows for a consideration of culture as a site of creativity, but at the same time, it insists on situating this creativity within the strictures of history and power. (28)

Victor Turner is an anthropologist whose thought on play is foundational to the study of ritual and play:

> Playfulness is . . . volatile, sometimes dangerous . . . which cultural institutions seek to . . . contain in . . . competition, chance . . . strength, in modes . . . such as theater, and in controlled disorientation, from roller coasters to . . . dancing . . . Play can be everywhere and nowhere, imitate anything . . . be identified with nothing . . . (31)

Finally, Michael Silk, Anthony Bush, and David L. Andrews have written on physical activity and body culture. For these scholars, the "physical" is:

> complex multilayered . . . product and producer of . . . overlapping systems and discourses (economic, political, aesthetic, demographic, regulatory, spatial). . . . The physical . . . is the site . . . the moment at which social divisions (. . . class, ethnic, gender, ability, generational, national, racial . . . sexual) are imposed, experienced . . . contested. We are thus driven . . . to understand . . . complexities, experiences . . . injustices of [corporeality] . . . (27)

The above definitions of culture, play, and the physical stimulate readers to engage with elaborate meanings and imagine various ways these manifest in society. Such is the work of cultural studies.

Explore!

- Read the above definitions. Restate each definition in your own words in a sentence or two. Provide a specific example from your own experience of each definition.
- Select one of the above quoted passages about culture, play, and the physical. Research the quotation's author(s) and conduct a search (through a library digital database or Google Scholar) of the author's research, publications, social media. Where was the author educated and in what field(s)? What are the author's most recent research interests and how does early work relate (or not) to current research? How have the authors contributed to exercise, sport, and physical culture studies?

Why Cultural Studies?

As a student of a kinesiology, you might wonder how cultural studies can help you to make a difference in the world—after all, the humanities do not seek "cures" of diseases, nor do cultural studies predict behavior, enhance performance, well-being, or lifespan as do the aims of fields such as physiology, biomechanics, occupational and physical therapy, coaching, and medicine. What is the use of cultural studies to a kinesiology graduate?

Foremost, the humanities and cultural studies ask us to understand the condition of humanity. What is it to be human in different times and places? It asks us to consider the wonder, the tragedy, the beauty, and diversity of humanity. Yet we are all the same. Engaged citizens of the world use cultural studies as enhanced, in-depth lens with which to view the world and human activity. Humanities knowledge is a foundation from which people converse and create, and sometimes that creation helps transform (change) culture.

The field of cultural studies is influenced by and probes ideas from fields as diverse as art, neuroscience, and architecture. Consider the following examples:

- Art can be used to reflect on sport and physical culture-related real-time experiences. Media, digital, fantasy, and marketed representations of these viewed on *YouTube* or gaming media may be appreciated and understood in terms not of win-loss, but of aesthetics, musical score, virtual experience, or comedic quality.
- Neuroscience is a field in which brain studies are at the top of government and medical priorities. A hot topic today is the dedication to a renewed understanding of the scientific/neural aspects of sport concussions and professional athlete suicides linked to head injuries. Cultural studies traditions, such as exemplified by the work of Alva Noë, remind us that "human experience is a dance that unfolds in the world and with others. You are not your brain (21)."
- Take note of the changes in sport stadia, now designed as giant media screens, with innovative materials, structural design, and vectors that move and enable interaction with athletes, spectators, shoppers, workers, the environment, and space. New corporations are even pioneering sport and play facilities in space and low gravity. The website of IPX Entertainment, a private corporation in Nevada USA, states that they are at work on forming a zero-gravity sports league and a space champions reality show that pits the best zero-gravity athletes against each other in contests in space.

What does it mean that even in exotic and novel geographies and architectures, sport, exercise, and body culture continue to be inscribed in traditional familiar modernistic ways?

Epistemology and Ontology

As mentioned in the opening sections of this chapter, some of the basic tools of cultural-interpretive studies and the humanities are critical reading, participating in and/or viewing performances and art works of all types, and conversation/debate. A university education prepares students to be active citizens of the world, and it is with these basic tools of the humanities that we should continue to challenge ourselves over a lifetime.

For example, over the course of your life, don't settle for habitually reading exclusively a particular literary genre or blog. In addition to your favorites, seek ever-more demanding and sophisticated advanced readings, display, performances, media, games, and ideas outside of your usual *epistemology* (way of knowing) and *ontology* (way of being). Build a digital or print library, an art collection, wear fashion that is uniquely and completely you:

> Shopping is a responsibility, an exercise of power. The food we eat, the clothes we wear, the objects we have in our homes form the very basis of our lives. The choices that we make about these things play a big role in determining who we are.... Shopping is sometimes exciting, sometimes neurotic, sometimes wasteful. But it's not frivolous. We use things and give them meanings. (13)

Ideas like that espoused by Thomas Hine help us to appreciate and even allow fashion or décor choices that disrupt or modify stereotypical notions of what a coach, therapist, gym, laboratory, physical education teacher, playground, and so on, should look like.

Peace and Community

A premise of the humanities/cultural studies is that as we view the world with the lens of cultural studies, transformation and understanding can come about in small ways. Through neighborly conversation, through individual small acts, through practices of self-reflexivity and critical analysis—all practices of cultural studies—humans can at the least stand side by side, realizing and empathizing with other worlds of understanding.

Sport, physical activity, exercise—these core foci of the epistemology and ontology of our field of study—seem to have promise for building human empathy and for helping communities foster peace and development. Indeed, of late, a myriad of initiatives such as the United Nations Sport for Development and Peace "Right to Play" have been devoted to building community. But it's not as simple as this when we use the lens of cultural analysis.

First, we can *critique/interrogate/deconstruct*, terms that are used in cultural studies to mean analyze, research, in-depth study. Gerald W. Creed interrogates "community" and argues that what a community is "is rarely specified," meaning that the term is so "commonsensical" that it seems not to "*need* defining" and "this is precisely why scholars need to pay attention to it." Community is not only about collectivity, but it also reinforces oppression, exclusion, violence, and genocide (6). So when we follow Creed and credit sport and physical culture with fostering nationalism, good citizenship, community, we can deconstruct the glorified role of sport in community building. Ponder this argument that goes against the idea of "sport for peace:"

> A predominant modern mythos embedded in popular and academic perceptions of sport decrees that ... playing on the youth football team builds character, that Palestinians and Israelis who skateboard or surf together are contributing toward world peace, and so on ... these and all such sport-embellished circumstances/settings/conditions are not about sport but are circumstances of any and all activities of public life ... However large sport allows humans to live, it is not sport itself that cures/heals societies, fosters development, and/or peace ... all sport does is place disparate individuals, communities, and nations next to each other (29).

Explore!

- Next time you hear "community" discussed in a university course or conversation, engage the speaker to consider the criticism that hand-in-hand with the upbeat notions of community come destructive and isolating features.
- Using the Internet, search the term "Olympism" and make a list of the meanings attributed to the term. Critique the various aims, definitions, functions, and promises that have been attached to the concept.

Critical Analysis and Self-Reflexivity

The cultural studies scholar seeks self-reflexivity, a trait of being aware of the sociocultural politics and historical origins of everyday life and actions in which one is engaged. Here is an illustration of an instance where self-reflexivity might have come in handy. One evening, ESPN broadcast the World Baseball Classic in Spanish instead of English. Many tweets immediately ensued, some defending the Spanish broadcast, but many others used derogatory racial slurs to complain. Read a report of the broadcast on the website, deadspin.com, written by one of their editors (warning: offensive language). Viewers who saw the telecast reacted to it at the deadspin.com site (http://deadspin.com/is-it-me-or-has-espn-been-taken-over-by-wetbacks-vie-5989829) among other places. As happens nowadays, larger news venues gathered extreme samples of tweets about the telecast and widely publicized them in articles reacting to the Spanish broadcast. It turned out that the author of one of the pejorative tweets headlined that evening was an athletic training graduate student in an American university's Department of Kinesiology. The student had tweeted hatred without self-reflexivity, without taking into account the history and culture of our country, or the speed and power of social media. What could have been a tiny moment to contribute to the good of society became the student's greater downfall.

Explore!

- On social media, Jaron Lanier's *You Are Not a Gadget: A Manifesto* offers apt advice. Select one pursuit recommended by Lanier in the direct quotations bulleted below and work on it throughout the semester. Report to the class what you did, along with the thought and creative process that went into your undertaking. That is, you do not have to actually present your website-blog-video-tweet to the class; instead, briefly describe what you undertook, exposing the seams of the processes of your project:
  - Create a website that expresses something about who you are that won't fit into the template available to you on a social networking site.
  - Post a video once in a while that took you 100 times more time to create than it takes to view.
  - Write a blog that took weeks of reflection before you heard the inner voice that needed to come out.
  - If you are twittering, innovate in order to find a way to describe your internal state instead of trivial external events, to avoid the creeping danger of believing that objectively described events define you, as they would define a machine (17).

Foundational Thought

Art, architecture, and neuroscience were identified earlier as fields of study that trade ideas with cultural studies of exercise, sport, and physical culture. Exercise, sport, and physical culture studies have also been influenced over the past half century by the literature and research of cultural anthropology, social history, literary criticism, and French philosophical thought:

- Roland Barthes wrote about sport in *What Is Sport?* (1).
- Pierre Bourdieu's ideas are used to analyze physical culture and social class (2).
- Michel Foucault's noteworthy books, interviews, and lectures investigate historical and societal processes that, in a famous passage, "invest, mark, train and torture the body; they force it to carry out tasks, to perform ceremonies, and to emit signs" (10).

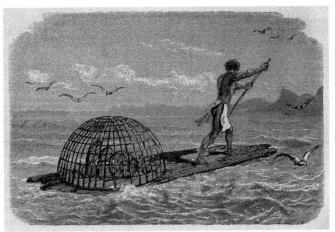

Figure 2.1. *Surfing has diverse global roots.*

What does all this connote? Culturalists understand that humans commonly think in terms of binaries—such as good-bad, black-white, fit-unfit, fast-slow. One part of the binary is thought to be positive (well, good, healthy) while the other might be subtly or unconsciously understood as "pathological"—negative, sick, deviant. As time passes, pathologies change. In one era, body odor, flat feet, and male chest hair are not matters of consideration in the least, but in another era, these cause embarrassment and create huge industries of remedies. It is not bad to think in binary terms, but we do need to be aware of what this binary thinking means in terms of how changing conceptions of self, family, and subculture are used to judge and understand others.

Orientalism, a book by Edward W. Said (24), has been influential to many disciplines, including physical culture studies. Said argued that in the developed West, there exists a binary, one side of which implies characteristics such as foreign, primitive, weak, less developed, effeminate, while the other side of the binary is judged as strong, healthy, manly, intelligent. For Said, the concept of orientalism is not only about Asia. Rather, it includes all manifestations of "otherness" that appear juxtaposed to white Western developed society. Applying Said's analysis to sport, we find that Western society celebrates a "narrative" (a story line, perhaps false or embellished, that societal members understand and circulate as truth) of a rich, long sport history, including invention of sport and teaching sport to "others" who are stereotyped to be too primitive or undeveloped to invent their own sport or have the stamina or work ethic to highly train and practice sport skills. If "others" do practice sport (such as early Polynesian surfing or contests of the Trobriand Islanders), the developed West often characterizes that sport as erotic or vulgar, outlaws it, and attempts to impose its European or American version of "civilized" sport.

Cultural anthropologist Susan Brownell argues that because of orientalism, China seemed to the West to be without a sport history even though Chinese sport practices have a long vibrant past (4). For many years, this belief prevented the International Olympic Committee from designating China as an Olympic Games host. As part of its (finally) successful bid for the 2008 Games, China had to emphasize its Western-like sport history in order to seem qualified to host the Games.

In another example of orientalism, white American males are said to be pioneers and heroes of sports like surfing. However, if the history of surfing is studied in depth, it is found that the ancient area of Peru, east and west coasts of Africa, Indonesia and also women and children were historically involved in surfing-like activities (Figure 2.1).

HEGEMONY AND THE UNSAYABLE

Hegemony, the power and dominance of particular beliefs, values, norms, practices, rule, symbol, style, is a theoretical aspect of culture that is widely studied by culturalists. Thinking about hegemony is a hallmark of critical analysis. Critical analysis enables one to be conscious of practices and beliefs that seem to be natural, and are deemed "right" or "true." Influenced by the work of canonical thinkers such as Antonio Gramsci and Foucault, and interrelated with the other concepts studied in this chapter such as binaries, orientalism and self-reflexivity, the paradigm (a model or concept) of hegemony investigates how "truth" and "knowledge" change historically and are influenced by language and social relations.

Styles, values, and beliefs surrounding physical culture and often taken for granted as natural or "the way it's always been," have a history. Consider for example the past 50 to 100 years during which time many scientists working in American physical culture erroneously believed that African Americans were "less buoyant" and thus less able swimmers because of supposed anatomical and biological differences. This same group was also believed to have relatively more "fast twitch" muscle fibers, thus making them biologically superior in short distance sprinting track events. The research featured in the documentary film *White Wash* (2012) clearly shows that centuries of slavery, segregation, and legal exclusion from water culture (swimming pools, swim instruction, beaches) as well as the abuse of slave owners who punished escaping slaves by drowning them, built a mythology about the dangers of water and prohibited African Americans from learning to swim. *White Wash* notes that today less than 2% of swimmers registered in the National Swim Association identify as black and 60% of African Americans report that they cannot swim. Think about ways that you can help change these statistics.

> After viewing the *White Wash* film in a university class, a student wrote, "I used to believe that black people didn't swim because it was something that we just didn't do. I remember trying every sport, but I was never encouraged to swim. After watching this video, I really want to learn how to swim and maybe even go surfing one day."

Other unquestioned "truths" disseminated by fields allied to kinesiology includes the idea that strenuous competition will harm female reproductive organs. Until 2014 women were banned from Olympic ski jumping because, as the president of the International Ski Federation warned, "This seems not to be proper for ladies from a medical point of view." Watch the 2005 MSNBC report by Rachel Maddow, "Why Girls Can't Jump," at www.youtube.com/watch?v=_Y_J9_NrXCM&playnext=1&index=21&list=PLB8D4F0B4F1515FED.

Pierre de Coubertin, celebrated as one of the founders of the modern Olympic Games, wrote of the Olympics as "the means of bringing to perfection the strong and hopeful youth of our white race, thus again helping towards the perfection of all human society" (32). This racist idea was once accepted as a premise of organized athletics, but even now de Coubertin continues to garner acclaim at Olympic Games opening ceremonies.

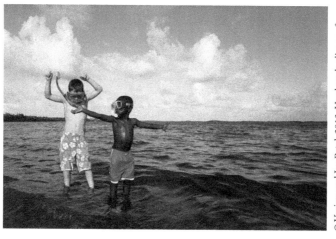

© Varina and Jay Patel, 2013. Used under license from Shutterstock, Inc.

Figure 2.2. *Erroneous myths about exercise and body culture can be erased at the level of everyday practices.*

These historically situated beliefs are not outrightly political or backed by force or authority. John Hargreaves, a pioneer in writing about sport and hegemony (11), reminds that hegemony is something that has power because we give it consent without question. Dominant groups and ideals maintain their authority and control without coercion. Sometimes a belief is so powerful that to question it is beyond the realm—the questioning is "unspeakable" or "unsayable" (12).

Hargreaves emphasizes that hegemony is "diffused" and continually circulates through society in matter-of-fact ways (11). Gender-related issues offer clear examples of hegemony. A student recounted that his girl-friend, an elite-level international competitive snowboarder, guided him down a difficult run. On the lift at the top of the mountain, before they started down, the lift operators and ski patrol quizzed the woman if she was "all right here?" Could she "handle the difficulty?" The hegemonic idea that sport is for males influenced the authorities to assume that the female was less athletically skilled then the male. What would you do if you found yourself in a similar situation?

> The work of an intellectual is . . . through the analysis that he carries out in his own field, to question over and over and over again what is postulated as self-evident, to disturb people's mental habits, the way they do and think things, to dissipate what is familiar and accepted, to reexamine rules and institutions . . . (9, 18)

Governmentality

Influenced by Foucault, Dr. Samantha King, a professor of kinesiology and health studies, wondered about "races for the cure" and "pink ribbon" campaigns that involve participants in walks, marathons, and other physical challenges that are paired with fundraising for cancer and disease-centered charities such as the Susan G. Komen for the Cure Foundation (Figure 2.3). While volunteerism and philanthropy are noble ventures, King argues that they involve "governmentality" (16).

People come to believe they are ideal citizens because they participate in charity event races. They devote extraordinary time and resources "training" for these races, purchasing athletic gear, consuming a myriad of pink-ribbon products, soliciting financial support from friends and family—all of which culminate in feel-good mass celebration athletic events that hide real suffering and societal/governmental faults/failures. Critics like King suggest that such personal devotion to "running for the cure" prevents citizens from engaging in communal efforts to amend laws or on collective social responsibility that effects changes in poverty, racism, or the cosmetics, foods, and industries that may *cause* cancer. In concentrating on individual body culture, exercise

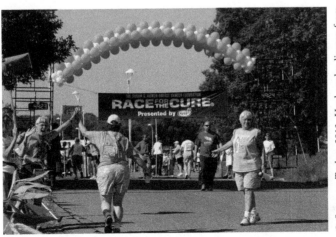

© Suzanne Tucker, 2013. Used under license from Shutterstock, Inc.

Figure 2.3. *Cultural critique of "Race for the Cure" in regard to governmentality.*

and sport—in other words, when we spend our time and resources working out/exercising for charities and "cures"—we no longer devote ourselves to instigating needed radical change in government, race relations, poverty, etc. This is governmentality.

Explore!

Students are encouraged to Watch *Pink Ribbons, Inc.*, (2011) http://firstrunfeatures.com/pinkribbonsinc/ a full length feature film that originated as a dissertation in kinesiology by Samantha King. King published her dissertation as *Pink Ribbons Inc.: Breast Cancer and the Politics of Philanthropy* (University of Minnesota Press, 2006), and this book inspired award-winning producer and director to create the film, *Pink Ribbons Inc.* Listen to an interview with King about her research and the film: http://will.illinois.edu/focus/program/beyond-the-pink-ribbon-the-politics-of-breast-cancer-civic-engagement-and-c

Body Culture

It is relevant to our field of study that it is through performances and actions of the body that society works. Historian Paul Connerton points out that societies remember certain things because they bodily perform them (5). C.L.R. James, in his classic treatise about cricket and culture observed that "We respond to physical action or vivid representation of it . . . because we are made that way . . ." (15). William McNeil's theory states that humans need the display of corporeal rituals in which humans move together (as in parades, sports) as an undergirding to society (19). For Brian Boyd, play helps humans "resist damage and loss," evolve "variety, emotions, intelligence, cooperation and . . . creativity itself" (3).

It is interesting that through their embodied performance, sport and exercise are prime vehicles of hegemony. But why? Hargreaves answers that sport, game, and play have universal appeal at the same time as being highly formalized with roles and rules. They are seemingly outside of "real" life, occurring in leisure time (11). When something appears to be free, fun, and natural such as 4- and 5-year-old girls wearing thick makeup and skimpy costumes as they cheer on boys playing in youth football leagues, hegemonic ideas about bodies, family, race, gender, and so on are displayed as "the way it is." To question or protest the unsaid gender divisions in Pop Warner football "Tiny Mite" Division seems trivial. Yet it is in raising questions in our communities and families that change begins to occur (Figure 2.4).

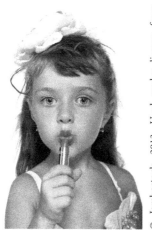 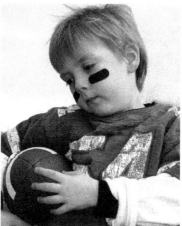

© Jambostock, 2013. Used under license from Shutterstock, Inc.

© Richard Paul Kane, 2013. Used under license from Shutterstock, Inc.

Figure 2.4. *Traditional visions of the body continue in today's physical culture.*

As in the Pop Warner football example, conventional critiques surrounding "women and sport" seek gender equity, focusing on how women are constrained by masculine cultural hegemony. But a cultural studies sensibility leads to a nuanced—and controversial—understanding of gender as described by an editor of a surf magazine. "Men and women surfers may not be equal. We've been blessed with different abilities, strengths, and appeal. Of course we'd love to see women right up there with men—equal exposure, clout, salaries—but there is something to be said for embracing the extraordinariness of being female" (14). Older cultural studies analyzed "the media" as a single repressive entity. Recent studies such as by Dr. Holly Thorpe magnify that media is not all encompassing, can be "enabling and productive," and that active participants in culture and sport "examine and make sense of the multiple and contradictory mediated discourses of femininity in the culture" (30).

SOCIOLOGY AND OUR FIELD OF STUDY

Cultural studies applied to exercise, sport, and physical culture within the discipline of kinesiology are relatively young as far as disciplines go (math and drama, for example, were considered academic subjects as early as 1000 B.C., with kinesiology and physical education having origins in early modernity) and are little studied in terms of their own sociology and anthropology. What are the obsessions of our fields of study? We can turn cultural critique to our disciplines and sub-fields themselves.

Examine your department or school's website. The director or head usually has a statement of welcome on the home page. Certainly most institutions of all types justify their objectives in mission or philosophy statements. When we assert in such expositions that we seek to address and enhance "quality of life" or to gain "new knowledge" concerning exercise and movement, what exactly do such statements entail? Consider this mission statement:

> The State . . . will first of all have to base its educational work not on the mere imparting of knowledge, but rather on physical training and development of healthy bodies.

The author of the quote is Adolph Hitler. These words are repeated in many variations from his *Mein Kampf* (*My Struggle*) and from other Nazi writers putting forward the rationale for the murder of nearly 17 million Jews, other religious groups, the disabled, ethnic minorities, and aged people. In an important essay for our field, Eric Segal shows "the road traveled from the modernist obsession with the physical" to the "extremist cultivation of the body as a symbol of racial superiority" is "frighteningly short" (25). Such is eugenics, a "science" that has the objective of producing fine offspring, especially in the human race.

Eugenics laws in the United States from the 19th century through the 1960s prevented marriage between those deemed mentally disabled, forced sterilization of criminals, and limited immigration of poor eastern European immigrants. These dehumanizing and racist practices have a history of ties with the sciences, pedagogy, and research that have to do with the physical, physical training, and education. *Fit: Episodes in the History of the Body* (1994), a documentary film that impacted kinesiology and sport studies, warns that "those who have the authority to define who is fit and who is not always include their own ideals and fears in their definitions."

William H. Sheldon, the originator of somatotype (body type) research that has been extensively used in kinesiology (formerly physical education), wrongly believed that the somatotype "appears to be the most deepseated, most general, and most overt expression of personality that a human being presents" (26). Sheldon's 400-page *Atlas of Men* is crammed with coldhearted animalistic descriptions of his human subjects' personalities that he based on measurement of their bodies:

> Sheep. Delicate limbed, fat-bodied, inoffensive browsers whose personal deportment is usually above reproach except that they eat too much and are too easily influenced . . . he does not amount to much. (26)

Sheldon's research took place over 60 years ago, but even today, courses and textbooks cover somatotypes without disputing Sheldon's specious viewpoints that masqueraded as science. Sport philosopher Heather L. Reid writes of our field of study, "the lab-coats and test-tubes bring an aura of intellectual respectability . . . but they objectify the athletic body more than ever. Now my body plays object not only to my mind, but also to scientists and technicians who regard it as an item to probe, measure and examine" (23).

Recently "active aging" and "health disparities" are common research themes in North American Departments of Kinesiology. Supported by important bodies, such as the National Institutes of Health (NIH), United Nations (UN), World Health Organization (WHO), and the Social Security Administration, it is customary for educators and researchers to direct their focus on strategies for older and/or people with health disparities to stay active and independent. For a deconstruction of the "active aging agenda" see Elizabeth Pike's work referenced here (22).

These research and funding initiatives forward a specific developed-modern-world-Western vision of "positive" health and "active" aging. Yet, in the historical-cultural context, other cultural-religious traditions accept aging and health disparities as human destiny, as possibly "redemptive:"

> Illness can lead to anguish, self-absorption, sometimes even despair and revolt. . . . It can also make a person more mature, helping him discern in his life what is not essential so that he can turn toward that which is. (From the *Catechism of the Catholic Church.* Ligouri MO: Ligouri Publications, 1994, sec. 1501)

Reflect for a moment on obesity, another recent preoccupation of our fields of research as well as of national and international policy. Margaret Carlisle Duncan, a cultural studies scholar, critiques "obesity public discourses" such as those presented by the "American Academy of Physical Education and Kinesiology . . . [that frame] obesity as an individual problem crying out for an individual solution" (8; see also 20). In her introduction to a special *Sociology of Sport Journal* issue devoted to studies of the sociology of obesity, Duncan explains:

> none of these authors is arguing that diseases associated with fat . . . are trivial or irrelevant. Such diseases clearly pose a danger to people's health. . . . Instead [we focus] on . . . public discourses that demonize fat, the sociocultural meanings of fat . . . taken-for-granted assumptions that fat is wholly bad, even egregious. (8)

Explore!

Examine your department or school's website and discuss it with your peers. Does it reflect your understanding of the department/college's aims? Suggestions for revision? Think about how you can personally carry forth the department's mission.

EXERCISE, SPORT, AND PHYSICAL CULTURE TO BE . . .

In kinesiology careers, we use the humanities to probe how labels, words, and even mission statements and lesson plans themselves have political-social power, how everything in culture has a history and a cultural context that informs how things are understood, valued, or perhaps forgotten. As you go into the world with a university degree, your vocation calls on you to voice questions, investigate evidence-based science gone wrong. We heed Norman K. Denzin's (one of the greatest sociologists of our times whose work has deep influence on cultural kinesiology) call to base our scholarship on "social justice, human rights, integrity, a belief in the dignity and worth of the person, compassion, love, and empowerment, resistance, dialogue" (7). Realize that how you communicate and relay your knowledge to others is not limited to the research paper or oral presentation. Unprecedented new and coming-onto-the-scene filmic, reading, and composition technologies offer modes of expression barely experimented with yet and open to your creative interventions.

In the next decade, the idea of a university, the conception of citizenship, the parameters of the body—and more—have the potential to be transformed by knowledge derived from kinesiology, an unimaginable revolution of a future promise. This is physical culture studies within kinesiology (perchance with new labels and identities), and you the reader are a pioneer of all that is to be or hoped for . . .

SUMMARY

The reader journeyed in this chapter through an overview of cultural interpretive studies and the humanities because these schools of thought can be used in, and have impacted, exercise, sport, and physical culture. We sampled significant ideas that assist in critical-cultural analysis, becoming familiar with some key thinkers such as Michel Foucault whose ideas have the capacity to reform exercise, sport, and physical culture studies. Recent important critiques, including those regarding obesity or that from Samantha King regarding governmentality, were covered in the chapter. Throughout the chapter, readers are inspired to develop and articulate ways of knowing and being (epistemology and ontology). Readers are urged to think about how cultural analysis and the humanities can be uniquely used in their own lives to affect social justice.

REFERENCES

1. Barthes, Roland, *What Is Sport?* Richard Howard, trans. New Haven and London: Yale University Press, 2007.

2. Bourdieu, Pierre, "Sport and Social Class," in Chandra Mukerji and Michæl Schudson, Eds. *Rethinking Popular Culture: Contemporary Perspectives in Cultural Studies.* Berkeley: University of California Press, 1991, pp. 357–373.

3. Boyd, Brian, *On the Origin of Stories: Evolution, Cognition and Fiction.* Cambridge, MA: The Belknap Press of Harvard University Press, 2009 (quotation p. 414).

4. Brownell, Susan, "Europe and the People without Sport History, or what Hosting the Olympic Games Means to China," in Brownell, *Beijing's Games: What the Olympics Mean to China.* Rowman & Littlefield Publishers, Inc., 2008, pp. 19–47.

5. Connerton, Paul, *How Societies Remember.* Cambridge University Press, 1989.

6. Creed, Gerald W., ed., *The Seductions of Community: Emancipations, Oppressions, Quandaries.* Santa Fe: School of American Research Press, 2006 (quotation p. 4).

7. Denzin, Norman K., *The Qualitative Manifesto: A Call to Arms.* Left Coast Press, 2010 (quotation p. 121).

8. Duncan, Margaret Carlisle, "Introduction: The Personal is the Political," *Sociology of Sport Journal,* 2008, 25, pp. 1–6 (quotations pp. 1, 3).

9. Foucault, Michel, "The Concern for Truth," in L.D. Kritzman (ed.) *Michel Foucault Politics, Philosophy, Culture: Interviews and Other Writing 1977–1984.* London: Routledge, 1988 (quotation p. 265 as originally cited in [18]).

10. Foucault, Michel, *Discipline and Punish: The Birth of the Prison.* A. Sheridan, trans. New York: Pantheon, 1977, original work published 1975 (quotation p. 25).

11. Hargreaves, John, *Sport, Power and Culture.* Cambridge: Polity Press, 1986 (quotations pp. 5–7; 10–15).

12. Harrison, Kathryn, "What's left unsaid. Review of Annie G. Rogers," *The Unsayable: The Hidden Language of Trauma. NYTimes.com.* (2006, August 13). Retrieved from <www.nytimes.com/2006/08/13/books/review/13harrison.html?pag>).

13. Hine, Thomas, *I Want That! How We All Became Shoppers: A Cultural History.* New York: Harper Collins, 2002 (quotation p. 208).

14. Irons, Jana, "Intro," *Salted: A Surf Magazine for Women,* Fall 2012, p. 12.

15. James, C.L.R., *Beyond a Boundary.* New York: Pantheon Books, 1963 (quotation pp. 203–204).

16. King, Samantha J., "Doing Good by Running Well: Breast Cancer, the Race for the Cure, and New Technologies of Ethical Citizenship," in Zach Z. Bratich, Jeremy Packer, and Cameron McCarthy, eds. *Foucault, Cultural Studies, and Governmentality.* State University of New York Press, 2003, pp. 3–11, 295–316.

17. Lanier, Jaron, *You Are Not a Gadget: A Manifesto.* New York: Vintage Books, 2010 (quotation p. 21).

18. Markula, Pirkko, and Richard Pringle, *Foucault, Sport and Exercise: Power Knowledge and the Self.* New York: Routledge, 2006 (quotation p. 178).

19. McNeill, William H., *Keeping Together in Time: Dance and Drill in Human History.* Cambridge, MA: Harvard University Press, 1995.

20. Murray, Samantha, "Pathologizing 'Fatness': Medical Authority and Popular Culture." *Sociology of Sport Journal,* 25(1), March 2008, pp. 7–21.

21. Noë, Alva, *Out of Our Heads, Why You Are Not Your Brain, and Other Lessons from the Biology of Consciousness.* New York: Hill and Wang, 2011 (quotation pp. xi–xiii).

22. Pike, Elizabeth, "The Active Aging Agenda, Old Folk Devils and a New Moral Panic," *Sociology of Sport Journal,* 28(2), 2011, pp. 209–225.

23. Reid, Heather L., *The Philosophical Athlete.* Durham, NC: Carolina Academic Press, 2002 (quotation p. 42).

24. Said, Edward W., *Orientalism.* New York: Vintage Books, 1979.

25. Segal, Harold B., *Body Ascendant: Modernism and the Physical Imperative.* Baltimore and London: Johns Hopkins University Press, 1998 (quotation p. 251).

26. Sheldon, William H., with the collaboration of C. Wesley Dupertuis and Eugene McDermott. *Atlas of Men: A Guide for Somatotyping the Adult Male at All Ages.* New York: Harper, 1954 (quotations pp. xv; 200). With appreciation to Caitlin Vitosky—Clarke for her research on this source.

27. Silk, Michael L., Anthony Bush and David L Andrews, "Contingent Intellectual Amateurism, or, the Problem with Evidence—based Research," *Journal of Sport and Social Issues,* 34(1), 2010, pp. 105–128 (quotation p. 112).

28. Springwood, Charles Fruehling, *Cooperstown to Dyersville: A Geography of Baseball Nostalgia.* Boulder CO: Westview Press, 1996 (quotation pp. 11–12).

29. Sydnor, Synthia, "On the Nature of Sport: A Treatise in Light of Universality and Digital Culture," forthcoming in Gary Osmond and Murray Phillips, eds., *Sport History in the Digital Era.* Champaign: University of Illinois Press (In Press).

30. Thorpe, Holly, "Foucault, Technologies of Self, and the Media: Discourses of Femininity in Snowboarding Culture," *Journal of Sport and Social Issues* 2008, 32, pp. 199–229 (quotation p. 200).

31. Turnerm Victor W., "Body, Brain, and Culture." *Zygon* 18(3) (September 1, 1983), pp. 221–245 (quotation pp. 233–234).

32. Young, David C., "How the Amateurs Won the Olympics," in *The Archaeology of the Olympics: The Olympics and Other Festivals in Antiquity.* Madison: The University of Wisconsin Press, 1988, pp. 55–75 (quotation p. 65).

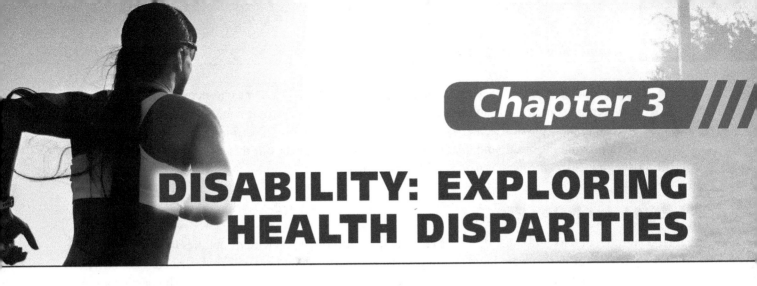

Chapter 3

DISABILITY: EXPLORING HEALTH DISPARITIES

 OUTLINE

 CHAPTER OBJECTIVES

1. Present an overview of major U.S. laws governing the status of persons with disabilities.
2. Describe the major models of disability.
3. Illustrate the prevalence and impact of disability in the United States.
4. Increase awareness of the health disparities experienced by persons with disabilities.
5. Describe determinants of health in persons with disabilities.
6. Demonstrate how physical activity promotion may alleviate health disparities among persons with disabilities.

A large proportion of the U.S. population has disabilities. Disability is not synonymous with poor health; however, persons with disabilities experience health disparities that could be partially alleviated by increasing their physical activity and fitness profiles. Therefore, kinesiology professionals can play a key role in improving the health and quality of life of these individuals, but this effort requires knowledge of critical issues that affect the lives of persons with disabilities.

LEGAL MANDATES

A large number of laws and court decisions regulate the status of people with disabilities in the United States. For the purposes of this chapter, however, only a few landmark federal laws will be described. The *Americans with Disabilities Act (ADA) of 1990*—last amended in 2008—is a federal law protecting the participation of people with disabilities in a broad array of life activities (1). ADA is a civil rights law consisting of five titles that prohibit discrimination against people with disabilities in employment (Title I), public entities (Title II), public accommodations (Title III), telecommunications (Title IV), and other life activities (Title V).

The *Rehabilitation Act of 1973* also prohibits discrimination against people with disabilities in programs conducted by federal agencies, in programs receiving federal financial assistance, in federal employment, and in the employment practices of federal contractors (3). This law offers people with disabilities—mainly those with severe disabilities—access to vocational rehabilitation and employment-related services. Section 504 of this act also increases educational opportunities for children and adults with disabilities, allowing for reasonable accommodations in schooling practices.

The *Individuals with Disabilities Education Act (IDEA) of 1990*—last amended in 2004—regulates how states and public agencies offer early intervention, special education, and related services to youth with disabilities from birth until the 21st year of age (2). IDEA mandates that all youth with disabilities have access to "a free, appropriate, public education in the least restrictive environment." Among other provisions, IDEA requires that public schools generate an Individualized Education Program (IEP) that outlines the services offered to each student with a disability. The IEP is developed by a team of knowledgeable persons, including the student's parents, and must be reviewed annually. This provision aims at increasing academic expectations for students with disabilities. Under this law, parents may request a hearing if they disagree with the proposed IEP. Currently, more than six million children receive special education under IDEA (7).

MODELS OF DISABILITY

The way disability is defined has large implications for health care and health promotion and, as a result, it has been a topic of debate among people with disabilities, disability advocates, researchers, and theorists. Drum (12) broadly identified four models of disability—Medical, Social, Functional, and Integrated—and discussed their implications for public health.

The *Medical model* reflects many medical practices. According to this model, disability is a problem inherent in the person and it is the direct outcome of disease, trauma, or other health conditions. Management of disability under this model aims at a medical cure. Disability is typically described in categorical terms (e.g., multiple sclerosis, cerebral palsy, Down syndrome). Such categorical classification allows for easy determination of eligibility for health care services (7). The Medical model, however, has been criticized by disability advocates because it tends to neglect social determinants of disability (12).

The *Functional model* emphasizes functional limitations arising from impairment. This model shares with the medical model the idea that disability exists in the person; however, it does not focus on identifying a medical cure to the impairment. Instead, the functional model concentrates on alleviating difficulties in functioning through appropriate strategies such as physical, occupational, and speech therapy. The functional model of disability reflects several U.S. laws where the definition of disability is based on limitations in major life activities—not simply on the presence of impairment (12). For example, this model is used in the ADA.

The *Social model* stands opposite to the medical and functional models. According to the social model, disability is socially constructed and arises from social oppression against people with impairments (12). In this model, disability is not an attribute of the person. Instead, it is an experience caused by architectural, social, and political barriers faced by persons with impairments. For example, a person with multiple sclerosis who needs a motorized wheelchair for ambulation may become disabled by social factors such as inaccessible buildings, negative attitudes, reduced opportunities for employment, low income, and limited access to the health care system. Under the social model, alleviating disability requires social change (12).

Integrated models have resulted from efforts to blend the positive aspects of the aforementioned models after accepting that disability is a multidimensional experience. One notable effort was based on the work of sociologist Saad Nagi, who identified four interacting components in the disablement process: (a) active pathology, (b) impairment, (c) functional limitation, and (d) disability (12). Later modifications viewed these facets as occurring sequentially and added a fifth dimension of societal limitations, accepting the idea that participation restrictions arise from social barriers (12).

An integrated model of disability is also endorsed by the World Health Organization and it is described in the International Classification of Functioning, Disability, and Health, better known as ICF (29). The ICF model views disability as an experience that arises from the dynamic interactions between a person's health condition and contextual factors—some found in the environment and some existing within the person (Figure 3.1). Examples of environmental factors are architectural concerns, technologies, services, policies, attitudes towards people with disabilities, and social relationships. Personal factors reflect a person's psychosocial attributes including age, sex, employment, income, education, attitudes, and self-efficacy among others. According to the ICF, disability has three interacting levels: (a) impairments, (b) activity limitations,

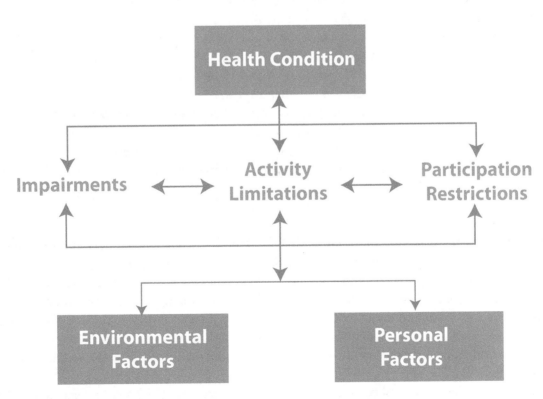

Figure 3.1.   *The ICF Model of Disability. Source: World Health Organization.*

and (c) participation restrictions (Figure 3.1). Impairments refer to loss or abnormality in body structure or function—either physical or mental. Activity limitations refer to difficulties in executing tasks. Participation restrictions are problems in involvement in life affairs. Parenthetically, it could be argued that low physical fitness and physical activity, both of which are common in people with disabilities (5, 19, 21, 25, 26, 28), may reside within impairments and activity limitations, respectively. In summary, the ICF model views disability as a multidimensional phenomenon arising from complex interactions between personal and environmental factors.

PREVALENCE AND IMPACT OF DISABILITY

A large number of people in the United States report having a disability. Different estimates for the prevalence of disability exist, reflecting differences between studies in defining disability. Using a set of criteria to define disability in the physical, communicative, and mental domains, the U.S. Census Bureau estimated that 18.7% of the U.S. population—approximately 56.7 million people—had a disability in 2010 (10). This estimate did not include people living in institutions such as nursing homes where residents are likely to live with a disability. Therefore, the actual proportion of the U.S. population having a disability may be higher than 18.7%. The prevalence of disability did not change significantly between 2005 and 2010. However, when adjusting for age, the proportion of non-institutionalized people with disabilities actually decreased from 18.6% to 18.1% (10). This means that the current disability prevalence is partially determined by the aging of the U.S. population.

It is widely accepted that more people live to old age compared to previous years. This trend is expected to continue (11, 22). Not surprisingly, the prevalence of disability increases with age with 70.5% of people aged 80 years or older report having a disability (Figure 3.2). A similar age-associated increase was found for the prevalence of self-reported severe disability and of the need for assistance with activities of daily living (Figure 3.2). Importantly, physical activity has been recognized as a means to reduce disability, extend years of independent life, and improve quality of life among older adults (22).

The prevalence of disability also varies as a function of race/ethnicity and sex (10). Although disability rates do not differ statistically between blacks and non-Hispanic whites (20.3 vs. 19.7%), both of these groups have lower rates of disabilities than Asians or Hispanics (13.0 and 13.12%, respectively). Notably, blacks have the highest rates of severe disabilities compared to all other groups. Disability is more common among women than men (19.8 vs. 17.4%). Age differences between races/ethnicities or sexes (e.g., there are more older women than men in the population) may partially contribute to differences in disability rates between these groups; however, they do not fully explain them (10). Furthermore, the age-adjusted prevalence of disability in the United States differs between various states with the highest rate occurring in West Virginia and the lowest in North Dakota (29.5 and 17.7%, respectively) (Figure 3.3). Consistent with the ICF model of disability, these findings collectively suggest that disability is a partial consequence of contextual factors within the person and in the environment.

Health conditions, however, also contribute to disability. Figure 3.4 shows the 11 most common conditions identified as the primary cause of disability among U.S. adults (27). Of interest to kinesiology professionals, the three most common disabling conditions are bone-, joint-, or heart-related, collectively accounting for about 42% of disability occurrence. Not shown in Figure 3.4 is a sex difference in arthritis/rheumatism—the number one condition leading to disability (19.0 and 24.3% for men and women, respectively), potentially contributing to the higher rates of disability among women. A healthy lifestyle that includes physical activity and proper nutrition may help in the management of the conditions included in Figure 3.4, potentially lowering disability rates.

The economic impact of disability in the United States is very large. In 2008, the federal government alone spent about 12% of its outlays—an estimated $357 billion—on programs for people with disabilities of working age (16). Federal programs for health care and income maintenance accounted for about 95%

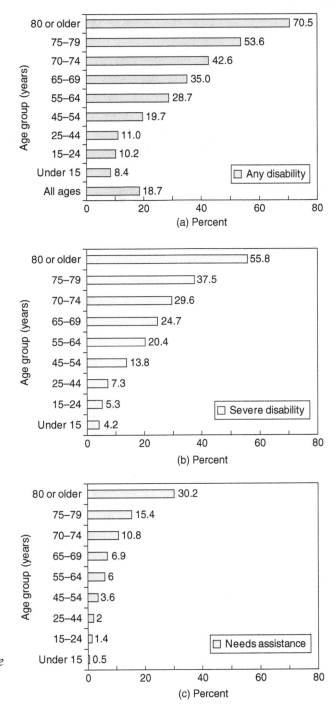

Figure 3.2. *Prevalence of any disability (A), severe disability (B), and need for assistance (C) as a function of age in the United States in 2010. Figure adapted from Brault (10).*

(about 47.5% each) of total federal expenditures (16). When adding state contributions to federal-state programs, the estimated total costs in 2008 were $428 billion (16). This represented an increase of 28% since 2002 after adjusting for inflation. It should be noted that the above figures do not include other expenditures made by cities or persons with disabilities, as well as indirect costs (e.g., missed work days, unemployment). Adults with disabilities are also more likely to be unemployed, to live in poverty, and to depend on public health insurance than adults without disabilities (5, 10). Arguably, physical activity professionals are in a position to alleviate the impact of disability and improve the health and function of people with disabilities through cost-effective lifestyle interventions.

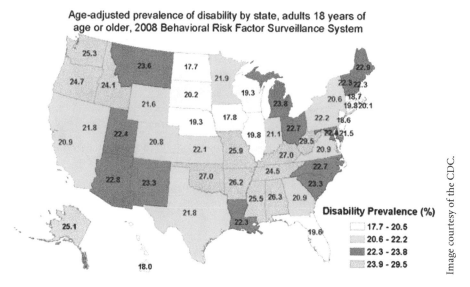

Figure 3.3. *Age-adjusted prevalence of disability among adults in the United States.*

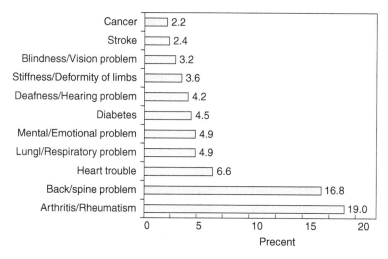

Figure 3.4. *Prevalence of most commonly reported disabling conditions among adults in the United States in 2005. Figure based on data as reported by the Centers for Disease Control and Prevention (27).*

HEALTH DISPARITIES

People with disabilities experience disparities in health (5, 13, 14, 28). They are more likely to report fair or poor health than people without disabilities (5). Furthermore, persons with disabilities have a higher number of health problems, broadly classified as associated, secondary, and comorbid conditions (14). *Associated conditions* are components of the primary disabling condition and are often not preventable. Examples of associated conditions are cognitive impairment and congenital heart defects in people with Down syndrome, spasticity in people with cerebral palsy, paralysis in people with spinal cord injury. In contrast, *secondary conditions* are physical or psychosocial health problems resulting from the primary disabling condition and are preventable. Examples of secondary conditions are fatigue or depression in a person with multiple sclerosis,

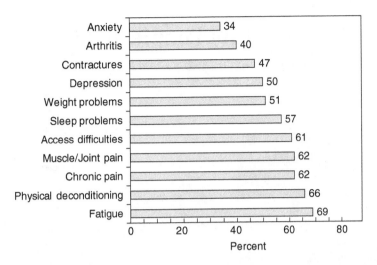

Figure 3.5. *Median prevalence of some secondary conditions. Figure adapted from Rimmer et al. (18).*

pain or pressure ulcers in a person with spinal cord injury who uses a wheelchair, obesity in a person with intellectual disability. Figure 3.5 shows some of the most prevalent secondary conditions among persons with disabilities (18). Notably, several of those could potentially be favorably managed by physical activity. Finally, *comorbid conditions* are health problems that develop independently of the primary condition. Examples of comorbid conditions are breast cancer in a woman with arthritis. The distinction between associated, secondary, and comorbid conditions is often not precise. From a clinical standpoint, how conditions are classified may have little impact on how they are managed. This classification, however, helps researchers identify factors contributing to the health disparities experienced by people with disabilities.

DETERMINANTS OF HEALTH

The determinants of health in people with and without disabilities are multifactorial as recognized by *Healthy People 2020*—a national agenda for improving health and alleviating health disparities among Americans (24). The *Healthy People 2020* agenda, which pays special attention to people with disabilities, employs an ecological framework—shown on Figure 3.6—where health outcomes arise from complex interactions between the physical and social environment, health services, individual behaviors, and biological/genetic factors (24). Included in this framework is a *social determinants of health* model that emphasizes the contribution of social factors to health. It has been proposed that social determinants, including socioeconomic, psychosocial, and community factors, affect health directly, but also indirectly through the mediating role of disease inducing or reducing behaviors and access to the health care system (6, 13). These theoretical frameworks imply that, apart from health conditions—discussed in the previous section—multiple other factors determine health in people with disabilities.

Social determinants may be partially responsible for the inferior health profiles of people with disabilities. As a population, these persons have lower levels of educational attainment, employment, and income than persons without disabilities (5, 10). They also experience higher rates of depression, anxiety, and social isolation; they have greater problems with transportation and accessibility; and they are less likely to attend social events (13). Complex interactions among these and other social determinants, such as age and sex, may cause health disparities in persons with disabilities.

Access to health care and lifestyle behaviors may also determine health in people with disabilities. Many of these persons, especially between the ages of 18 and 44 years, report that they do not have a usual place of medical care, although proportionally this is not different from that of people without disabilities (5).

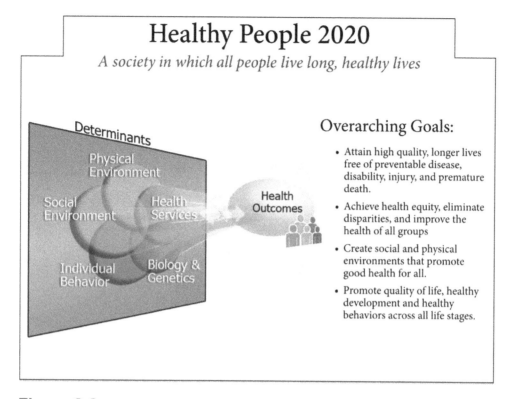

Figure 3.6. *The Healthy People 2020 theoretical framework. Figure downloaded from www.healthypeople.gov*

Persons with disabilities also have lower access to private health insurance, possibly because they are less likely to be employed. As a result, they depend to a greater extent on public health insurance programs. They are also more likely to make lower use of some preventive services such as pap smear tests or mammograms (5). Furthermore, persons with disabilities have lower physical activity levels than those without disabilities and are more likely to smoke and be overweight or obese (5, 26, 28). Access to health care and lifestyle behaviors have been theorized to have an impact on health through complex interactions with social determinants (6). The relationships among these factors may help explain the health disparities experienced by persons with disabilities (13).

PHYSICAL ACTIVITY AND PHYSICAL FITNESS

The health profiles of persons with disabilities may be improved by increasing their physical activity and physical fitness levels (26). Physical activity is any bodily movement produced by the skeletal muscles that increases energy expenditure (9). Indisputably, physical activity improves the physical and psychosocial health profiles of people with and without disabilities (26). To achieve health benefits, people should attempt to meet the Physical Activity Guidelines for Americans issued by the U.S. Department of Health and Human Services (23). Specifically, it is recommended that, each week, adults perform 150 minutes of moderate intensity or 75 minutes of vigorous intensity aerobic activity, or an equivalent combination of moderate and vigorous intensity activity. This amount should be accumulated in bouts of at least 10 minutes in duration. Furthermore, adults should engage in muscle strengthening activities at least two days per week. Children and adolescents should be active for 60 minutes each day mostly in moderate or vigorous intensity activity. As part of these 60 minutes, youth should also perform muscle and bone strengthening activities at least three days per week. The above guidelines also apply to people with disabilities who are able to meet these recommendations. People with disabilities who are not able to meet the guidelines should be as active as their abilities allow

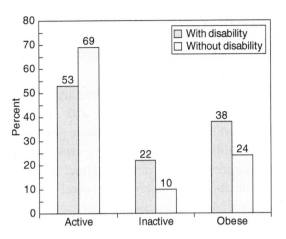

Figure 3.7. *Prevalence of activity, inactivity, and obesity among adults with and without disabilities in the United States. Physical activity data are from 2009, whereas obesity data are from 2010. Figure based on data available at the Disability and Health Data System of the Centers for Disease Control and Prevention (http://dhds.cdc.gov).*

and avoid inactivity. Importantly, it is recommended that people with disabilities and people with chronic health conditions consult their health care providers in determining the proper type and amount of physical activity for them.

Unfortunately, the physical activity levels of persons with disabilities are lower than those of persons without disabilities (5, 19, 25, 26, 28). Figure 3.7 shows that a smaller proportion of persons with disabilities meet the guidelines for health promoting physical activity and a greater proportion does not engage in physical activity compared to persons without disabilities. Arguably, the low physical activity levels of persons with disabilities may be a cause of the health disparities they experience (18, 19, 21). Therefore, promoting physical activity in people with disabilities may improve their health.

Physical fitness is the ability to effectively perform muscular work and it increases by participating in regular physical activity and exercise (9). Physical fitness is a construct with many components, some of which are considered responsible for improving health and lowering the risks for mortality and morbidity (9). Traditionally, health-related physical fitness includes five components: (a) cardiovascular endurance, (b) body composition, (c) muscular strength, (d) muscular endurance, and (e) flexibility (4). Some theorists, however, have proposed an expanded view of health-related physical fitness as additional attributes are found to have a relationship with health (9). Examples of additional components under this view include motor fitness, encompassing agility, balance, coordination, and speed of movement; and metabolic fitness, encompassing glucose tolerance, insulin sensitivity, lipid metabolism, and substrate oxidation (9).

Physical fitness is generally lower in people with disabilities, likely predisposing them to higher risks for mortality and morbidity (8, 21). Low physical fitness may also decrease mobility, independence, and employment, especially in occupations requiring physical labor and overall participation in social situations. Different impairments may affect different aspects of fitness. For example, a person with cystic fibrosis may have low cardiorespiratory fitness, someone with multiple sclerosis may have low musculoskeletal fitness, and a person with Parkinson's disease may have low motor fitness. Especially worrisome is the adverse body composition profile of persons with disabilities. As shown in Figure 3.7, obesity is more prevalent among these persons compared to persons without disabilities. It should be considered that people with disabilities may achieve very high levels of physical fitness and performance as demonstrated by elite athletes with disabilities. As for physical activity, promoting physical fitness in persons with disabilities may improve their physical and psychosocial well-being.

DETERMINANTS OF PHYSICAL ACTIVITY AND FITNESS

Physical activity professionals have a critical role to play in alleviating health disparities in persons with disabilities. Achieving this goal should start with the identification of factors that predispose them to low physical activity and physical fitness. This may be facilitated by using the ICF model of disability (Figure 3.1).

According to this theoretical model, low physical activity and physical fitness may be thought as residing within activity limitations and impairments, respectively. Therefore, this approach suggests that the physical activity and physical fitness profiles of persons with disabilities are influenced by factors within the person *and* factors in the environment (Box 3.1).

The health status of persons with disabilities may contribute to their low physical activity and physical fitness levels (19). As mentioned above, people with disabilities show high rates of associated, secondary, and comorbid conditions, which may present barriers to physical activity and exercise participation. Physical fitness in particular may be influenced by different impairments in physiologic function, such as pulmonary, cardiovascular, muscular, or metabolic dysfunction. Functional level and participation profiles of persons with disabilities may also contribute to a low level of physical activity and fitness. Another determinant may be the age profile of people with disabilities. Physical activity and physical fitness decline with aging (15) and, as discussed above, many people with disabilities are of older age. Psychosocial contributors likely include attitudes toward physical activity, knowledge related to healthy lifestyles, education, income, employment, and self-efficacy. Many of these factors are impacted by disability. The aforementioned factors may also interact with other personal attributes such as sex, race, and ethnicity, collectively contributing to the adverse physical activity, fitness, and—ultimately—health profiles of persons with disabilities.

BOX 3.1 Identifying Barriers to Physical Activity for Persons with Disabilities Based on the ICF Model

Barriers to Physical Activity

- Within the Person
  - Health problems
    - Associated conditions
    - Secondary conditions
    - Comorbid conditions
  - Older age
  - Low fitness levels
  - Psychosocial factors
    - Low education
    - Low employment levels
    - Low income
    - Low knowledge on healthy lifestyle
    - Negative attitudes toward physical activity
    - Low self-efficacy

- Environmental
  - Lack of accessible, inclusive, and properly designed programs
  - Lack of knowledgeable kinesiology professionals
  - Transportation difficulties
  - Social exclusion
  - Negative attitudes toward people with disabilities
  - Competing family responsibilities
  - Parental education and income

It is also very likely that the social and physical environment contributes to their physical activity and fitness levels (19). Social exclusion; negative attitudes toward them; transportation problems; lack of knowledgeable of exercise professionals; and a lack of accessible, inclusive, and appropriately designed physical activity programs present barriers to physical activity for people with disabilities (19). More than likely, personal and environmental factors interact in complex ways, collectively contributing to lower the physical activity and fitness levels of persons with disabilities.

HEALTH AND PHYSICAL ACTIVITY PROMOTION

Health professionals who are aware of the above factors may more effectively promote physical activity and health in persons with disabilities. Some theorists argue that effective health promotion programs should be physically, socially, and economically available to people with disabilities who should also contribute to the development and implementation of such programs (17). Health promotion programs should achieve measurable objectives and have a strong theoretical framework. Examples of available frameworks are (a) the transtheoretical model, based on the idea that a person's level of readiness for change impacts the likelihood of changing behavior; (b) social cognitive theory, emphasizing the role of the social environment, the person's cognition, and the person's present behavior in determining future behavior; and (c) ecological models, stressing that behaviors arise from the interactions between personal and environmental factors (17). In accordance with the ecological approach, Rimmer and Rowland suggested that removing barriers to health promotion in people with disabilities can be achieved by concomitantly empowering them and enabling the environment (20).

Kinesiology professionals are in a unique position to ameliorate disparities in health and lifestyle behaviors by developing effective community-, school-, or home-based physical activity programs. Well-designed programs may contribute to the management of associated conditions, prevent secondary and comobid conditions, and create lifelong healthy lifestyles. To achieve these goals, physical activity promotion should be multidimensional. It should be adapted to the physical, cognitive, and psychosocial health profiles of persons with disabilities. It should empower them by offering knowledge on physical activity and health and consider their needs for enjoyment and participation. Furthermore, the environmental contexts in which physical activity occurs must be considered—physical activity programs should be accessible, inclusive, and constructed in a way that values the lives and experiences of persons with disabilities (19).

Well-designed physical activity programs for persons with disabilities should also be based on empirical evidence. Adequate evidence supports that physical activity programs effectively improve the health of persons with disabilities and that the benefits of physical activity outweigh its risks (26). More research, however, is needed in establishing the strength of the relationship between physical activity and health in persons with disabilities. Furthermore, the exact frequency, intensity, and duration of physical activity that improves health across people with different types and levels of impairments must be determined with further research (26). Improving the empirical knowledge base requires the collaboration of many research centers around the country and of researchers with different backgrounds. Importantly, the quality of research on physical activity and health may increase if people with disabilities contribute to the development of the research agenda. They know firsthand what the critical issues in their lives are and can help researchers in identifying important research questions and hypotheses.

CAREERS

Effectively promoting physical activity and health in persons with disabilities requires the collective effort of professionals with diverse backgrounds. The following is a short list of professionals who can address their physical activity and health needs. Notably, these occupations are available for kinesiology students, in most cases, with additional training.

- Adapted Physical Activity Specialists
- Clinical Exercise Physiologists
- Fitness Professionals
- Nurses
- Physical Therapists
- Occupational Therapists
- Primary Care Physicians
- Rehabilitation Specialists
- Researchers
- Strength and Conditioning Specialists
- Therapeutic Recreation Specialists

DISABILITY ORGANIZATIONS

There are many national and international organizations that contribute to the development and dissemination of knowledge related to health and physical activity promotion for people with disabilities. Below is a short list of select organizations in alphabetical order.

- American Association for Health and Disability (www.aahd.us)
- American Association on Intellectual and Developmental Disabilities (www.aaidd.org)
- American College of Sports Medicine (acsm.org)
- American Public Health Association (www.apha.org)
- Centers for Disease Control and Prevention (www.cdc.gov)
- Christopher & Dana Reeve Foundation (www.christopherreeve.org)
- International Federation for Adapted Physical Activity (www.ifapa.biz)
- National Center on Health, Physical Activity, and Disability (www.ncpad.org)
- National Institute on Disability and Rehabilitation Research (www2.ed.gov/about/offices/list/osers/nidrr)
- National Institutes of Health (www.nih.gov)
- Special Olympics (www.specialolympics.org)

SUMMARY

A vast array of legislation, including the ADA of 1990, the Rehabilitation Act of 1973, and the IDEA of 1990, protects the rehabilitation, educational, and civil rights of people with disabilities in the United States. More recent models view disability as an experience that arises from interactions between personal and environmental factors. Disability affects a large portion of the U.S. population, especially older adults. People with disabilities experience health disparities. Knowledgeable kinesiology professionals are in a position to improve the health status of persons with disabilities through appropriately designed physical activity programs.

REFERENCES

1. Americans with Disabilities Act of 1990. 1990.

2. Individuals with Disabilities Education Improvement Act of 2004. 2004.

3. Rehabilitation Act of 1973. 1973.

4. ACSM. *ACSM's Guidelines for Exercise Testing and Prescription. 8th ed.* Baltimore: Lippincott Williams & Wilkins, 2009.

5. Altman, B., and A. Bernstein, *Disability and health in the United States, 2001–2005.* Hyattsville, MD: National Center for Health Statistics, 2008.

6. Ansari, Z., N. J. Carson, M. J. Ackland, L. Vaughan, and A. A. Serraglio, "A public health model of the social determinants of health." *Soz Preventivmed* 48 (2003): 242–251.

7. Bersani, H., and L. M. Lyman, "Governmental policies and programs for people with disabilities." In: *Disability and Public Health,* edited by C. E. Drum, G. L. Krahn, and H. Bersani. Washington, D.C.: American Public ealth Association, 2009, pp. 79–104.

8. Blair, S. N., and M. J. LaMonte, "Physical activity, fitness, and mortality rates." In: *Physical Activity and Health,* edited by C. Bouchard, S. N. Blair, and W. L. Haskell. WL. Champaign, IL: Human Kinetics, 2007, pp. 143–160.

9. Bouchard. C., S. N. Blair, and W. L. Haskell, "Why study physical activity and health?" In: *Physical Activity and Health,* edited by C. Bouchard, S. N. Blair, and W. L. Haskell. Champaign, IL: Human Kinetics, 2007, pp. 3–19.

10. Brault, M. W. *Americans with disabilities: 2010.* Washington, DC: 2012.

11. DiPietro, L. "Physical activity, fitness, and aging." In: *Physical Activity and Health,* edited by C. Bouchard, S. N. Blair, and W. L. Haskell. Champaign, IL: Human Kinetics, 2007, pp. 271–285.

12. Drum, C. E., "Models and approaches to disability." In: *Disability and Public Health,* edited by C. E. Drum, G. L. Krahn, and H. Bersani. Washington, DC: American Public Health Association, 2009, pp. 27–44.

13. Drum, C. E., G. L. Krahn, J. J. Peterson, W. Horner-Johnson, and K. Newton, "Health of people with disabilities: Determinants and disparities." In: *Disability and Public Health,* edited by C. E. Drum, G. L. Krahn, and H. Bersani. Washington, DC: American Public Health Association, 2009, pp. 125–144.

14. Field, M. J., and A. M. Jette, *The Future of Disability in America.* Washington, DC: The National Academies Press, 2007.

15. Katzmarzyk, P. T. "Physical activity and fitness with age among sex and ethnic groups." In: *Physical Activity and Health,* edited by C. Bouchard, S. N. Blair, and W. L. Haskell. Champaign, IL: Human Kinetics, 2007, pp. 37–47.

16. Livermore, G., D. C. Stapletonand M. O'Toole, "Health care costs are a key driver of growth in federal and state assistance to working-age people with disabilities." *Health Aff (Millwood)* 30 (2011): 1664–1672.

17. Peterson, J. J., L. Hammond and C. Culley, "Health promotion for people with disabilities." In: *Disability and Public Health,* edited by C. E. Drum, G. L. Krahn, and H. Bersani. Washington, DC: American Public Health Association, 2009, pp. 145–162.

18. Rimmer, J. H., M. D. Chen, and K. Hsieh, "A conceptual model for identifying, preventing, and managing secondary conditions in people with disabilities." *Physical Therapy* 91 (2011): 1728–1739.

19. Rimmer, J. H., and A. C. Marques, "Physical activity for people with disabilities." Lancet 380 (2012): 193–195.

20. Rimmer, J. H., and J. L. Rowland, "Health promotion for people with disabilities: Implications for empowering the persons and promoting disability-friendly environments." *American Journal of Lifestyle Medicine* 2 (2008): 409–420.

21. Rimmer, J. H., W. Schiller and M. D. Chen, "Effects of disability-associated low energy expenditure deconditioning syndrome." *Exerc Sport Sci Rev* 40 (2012): 22–29.

22. Robert Wood Johnson Foundation. *National Blueprint: Increasing Physical Activity Among Adults Age 50 and Older.* Princeton, NJ: Author, 2001.

23. U.S. Department of Health and Human Services. *2008 Physical Activity Guidelines for Americans.* Washington, DC: Author, 2008.

24. U.S. Department of Health and Human Services. *Healthy People 2020*. Washington, DC: Author, 2010.

25. U.S. Department of Health and Human Services. *Physical Activity Among Adults with a Disability–United States 2005*. Washington, DC: Author, 2007.

26. U.S. Department of Health and Human Services. *Physical Activity Guidelines Advisory Committee Report, 2008*. Washington, DC: Author, 2008.

27. U.S. Department of Health and Human Services. *Prevalence of Most Common Causes of Disability Among Aduts–United States 2005*. Washington, DC: Author, 2009.

28. U.S. Department of Health and Human Services. *The Surgeon General's Call to Action to Improve the Health ans Wellness of Persons with Disabilities 2005*. Rockville, MD: Author, 2005.

29. World Health Organization. *International Classification of Functioning, Disability and Health*. Geneva: World Health Organization, 2001.

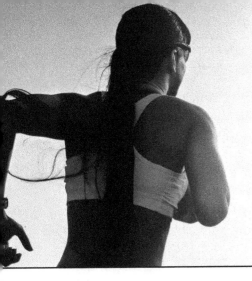

Chapter 4

PROFESSIONAL CONCERNS

OUTLINE

OBJECTIVES

1. Identify Flexner's six criteria that qualify an occupation as a profession.
2. Distinguish between a nonprofessional occupation and a professional occupation using the profession pyramid.
3. Identify the distinguishing characteristics of disciplines and professions.
4. Explain role delineation and professional encroachment.
5. Explain the difference between certification and licensure.
6. Explain the value of certification and licensure to professional activity.

This text postulates the thesis that kinesiology is transdisciplinary. That is, it functions in academics as a conglomerate field of study comprised of many disciplines. Introductory books have previously treated exercise physiology, biomechanics, and the other fields of kinesiology as *subdisciplines*. This approach minimizes the importance and growth of these disciplines and neglects the fact that kinesiology has evolved into something more than a unidisciplinary field. Rather, it has become "trans" disciplined, bridging the gap between the parent disciplines from which kinesiology draws its science. As a result, a coalescing into a unified whole has occurred in much the same way business administration functions for disciplines such as management, marketing, finance, and accounting (among others). This text, therefore, presents the *disciplines* and *professions* of kinesiology, deliberately elevating each in rank so that the transdisciplined field stands out in stark contrast to its many constituent parts, each having become far more than a mere subdiscipline. It is with this construct in mind that professional issues are next considered.

WHAT IS A PROFESSION?

Is kinesiology a profession or a discipline? Is clinical exercise physiology a professional field? Is exercise psychology? What about physical therapy or occupational therapy or sport management? These are important questions because kinesiology students sometimes struggle to understand the nature of the field they are entering. Neither is the issue an exercise in semantics, for there are real and substantial differences between what may be labeled an academic discipline versus a profession.

A professional is someone who is characterized by and conforms to the technical and ethical standards of a profession. The allied health reference text, *Miller-Keane Encyclopedia & Dictionary of Medicine, Nursing, & Allied Health*, defines a profession as: "A calling or vocation requiring specialized knowledge, methods, and skills, as well as preparation . . . in the scholarly, scientific, and historical principles underlying such methods and skills. A profession continuously enlarges its body of knowledge and functions autonomously in formulation of policy."

Early use of the term *professional* meant a commitment to a certain way of life. The verb, *profess*, meant to be received formally into a religious community such as a monk who took monastic vows in a religious order. It implied a public avowal to follow a path of high moral ideals. By the late 17th century the word became more secular in meaning and expanded beyond religion to include those who were qualified to pursue a vocation or calling. Traditionally, there have been three clearly identified professions—law, medicine, and the clergy. They required knowledge, shared values and wisdom, and a *fiduciary* relationship with others. Fiduciary refers to the trust a client has in the professional and the solemn responsibility a professional has to his or her clients.

Early in the 20th century, Abraham Flexner wrote specifically about whether social work was indeed a profession (3). He listed six criteria that qualified an occupation as a profession:

1. Intellectual pursuit and responsible actions
2. Knowledge base derived from science and research
3. Practice involves the use of practical skills—not solely academic
4. Representative professional organization
5. High level of communication with members in good standing
6. Altruism

Writing about health care, Purtilo and Cassel (5) mention five critical characteristics that somewhat parallel Flexner's much earlier list:

1. Self-governed autonomy (no corresponding item in Flexner's list)
2. Social value (no corresponding item in Flexner's list)
3. Specialized knowledge (items 2 and 3 in Flexner's list)
4. Representative organization (item 4 in Flexner's list)
5. Lifetime commitment (item 6 in Flexner's list)

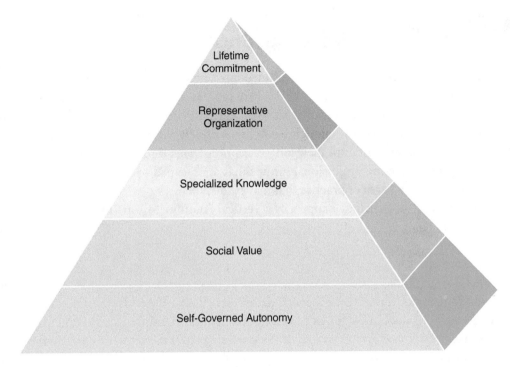

Figure 4.1.   *The professional pyramid.*

For an occupation to be fully actualized as a health profession, Purtilo and Cassel declare that all five of these characteristics should be present. Figure 4.1 shows how these characteristics are related in a hierarchical fashion. As you ascend to the top of the pyramid, each characteristic becomes less valued in terms of its importance to the professional status of the group. However, if one layer is removed the whole becomes less stable and the premise starts to crumble.

Autonomy

The base of the pyramid, like any structural foundation, is critical to the claim of professional status. Self-governed autonomy refers to the freedom of a profession to act independently by using sound judgment in practice. Implicit in self-governed autonomy is the need for control *of* the profession by individuals *in* the profession.

An autonomous profession is one in which the practitioner has the qualifications, responsibility, and authority for the provision of services that fall within his or her scope of practice. Autonomy connotes self-government. Therefore, it contrasts with the term *hegemony*, which means the domination of one group by another. This means that when a so-called health care profession dominates the practice of another, the one dominated is not autonomous and can hardly claim the mantle of profession. Domination can occur in a legal sense when one group's licensing law clearly establishes the "right of practice" in an area that another group aspires to. Domination can also occur less formally as in the everyday work setting (see the case study for an example).

Autonomy does not mean complete freedom from all monitoring and regulation. Even the most entrenched professions are closely scrutinized and their practices repeatedly reviewed by bodies established by federal and state statutes, by accrediting agencies, by consumer groups, and by peers in the same profession. With the growing involvement of government agencies and corporations in underwriting the costs of human services, and with the growing trend for challenging professional competence through litigation, there is an ever-increasing abridgment of the independence of all professions. Professions, then, do not claim immunity from external review and regulation. Rather, professions declare the responsibility for formulating standards of independent practice, for the definition of the appropriate scope of its professional practices, and for the development of individual and institutional standards for the delivery of services.

CASE STUDY: Professional Encroachment

The definition of encroachment is to trespass or intrude, to advance beyond the proper, original, or customary limits. This happens all the time in health care practice even in the face of licensing laws where there is a narrow description of professional responsibilities. Usually, though, it is the narrow description that causes the problem because enough flexibility is usually there for licensed professionals to add additional tasks and responsibilities to their job descriptions. This leads to professional frustration and may even cause lawsuits among professional groups that are deemed to be professional peers, but that nevertheless compete for an area of practice that may be disputed.

Encroachment usually does not happen in a vertical (bottom to top) manner. For example, one would be hard-pressed to find a case where physical therapy is encroaching on the medical profession. The reason is simple. It would be suicide for physical therapists to do so. However, the opposite (top to bottom encroachment) happens all too often. Here is a case in point.

I was once a young "practicing" clinical exercise physiologist directing inpatient and outpatient cardiac rehabilitation programs in a major medical center in my home state. Having a master's degree at the time and being well prepared in the job of providing therapeutic exercise rehabilitation to patients, I was nevertheless taken aback one day when one of the cardiologists came into our clinic and proceeded to instruct me on what to do with his patient in subsequent rehab sessions to which he would be referring him. The patient had just undergone cardiac catheterization to determine the level of atherosclerotic blockage in his coronary arteries.

Said the doctor, "I want my patient on a 5 MET activity prescription. I don't care what type of ergometer, just do not exercise him more than 5 METS."

I have used this example over the years to advise students in two ways: (a) Be prepared as best you can for the job because if I had looked at the doctor with a vacuous expression signifying that I had no idea what he meant, I would have probably been fired, and (b) specialized knowledge is very important for understanding what is and is not to be considered a profession. Let's focus on number two.

There are many things that can be taken away from this example, but for the purposes of this chapter this case study is meant to illustrate the point that professionals have specialized knowledge that others do not have and that is used in professional practice. Ask yourself the question, what specialized knowledge does a clinical exercise physiologist have that others (perhaps nurses, physicians, and physical therapists) do not? Surely part of the answer must be the ability to write exercise prescriptions for patients with chronic diseases using the fundamental principles of exercise physiology. Now, what did that doctor do? The answer is that he *coopted* my specialized knowledge and told me how to use it, instructing me at what intensity to exercise his patient. *(As a side note, how did he know that a 5 MET intensity was proper for his patient? Without performing a graded exercise test (none was performed), there is no way to know whether 5 METS would be too heavy a load or too light!)* Now, I'm not saying that physicians should not know what a MET is and how to use it for exercise intensity prescription in cardiac rehabilitation. Most don't, in fact, but the fact that this cardiologist could talk *my* "professional language" and was able to *order* me in *my* "professional setting" speaks volumes about the state of clinical exercise physiology at the time (ca. 1984). The state of clinical exercise physiology as a "profession" remains largely unchanged today (2).

Authority to function autonomously within the scope of practice of a profession is signified when members of that profession:

1. are a point of entry for services that fall within its scope of practice.
2. select the appropriate candidates for those services.
3. determine appropriate diagnostic methodology and suitable approaches to and duration of treatment.
4. effect referrals for services to be provided by other members of the profession as well as by members of other professions.

These characteristics should be manifested in the delivery of services. When any are curtailed, clients or patients may be deprived of needed services or the quality of whatever services are provided may be impaired.

Recognition of a profession's authority must be immediately followed by recognition of that profession's responsibility. Responsibility may be generally defined in two respects: *legal responsibility* and *ethical responsibility*. An essential characteristic of a profession's autonomy is that its members bear individual legal responsibility for all of their practices. When professionals are employed by institutions or other individuals or organizations, the legal responsibility may be shared, but the professional is never absolved of individual responsibility. In many instances, members of the profession may also share legal responsibility for services delivered by students and by the professionals and the paraprofessionals they supervise. Therefore, professionals are personally responsible for instances of malpractice or negligence before the courts and licensing bodies.

Ethical responsibilities extend well beyond legal responsibilities. They include assuring the quality of services, offering consumers freedom of choice and providing whatever information is needed for making informed choices, and maintaining salutary inter- and intra-professional relationships insofar as is consonant with consumers' best interests. Ethical responsibilities are always incumbent on individual professionals. They are never transferred to employers, administrators, or supervisors to whom a professional is answerable.

SOCIAL VALUE

The claim to professional status is also made with regard to the service provided to society. Social value means that society benefits from the practice rendered by the professional. There must be a threshold level of social value that is evident for an occupation to be classed as a profession. Each of the early professions had a great deal of social value when you consider the need to escape legal difficulties, or to regain health, or when spiritual issues are at stake.

But is membership to the exclusive club labeled *profession* limited only to these three, or are there other occupations today that have enough autonomy and social value to cross the professional threshold? Considering the way Purtilo and Cassel delimit the term, the answer is clearly *yes*.

Before continuing with the idea of social value, however, the difference between profession and discipline should be compared and contrasted. The mutually beneficial relationship between the disciplines and related professions of kinesiology is illustrated in Figure 4.2. The disciplines of kinesiology (Sport Philosophy, Sport History, Sport Sociology, Exercise Physiology, Sport Nutrition, Physical Activity Epidemiology, Applied Anatomy, Biomechanics, Exercise and Sport Psychology, and Motor Behavior) are presented in separate chapters in Part Two of the text. These disciplines (and others throughout academia) function by providing definitions and descriptions of observed phenomena and establishing cause/effect relationships of variables. These are research-based concerns that add to the body of knowledge of the discipline.

Professions, however, are not primarily concerned with generating new knowledge (although research in professional fields is certainly a valuable function), but rather with using the knowledge created by disciplines to establish a more valid basis of practice. The knowledge derived from disciplinary research is translated into

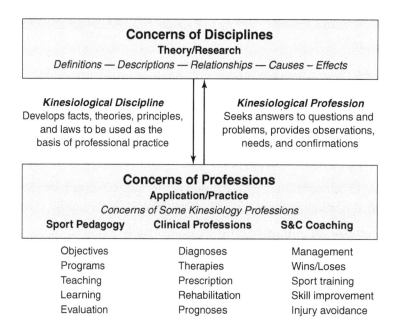

Figure 4.2. *The relationship between an academic discipline and a related profession is symbiotic, the flow of information occurring in both directions.*

practice by the profession. In turn, professions function as guides for the disciplines, often leading them to alter a theory based on observations made in the day-to-day practice of the profession. The comments of Abernethy and co-workers are important to understanding the interrelationship between discipline and profession (1):

> The principal function of a discipline is therefore to develop a coherent body of knowledge that describes, explains and predicts key phenomena from the domain of interest. In contrast, professions, as a general rule, try to improve the conditions of society by providing a regulated service in which practices and educational/training programs are developed that are in accordance with knowledge available from one or more relevant disciplines. Disciplines therefore seek to understand subject matter and professions to implement change based on this understanding.

The professions of kinesiology work from a foundational knowledge of human movement. These professions (Physical and Occupational Therapy, Clinical Exercise Physiology, Therapeutic Recreation, Athletic Training, Sport Pedagogy, Sport Management, Recreation and Leisure, Health-Fitness, and Strength and Conditioning Coaching) are presented in separate chapters in Part Three of the text.

It is easy to see the social value associated with the three traditional professions mentioned above, but what of the professions of kinesiology? Is there intrinsic social value in sport pedagogy, for example, or athletic training, or clinical exercise physiology? The answer to these questions rest in what these professions bring to the table, but instead of examining each of the 10 professions presented in this book, for brevity sake, it is better to step back and look at the overall field.

Recall that the meaning of kinesiology is the study of movement. Is there intrinsic social value in that? As we have seen in Chapter 1, movement has a fundamental role in human existence precisely because it is an attribute intricately interwoven to what it means to be human. Abernethy and co-workers (1) elaborate:

> The study of human movement is important in and of itself as movement is a central biological and social phenomenon. The study of human movement is central to the understanding of human biology as movement is a fundamental property, indeed indicator, of life (remembering that biology is literally the study of life). Human movement offers a valuable medium for the study of biological

phenomena fundamental to developmental changes across the lifespan (changes that occur with aging as a consequence of internal body processes), to adaptation (changes that occur as an accommodation or adjustment to environmental processes) and to the interactions of genetic and environmental factors (nature and nurture) that dictate human phenotypic expression.

The study of movement is socially and culturally warranted and is an important component of the professional practice of many fields falling outside the realm of kinesiology. Practitioners in fields such as nursing, medicine, and engineering/ergonomics, for example, should have a thorough understanding of human movement. So, the answer to the question posed earlier is that there is great social value in studying movement, physical activity, exercise, and sport, all of the traditional components of kinesiology. To move is to be alive, to be human, which makes academic preparation in any of the fields of kinesiology worthwhile.

Specialized Knowledge

Specialized knowledge assumes that the profession has intellectual ownership of a body of knowledge that sets them apart from others. A body of knowledge represents the complete set of concepts, terms, and activities that make up a professional domain as defined by the relevant professional association. The body of knowledge is the sum total of all the research and scholarship in a discipline, and because new research is constantly being performed the body of knowledge changes and expands. Professional associations define the technical knowledge required for acceptance into the profession—often through academic, experience, and related requirements. This body of knowledge is specific and generally poorly understood by other professions and society at large, making it necessary for professionals to work without supervision and be technically autonomous. Professionals accept responsibility and liability for their work, which necessitates a high degree of trust that they govern themselves with the public interest being paramount. Refer back to the case study presented earlier, and using Purtilo and Cassel's criteria, ask the question, is clinical exercise physiology a profession?

The practice of a profession requires the exercise of reasoned judgment in the application of this specialized knowledge. Professionals are frequently required to make judgments based on knowledge and understanding of a situation. Often, there are a variety of factors and several acceptable solutions when solving problems. Decision makers must be able to identify and evaluate possible alternatives, considering that many people can be significantly affected by the decisions made by the professional.

Representative Organization

A professional organization is essential to provide standards, regulations, structure, and a means of communication for members of the profession. Through practice laws, governments grant the privilege of self-governance and the associated responsibility to regulate professional matters to selected professions. Members of self-governing professions accept legal and ethical responsibility for the work they do and hold the interest of the public and society in the utmost regard. This protects society and encourages pride of workmanship, productivity, individual responsibility, self-discipline, ethical standards, and public interest.

The representative organization institutes standards to ensure that members are responsible and accountable for practicing in a skilled and ethical manner. Self-regulation and mutual accountability must be stringent to merit societal trust in accordance with their fiduciary responsibility. Technical and professional standards of conduct are set, revised, maintained, and enforced by associations and often address the following issues:

- Certification and licensure: ensuring that only properly qualified members are allowed to practice
- Code of ethics: protecting the public against unethical and incompetent practitioners
- Technical requirements: ensuring that professionals protect public safety and well-being

- Continuing competence: requiring professional development and adherence to standards and guidelines
- Regulation and control: enforcing against non-licensed and non-qualified persons
- Discipline: sanctioning members who fail to comply with proper standards of practice and ethics.

Lifetime Commitment

Professionals are often dedicated individuals committed to their community through the practice of their profession. For professionals, there is a public interest bias that takes precedence over self-interest. This often manifests as a duty to public service, what Flexner calls *altruism* in his list of professional attributes.

> Altruism is giving without expectation of compensation or return of any kind.

An example of professional altruism is when a lawyer takes a case free of charge (*pro bono*) or when a physician sees an indigent patient and waives his fee. Professionals should continually strive to give back to society through service that draws on professional expertise. They should participate in activities that contribute to the community at large and be willing to donate their time and expertise.

Professionalism is a passion for personal responsibility, devotion to a life of service, a commitment to a mission, and an openness to new ideas and alternatives. In contrast, technicians (or *paraprofessionals*) define their role much more narrowly. They see no larger purpose, set their sights low, and know enough about their work without having a holistic view of it.

> A paraprofessional is a person to whom a particular aspect of a professional task is delegated, but who is not licensed to practice as a fully qualified professional. They work alongside the professional.

The six characteristics of professional style—a professional way of being—are summarized below:

1. Ethical: moral standard of conduct
2. Altruistic: regard for and devotion to the interest of others, unselfish
3. Responsible: accountable, answerable, trustworthy, and able to respond
4. Theoretical: systematic and abstract principles of professional action
5. Committed: a lifetime of devotion
6. Intellectual: responsible for continuous development of professional knowledge and skills (learning is not a task, but a way of living and being)

OVERVIEW OF CERTIFICATION AND LICENSURE

The Centers for Disease Control and Prevention and the American College of Sports Medicine in 1995 published joint recommendations for physical activity and public health. In that same year, the President's Council on Physical Fitness and Sports announced a multi-million-dollar budget to promote youth sports and physical activity. After these developments, the U.S. Surgeon General announced an endorsement that all Americans would benefit from regular physical activity, and the U.S. Department of Agriculture included a statement about regular physical activity in its publication, *Dietary Guidelines for American Adults*. In the almost 20 years since these statements brought exercise to the forefront of public awareness as a necessary component of disease prevention, its role in the future of public health has been solidified. A corollary to this, however, is the need to have qualified individuals at the forefront of public interaction. The process of certification, licensure, and registration ensures this.

Certification

Certification is the process by which an individual is evaluated and recognized as meeting certain predetermined standards through successful completion of a valid and reliable examination. Certification is usually administered by a nongovernmental agency such as a professional organization and is a voluntary process on the part of the individual. However, as expectations among employers and governmental agencies increase, certification is often desired and/or required for employment.

There is an increased public awareness of the role that physical activity and exercise play in producing health. Because of this there is an even greater need to demonstrate practitioner competence by requiring certification of exercise professionals. Certification helps the individual demonstrate knowledge and proficiency and is an important part of professional preparation for careers in kinesiology, assisting employers in at least three ways:

1. Identifying levels of expertise among candidates for employment
2. Providing rationale for advancement
3. Enhancing confidence among consumers, clients, and/or patients in their organization

Certification has increasingly become a condition of employment, retention, and/or advancement and may benefit the employee by increasing opportunities for better jobs, a greater level of credibility, expanded competence and qualifications, more self-confidence, and greater income.

Licensure

Licensure is the granting of permission by a government agency to an individual to engage in a practice or activity that would otherwise be illegal. Types of licensure include issuing licenses for medical professionals (physicians) and allied health professionals (nurses, physical therapists, occupational therapists). Licensure is usually granted on the basis of education and examination criteria rather than performance. For example, physicians take board exams after going to medical school in order to obtain a legal license to practice medicine. Licensure is usually permanent, but a periodic fee, demonstration of competence, and/or continuing education may be required.

The difference between certification and licensure is that people who are licensed can legally practice a regulated profession, whereas people who are certified may not have legal authority to practice unless the state recognizes the certification as the licensure requirement. There is an effort to move toward licensure for some of the kinesiology professions (clinical exercise physiologists, athletic trainers, and health-fitness specialists).

Licensing is a state issue, not a national issue. Only states can pass laws requiring licensure. Although many national organizations endorse state licensure, the licensing of a professional and the requirements for licensure must come from within the state. Certification, however, is a national issue governed only by the organization from which it is developed. Therefore, regulation of certified individuals comes from within the certifying agency. In many instances, however, a certification program is used as a licensing examination. See the sidebar for the case in Louisiana, which in 1996 became the only U.S. state to license clinical exercise physiologists (4).

SUMMARY

A profession manifests five characteristics: autonomy, social value, specialized knowledge, representative organization, and lifetime commitment. Professionals have a societal bias rather than a personal bias and are responsible legally and ethically for the practice of their profession. The public good is guaranteed when practitioners are certified and/or licensed to practice.

The Case of Louisiana

Louisiana uses as its licensing examination the Exercise Specialist certification of the American College of Sports Medicine (ACSM). To qualify for a license as a clinical exercise physiologist in Louisiana, the following conditions must be met: (1) be at least 21 years of age, (2) be of good moral character . . . , (3) be a citizen of the Unites States or possess a valid and current legal authority to reside and work in the United States . . . , (4) have successfully completed a Master's of Science degree or Master's of Education degree in an exercise studies curriculum at an accredited school, which, at the time of the applicant's graduation, is approved by the American College of Sports Medicine or the board, (5) be certified as an Exercise Specialist by the American College of Sports Medicine, having taken and successfully passed the ACSM certifying examination, as administered by ACSM or by the board . . . , (6) have successfully completed an internship of 300 hours in exercise physiology under the supervision of a licensed exercise physiologist.

In this particular case, Louisiana adopted the ACSM Exercise Specialist certification as its own licensing examination, because there are no legal requirements for the state to prepare and provide its own licensing examination. Therefore, there is an alliance of sorts between a national certifying agency (which has no licensing authority) and a state that can issue a license. The ACSM Exercise Specialist certification program satisfies the Louisiana State Board of Medical Examiner's requirements for the licensed clinical exercise physiologist. Other professional organizations have similar relationships. The American Dietetic Association Registry Examination, for example, is often used as the qualification examination in states where the practice of dietetics is regulated by licensure.

For example, the Louisiana Clinical Exercise Physiologist Licensing Act provides that, under the supervision of a physician, the clinical exercise physiologist can administer a graded exercise test. The law (although this may not have been the intention) reads, " . . . in a cardiopulmonary rehabilitation program . . . " Does this mean that only the clinical exercise physiologist can administer a graded exercise test, or can a health and fitness professional administer a test to that same person (with or without disease) outside of a cardiopulmonary rehabilitation program? Likewise, if a hospital or medical center does not offer a structured cardiopulmonary rehabilitation program, can a professional (physical therapist or registered nurse) other than a clinical exercise physiologist administer the same test? Unless previously governed by legislation, these questions can only be answered at the local site, taking into consideration all of the circumstances surrounding the actions in question (4).

REFERENCES

1. Abernethy, B., V. Kippers, L. T. Mackinnon, R. J. Neal, and S. Harrahan, *The Biophysical Foundations of Human Movement.* Champaign, IL: Human Kinetics, 1997.

2. Brown, S.P. "The professionalization of exercise physiology: A critical essay." *Professionalization of Exercise Physiology* (online) 3(6)(2000).

3. Flexner, A. "Is social work a profession?" *School and Society* 1 (1915): 901–911.

4. Louisiana Clinical Exercise Physiologists Licensing Act, R.S. 37: 3421–3433. Department of Health and Hospitals, Board of Medical Examiners. *Louisiana Register* 23(4)(1997): 405–412.

5. Purtilo, R. B., and C. K. Cassel, *Ethical Dimensions in the Health Profession.* Philadelphia: W.B. Saunders Company, 1993.

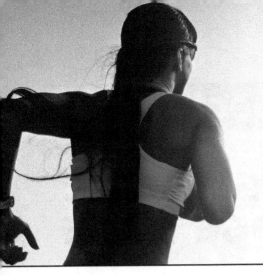

PART TWO

THE DISCIPLINES OF KINESIOLOGY

Prior to the 1960s, most of the disciplines covered in this text were taught as part of traditional physical education curricula. However, in this tumultuous decade, graduate physical education came under fire, resulting in a reexamination of the field and greater specialization. This specialization amounted to a philosophical shift toward the basic and applied sciences as a springboard to a more methodical study of physical activity, exercise, and sport. As an outcome of this introspective movement, the new field of exercise science had emerged. At the same time, the academic study of sport using the tools of other parent disciplines began to take shape and would later be termed sport studies. The outcome was a gradual shift to a renaming of the field, with kinesiology now the most prominent title of academic departments studying exercise, physical activity and sport.

Section 1 ///

HUMANITIES/SOCIAL SCIENCE KNOWLEDGE BASE

The three disciplines covered in Section 1 of the text are important to an understanding of the social forces affecting our behavior as we participate in exercise and sport or study it as kinesiology students. Chapter 5 presents an overview of sport philosophy by covering the meaning of philosophy and the insights that can be gained by asking philosophical questions related to sport. Chapter 6 discusses the field of sport history by illustrating how a historical perspective can help us better understand topics such as sport participation patterns observed in society today. Chapter 7 focuses on sport sociology by noting how issues such as performance-enhancing drug use can be better addressed and how fields such as coaching and strength training can benefit from using a sociological perspective.

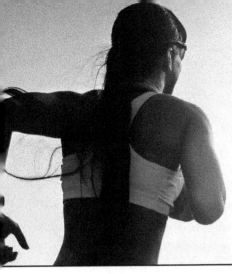

Chapter 5 ////

SPORT PHILOSOPHY

OUTLINE

OBJECTIVES

1. Define philosophy and understand the key ideas of philosophical inquiry and analysis.
2. Recognize the distinctive methods that philosophers use to understand sport.
3. Identify practical examples of philosophical issues in sport including
4. Recognize how the philosophy of sport adds to our understanding of sport, play, games, and physical activity.

The recent admission of widespread performance enhancing drug (PED) use by American cyclist Lance Armstrong (Figure 5.1) generated considerable media attention and a catastrophic fall from grace in the eyes of the public. Many of the most intensely debated questions in the doping scandal centered on issues of ethics, values, fairness, and the win-at-all-costs mentality of high-performance sport. Not only did Armstrong's admission strike a blow for the idea of fair play in competition, it also struck at the idea of holding up sporting personalities as paragons of virtue and people who inspire us to reach for our goals. Moreover, as additional information came to light, it became clear that doping in the sport of cycling was widespread and deeply embedded in the fabric of the sport. To add insult to injury, many people supported Armstrong and his athletic pursuits due to his incredible story: from death's doorstep, with a less than 50% chance of recovery from advanced testicular cancer to becoming one of the most decorated cyclists in the history of the sport, winning an unprecedented seven consecutive Tour de France titles. As the founder and public face of the Livestrong Foundation, an organization he established that according to his website (www.livestrong.com) was created to "fight to improve the lives of people affected by cancer," Armstrong had become a hero of almost mythic proportion. However, to some inside and outside of the sport of cycling, this run of success seemed almost too good to be true, especially considering that almost every major rival of Armstrong's had either tested positive for or was under the suspicion of using performance-enhancing drugs to achieve sporting success. As it turned out, by Armstrong's own admission, the fairytale career and the rewards that go with it, was built on a lie.

The case of Armstrong, while not unique, offers us a crash course in some of the key issues the discipline of sport philosophy addresses. Some of the critical questions in the Armstrong affair include:

- Is it ever acceptable to break or bend the rules in order to achieve sporting success?
- Do PEDs give athletes an unfair advantage over their competitors?
- Are the potential long-term health risks of PED use worth the short-term rewards?
- If all of your competitors are using PEDs, doesn't that *level* the playing field?
- Are sport stars expected to be paragons of virtue and role models for children and adults alike?
- What even counts as performance enhancement in the first place?

As we will see in this chapter, the Armstrong case can be productively evaluated through the lens of sport philosophy. But what is sport philosophy in the first place? Simply put, sport philosophy utilizes the concepts and ideas of philosophy and the methods of philosophical inquiry and focuses its attention on sport, play, games, and physical activity. Moreover, sport philosophy is concerned with the nature and purpose of sport and physical activity.

Before we explore the basic tenets of sport philosophy as a discipline within kinesiology, it will be helpful to turn our attention to understanding what philosophy is in general. We will then look at the development of sport philosophy as a distinct discipline. It will also be important to examine some contemporary examples

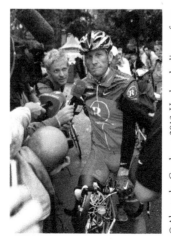

Figure 5.1. *Speculation about performance enhancing drug use has hounded cyclist Lance Armstrong for years.*

© Alexander Gordeyev, 2013. Used under license from Shutterstock, Inc.

BOX 5.1 What Counts as Gaining an Unfair Advantage?

To illustrate the ambiguity of what counts as performance enhancement in sport, consider the case of endurance athletes like cyclists, runners, and cross-country ski racers. Sport science has suggested that an endurance athlete can gain a performance boost by increasing his or her red blood cell count, thus increasing the ability to transport oxygen to the muscles and allow the athlete to work harder and recover faster. So how can you increase your red blood cell count? In fact, there are at least four ways to accomplish this goal: (1) train at altitude, (2) sleep in a hypoxic tent that mimics the condition of high altitude, (3) inject a substance that facilitates the production of red blood cells (erythropoietin or EPO), or (4) withdraw your own blood and then strategically retransfuse the blood ahead of a targeted competitive goal in order to supercharge the blood. Interestingly, from a philosophical point of view, the first two of these techniques are perfectly legal and last two of these techniques, if discovered, could lead to a ban of up to two years from competition. How do we determine what techniques and substances are okay to use and which ones are cheating (Figure 5.2)? One aim of philosophy is to help clear up these kinds of uncertainties.

in the world of sport where sport philosophy can contribute to our understanding of what is at stake. Finally, some conclusions will be drawn about how sport philosophy helps kinesiology students learn to understand and appreciate human movement and physical activity.

WHAT IS PHILOSOPHY?

The word *philosophy* comes from the Greek words *phileo,* meaning "to love" or "to befriend," and *sophia,* meaning "wisdom." Thus, philosophy literally means the love of wisdom. Socrates (Figure 5.3) is generally thought to be one of the founders of Western philosophy, and indeed it was Socrates who famously declared that *the unexamined life was not worth living.*

The importance of examining the world and our purpose in it remains one of the most fundamental ideas that continue to guide the field of philosophy in general and the discipline of sport philosophy in particular. Broadly speaking, philosophy is concerned with ideas and understanding. Philosophers are curious about the meaning of the world. More importantly, however, philosophy gives us the tools to articulate *why* people hold certain beliefs. Indeed, being able to present a reasonable and rational argument for your beliefs is one of the main objectives of philosophy. Although sometimes it is seen as being detached from the real world,

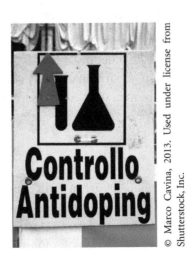

Figure 5.2. *Cat and mouse: How effective are efforts to catch doping athletes?*

© Marco Cavina, 2013. Used under license from Shutterstock, Inc.

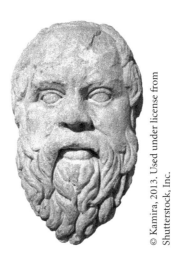

Figure 5.3. *Ancient Greek Philosopher, Socrates: 469–399 B.C.*

© Kamira, 2013. Used under license from Shutterstock, Inc.

philosophy does not simply deal in the hypothetical and murky. In many respects, it is exactly because we apply a philosophical analysis that we are able to boil down vexing social questions to their core elements and thus provide a platform to make reasoned and informed decisions.

Andrew Holowchak rightly notes, "Philosophic argument attempts to clarify matters by ridding everyday language of ambiguity and vagueness. What is the payoff? A better understanding of the issues and perhaps even a solution to some stubborn problem" (2). So while philosophers do reflect on serious questions, often this process of interrogation serves a vital purpose. In the field of kinesiology, for example, could you make a compelling case for the value of exercise and physical activity? As students of kinesiology, you may be called upon to present a reasoned and convincing argument for a policy or position that could impact the lives of people in your community. Among other things, philosophy helps to fine-tune these skills. In the same way you might practice to become more proficient at an athletic skill, you must also train your "philosophical muscles" to maximize your potential. The good news is that you are not starting from scratch.

Have you ever wondered about the nature of reality, struggled with a big decision, argued a political point of view with a friend or family member, or grappled with the question, should baseball players who used PEDs be enshrined in the Hall of Fame? If the answer is yes, then you are, more likely than not, engaging in philosophical thinking. However, the mere fact that we think about these kinds of issues does not necessarily make us philosophers, but it does help us to gauge what Kretchmar calls our "philosophical readiness," or put another way, our willingness to consider philosophical explanations and use philosophical tools in the search for answers to the questions stimulated by our curiosity of the world around us and our place in it (3).

Branches of Philosophy and General Topics of Inquiry

In many respects, philosophy can be understood as a metadiscipline. In this way, it is often argued that philosophy can provide foundations for the other disciplines, or at least tell us what is the job and nature of other disciplines. As to kinesiology, philosophy can help us shed light on issues related to physical activity and human movement. Historically, philosophy is often divided into several branches of inquiry that help us better understand the world.

Metaphysics

Some of the big-picture questions like the nature of reality and the nature of being are addressed in the branch of philosophy called *metaphysics*. While literally meaning "beyond physics," metaphysics has been a notoriously hard branch of philosophy to define. In a modern context, metaphysics helps us distinguish one thing from another, often by using description. So, in kinesiology, for example, if we were to ask if *play* is a valuable form of human movement (a question of value that will be explained below), a metaphysician might ask the *prior* question, "What *is* play?" In this sense, metaphysics and metaphysical questions help us understand the essence of existence.

Some of the earliest work in sport philosophy wrangled with the metaphysical question: What is sport? While this may seem like a silly question, have you ever thought about what should be included in sport? Is cheerleading a sport? What about golf, soccer, curling, baseball, or auto racing? The early attempts to answer these questions relied on what is often known as a *formalist* account. In a formalist account of sport, one must provide a clear and exhaustive set of conditions that, if met, would allow us to say if an activity should or should not be considered a sport. Exploring this question from a metaphysical point of view allows us to distinguish things that we often call games, like Monopoly, from things that we typically call sports, like American football. Can you think of characteristics that help to differentiate the two? If you can, you are doing metaphysics.

Epistemology

Philosophical inquiry that examines the questions—what do we know and to what degree can the things we *think* we know be true?—falls under the branch of philosophy known as epistemology. Epistemology deals with the question of what do we know with certainty. To what degree, for example, do my biases and subjectivity cloud my perception of the world? Put simply, epistemology is interested in *ways of knowing*. For example, can we only know what we are able to test and prove through the scientific method or does subjective knowledge count for some of our understanding of the world? In philosophy, we might ask whether knowledge is innate or whether knowledge is acquired through experience and measurement. In fact, these two positions roughly outline major traditions in epistemology know as *rationalism* and *empiricism*.

Rationalists believe that reason is the primary source of knowledge and that, as such, it is an innate human quality. In this view, what one knows is what one is able to clearly reason, since we are often tricked by our senses. In this way it is not just what you can experience and quantify that should count as knowledge, but what you are able to reason that counts as truth. Empiricists, on the other hand, doubt that a person can rely only on what can be measured, observed, and verified through the senses or through the use of precise measurement devices. The way we are able to gain an understanding of the world of sport and physical activity may certainly be evaluated through an epistemological lens. How much do we know about the world through thinking and how much do we know about the world through measuring it? In kinesiology, this is often expressed as the *mind-body* problem. A more contemporary evaluation of human movement by kinesiologists often acknowledges that both the mind and the body figure importantly in our knowledge of sport, play, and physical activity.

Axiology

Examinations about the value of things (like the value of play in the example above) fall into the branch of philosophy known as axiology. The following questions are axiological. What is a meaningful life? How does physical activity help contribute to a good life? Is a cooperative or a competitive orientation to sport more meaningful? Is sport art? Clearly there are sports that depend on an artistic evaluation in competition, such as figure skating, but does that mean that skating *is* art?

Axiology is concerned with how we assign and assess value and meaning in art, in life, or in sport. In general, questions of value are often boiled down to a few key notions. One idea has to do with intrinsic values while the other is concerned with extrinsic value. Intrinsic value is concerned with the value of something in and of itself while extrinsic value is best thought of as a means to an end. In kinesiology, an issue that, at its core, is axiological in nature has to do with exercise adherence. We know that exercise can provide tremendous benefits across the life span, but how can we help to facilitate exercise, particularly in sedentary and at-risk populations? An extrinsic view might say that losing weight or looking good can be strong motivation in taking up an exercise program. On the other hand, an intrinsic perspective might suggest that exercise (beyond these external benefits) will most likely be carried out long-term if we do it because it is valuable in and of itself. Perhaps a combination of these perspectives will garner optimal results, but recognizing that these two ideas are questions of value and, as such, necessarily axiological in nature, is the domain of sport philosophy.

Ethics

How ought we to behave? What is the nature of right and wrong? The branch of philosophy known as ethics considers issues of right and wrong actions, guidelines that impact our behavior, the code of ethics in our jobs or professional settings, and personal and professional obligation to others. While the field of ethics can delve into theoretical questions about the nature of morality, practical or applied ethics deals with real-world, day-to-day issues in our personal and professional lives.

Consider the example of Lance Armstrong from the beginning of the chapter. Can you think of any ethical questions that might be raised with respect to his use of PEDs to gain a competitive advantage in bicycle races? Is it cheating if everybody is using PEDs? Are these kinds of systematic rule violations, as Morgan (4) has suggested, simply a logical consequence of the high stakes, market-driven direction (at the pro and college level) sport has been moving in over the past few decades? Is it morally permissible to take money based on a performance that was the result of illegal drug use? Does intent matter more than the result of a particular action? Indeed, much of the contemporary work that is done in sport philosophy deals with ethical questions. To be sure, questions about fairness, cheating, breaking the rules and professional conduct on the job all fall within the philosophical domain of ethics.

What Is Philosophical Thinking?

Now that we have briefly explored what philosophers study, let's turn our attention to how they *do* philosophy. It might be clear by now that philosophy, unlike many of the other subjects you have encountered, depends less on data collection and analysis and more on reason, logic, and the clarity of one's argument. Therefore, one of the important skills any budding philosopher should hone is the ability to reason. According to Kretchmar (3), there are at least three main types of reasoning used by sport philosophers: inductive, deductive, and descriptive. These approaches are not mutually exclusive. In fact, a combination of elements of each type of reasoning often yields important insights into our topic of study.

The scientific method is the systematic process of acquiring knowledge whereby theories or hypotheses are either confirmed or shown to be false. The *Oxford English Dictionary* defines the scientific method as "a procedure that has characterized natural science since the 17th century, consisting in systematic observation, measurement and experiment, and the formulation, testing and modification of hypotheses." This method of acquiring knowledge is called scientific, because it is based on empirical and measurable evidence subject to specific principles of both inductive and deductive reasoning.

Inductive Reasoning

Inductive reasoning moves from a limited number of specific instances to more general conclusions about the class that a thing belongs to. In other words, one typically moves from concrete examples to more abstract (although fairly likely) conclusions. From this point of view, inductive reasoning in a philosophy often starts with a general observation or expression of particular ideas and moves to a broad conclusion based on those distinct observations or arguments. For example, say you were trying to define what physical activities count as a sport, using inductive reasoning, you might begin to list many activities that are thought to be sports (judo, baseball, soccer, distance running, rugby, etc.) and then identify the specific characteristics each have in common and that also set them apart from other activities, like walking to class or hiking on a trail. So long as your examples are neither too broad (anything that involves physical movement) or too narrow (must involve a ball), you may be able to draw useful conclusions about which activities can be called sports.

Deductive Reasoning

Deductive reasoning, on the other hand, moves from general claims or premises and then draws specific conclusions. Broadly speaking, the notion of deductive reasoning also suggests that the conclusion one draws is more likely to be true since, in a deductive argument, the premises (or facts) are intended to provide such strong support that it would be nearly impossible to draw any other conclusion.

Turing back to our sport example, let's say you start with the premise that for something to be considered a sport, it must incorporate obvious physical skill. Using poker as an example, is the previous statement still true? It is pretty clear that poker requires a great deal of skill and strategy in order to be successful, but does it require *obvious physical skill*? If it does not, based on our original premise, then we cannot include poker in the list of things we call sport. It should be clear in this example that the validity of your conclusions in deductive reasoning is only as sound as the truth of your premises in the first place.

Descriptive Reasoning

Descriptive reasoning, in general, entails examining one instance or example of an event and then faithfully and exhaustively describing its most fundamental attributes. One way to do this kind of descriptive work is to provide a detailed and often nuanced explanation of a particular experience. Let's turn to an example from kinesiology to better illustrate this concept.

Descriptive reasoning is often used in the philosophical tradition known as phenomenology. One way to understand the idea is to say that, in general, phenomenological thought focuses on "lived" experiences as understood from the first-person perspective. With this in mind, a great deal of the work done within this tradition is descriptive in nature. For example, have you ever tried to explain to somebody, as thoroughly as possible, how to perform a sporting skill, what it is like to perform a perfect jump shot in basketball, or what it feels like to perform a complex motor skill like climbing a rock face or performing a tumbling routine in gymnastics? Descriptive reasoning would argue that not only is it important to be able to articulate those activities by way of exacting and detailed explanation, but that we can know the essence of a physical activity—and therefore think about its greater meaning—through such an intellectual enterprise. In this way, descriptive reasoning is especially useful, from a philosophical perspective, for helping to understand one's firsthand experience of moving through time and space.

WHAT IS SPORT PHILOSOPHY?

As mentioned in the opening of the chapter, sport philosophy uses the framework and tools of its parent discipline, philosophy, in order to investigate and understand key ideas in kinesiology. Sport philosophy is considered one of the core disciplines of kinesiology, and many undergraduate and graduate programs include a class or classes that explore some of the key ideas described in this chapter. However, beyond just looking at kinesiology issues through one or more of the branches of philosophy described earlier, sport philosophy has evolved into a discipline unto itself. In some ways, it could be said that the unique characteristics of sport and physical activity helped sport philosophy to move beyond its parent field of philosophy and, in fact, helped to contribute to it.

Brief History of Sport Philosophy

Kretchmar provides a useful overview of the history and development of the field of sport philosophy (3). While there is no doubt that people have been discussing the value and meaning of human movement since at least the time of the ancient Greeks, the systematic look at sport through a philosophical framework can be said to have begun in late 1960s. The first meeting of the Philosophic Society for the Study of Sport (PSSS) took place in 1972, and the organization quickly established the *Journal of the Philosophy of Sport* in 1974. This journal remains one of the premier venues for the intellectual exchange of important ideas in the field and should be the first stop when researching a sport philosophy–related topic.

Classic and Contemporary Questions in Sport Philosophy

What is the nature of sport, play, and game?

Can sport be considered art?

What is fairness and sportspersonship?

Should violent sports like MMA or American football be banned?

Are female athletes of the same rank as male athletes?

Does sport affect or reflect social morals and values (both in individuals and in society)?

Should certain drugs be banned from sport?

What place does winning have in sport?

Can sport help to frame a meaningful life?

Can I come to know myself better through sport participation?

Can physical activity provide a way of knowing more about the world around me?

Has the free-market helped or hurt amateur and professional sport?

Is it fair for transgendered athletes to compete against athletes of their reassigned sex?

Among the key early figures in the development of sport philosophy as a bona fide discipline in kinesiology were Paul Weiss, the inaugural president of the PSSS, along with Warren Fraleigh, Seymour Kleinman, Hans Lenk, Ellen Gerber, Scott Kretchmar, and Klaus Meier. Due to their commitment, strong leadership, and small but dedicated membership, the PSSS established the foundation upon which the discipline still rests. While the PSSS was evolving, it was undoubtedly experiencing not only growing pains, but more fundamental criticism from within the ranks of the traditional realm of philosophy. As a discipline struggling to define itself both within and outside of the tradition of philosophy, many of the early scholars in the field found themselves striving to have their work taken seriously beyond the ranks of their fellow PSSS members.

Within the field of kinesiology today, sport philosophy as a stand-alone degree concentration is quite rare. While the number of graduate programs currently offering advanced degrees in sport philosophy is few, most programs at the undergraduate level do incorporate sport philosophy classes within their core curriculum. Many kinesiology curriculums introduce some of the classic issues in sport philosophy in addition to many of the practical and professional ethical issues in the field. In this way, philosophy is obviously seen as a core viewpoint in the field of kinesiology.

In the early days of the sport philosophy, some of the central questions academics asked had to do with defining sport, articulating the concept of fair play and sportsmanship, and aesthetic questions about the value of sport as an artistic form. A quick look at the current work being done in sport philosophy will show a move from the more theoretical and ideological to the more practical and applied. Currently, issues such as the use of performance-enhancing drugs, the ethical considerations of youth contact sport participation, disability sport and fairness, sport and violence, and the use of technology in sport constitute a significant contribution to the academic literature.

Current Issues in Sport Philosophy

Violence in Sport

Mixed Martial Arts (Figure 5.4) is a combat sport that includes a combination of striking (boxing and kickboxing) and grappling (wrestling, judo, and Jujitsu). The sport has been skyrocketing in popularity over the past 10 years, but it has been fraught with controversy. Indeed, former U.S. presidential candidate John McCain once famously decried MMA as "human cockfighting." While its reputation has certainly been overhauled since the

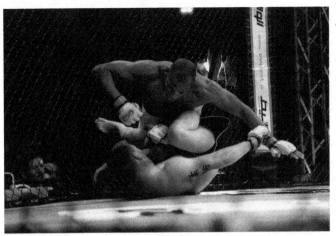

© Ehab Othman, 2013. Used under license from Shutterstock, Inc.

Figure 5.4. *The controversial sport of Mixed Martial Arts.*

mid-1990s when McCain made that statement, not everyone has a favorable opinion of the sport. Like boxing before it, one of the key questions you could pose about MMA today is, Just because the sport is popular and/ or profitable is it morally acceptable? As an exercise in sport philosophy, we will take a look at a few of the arguments used to ban violent sport and then subject them to philosophical scrutiny. It is important to note that the purpose of this exercise is not to convince you of one side or the other of the issue, but rather, if you are going to hold a position, you must defend it through critical thinking and rational argumentation.

What are the main arguments one could make for banning MMA? One argument that obviously springs to mind, especially if you have seen a particularly spectacular knockout of an MMA combatant, is to protect the safety of the athlete. Without question, athletes are at risk when the cage door locks behind them and the bell rings to sound the beginning of a match. It seems reasonable that we should restrict athletes from making decisions that will likely cause them great harm and in rare cases, even death. However, using Simon's classic work on the moral permissibility of boxing, we can argue that while it is quite true that prohibiting athletes from participating in MMA bouts would certainly prevent them from possible harm, the same could be said of stopping someone from running an ultra-marathon, skateboarding in an empty pool, or chewing tobacco (5).

The philosophical concept at issue here is called *paternalism* (5). Paternalism is best described as the interference of an individual's liberty (or free will choices) by an outside entity for what is said to be his or her own good. The classic argument against paternalism was posited by John Stuart Mill (1806–1873) in his treatise, *On Liberty*. According to Mill, it is far worse, as long a person understands the consequences of his or her actions, to restrict somebody from doing something that may knowingly cause him or her injury than it is to let that person make a decision that could result in harm. In other words, as long as my choices do not prevent you from freely choosing to do something, there is no justification to interfere with my choice based on what you think is best for me.

Let's return to MMA. Using this free-will argument, we are never justified in telling a mentally competent adult what he or she can or cannot do, even if the choice will obviously cause that person potential harm or injury. So the burden, it seems, is on deciding if both athletes in an MMA fight understand that they are at risk for great harm. If they do, then, "let's get it on."

So while he would argue we are not justified in paternalistically restricting participation in MMA, Simon makes a pretty interesting second argument for its prohibition. If we can prove that the athlete does not really understand the consequences of his actions or that he will, at some point in the future (as a result of damage sustained by participating in MMA), be in such a position as to compromise his ability to freely choose (due to cognitive impairment), we may have a stronger case for restricting participation. In this case, we may be justified to intervene on paternalistic grounds. Simon ends his argument by suggesting that, while there is no compelling justification for banning boxing outright, there is certainly a case to be made for significantly restricting what is allowed in the sport. If, he concludes, that repeated blows to the head will eventually impact a person's ability to make rational decisions, we are warranted in eliminating or otherwise significantly restricting head-shots or requiring athletes to, at minimum, wear protective equipment.

The idea in presenting this issue is not so much that you pick a side either for or against MMA, but rather that you can see how the application of philosophical concepts, such as liberty, free-will, and paternalism, help to zero in on the issues at hand. If anything, a philosophical examination leads to more initial confusion about something we thought we had a strong opinion about, but in the end, we are often in a much better position to defend our point of view after subjecting the issue to a philosophical interrogation.

Spotlight Activity in Sport Philosophy: Making the Case: What Role Should Sport Play in Society?

Read Chapter 2 in Drewe's *Why Sport?: An Introduction to the Philosophy of Sport* (1). Identify the following key concepts and prepare to integrate them into the following activity:

- What role should sport play in society?
- What is the difference between intrinsic vs. instrumental values?
- What is competition? Is it always about crushing your opponent?
- Is sport worth the price we pay and are there downsides of sport today?

Problem: The city's budget needs to be passed and youth sports are on the chopping block! As kinesiology majors, you are uniquely positioned to offer some perspective to decision makers and other community stakeholders about the negative implications of such a resolution.

Preparation: In consultation with your team (no more than three to four students), stake out a philosophical justification for continuing to promote and fund youth sport and present it to the city council.

- Your team will have 20 minutes to prepare and craft a statement , so you must work efficiently!
- Use a sheet of paper or your computer to jot down ideas, thoughts, notes, concept maps, etc.
- Write a clear and concise statement that makes your case as convincingly as possible.

Action: Your team will have no more than 2 minutes to state your case. Be sure to write your ideas in a clear and concise position statement of no longer than one double-spaced page.

Note: As aspiring sport philosophers, it will be important to define your terms, identify the intrinsic/instrumental values unique to sport, and articulate the consequences of eliminating sport from society.

SUMMARY

Sport and physical activities are an important part of society (Figure 5.5). As kinesiology students, it will be essential for you to clearly and effectively argue for the intrinsic and extrinsic value of lifelong fitness. Not only can strong arguments be made for the value of regular physical activity, but that our participation in sport, play, and games can also be a pathway to deeper understanding of ourselves and the world around us. Sport philosophy provides us with the perspectives and techniques to carefully scrutinize the crucial issues in the field and helps us to better communicate those issues to public and professional entities. There is no doubt that questions philosophers ask often seem only to lead to more questions, but the hope is that by cultivating your intellectual curiosity and fine-tuning your philosophical thought processes, you will be able to adequately address the serious challenges you will face as professionals in the field of kinesiology.

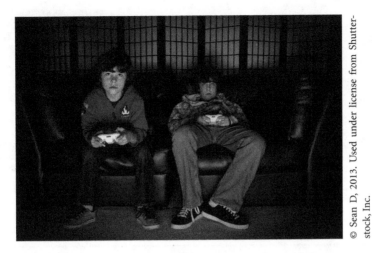

© Sean D, 2013. Used under license from Shutterstock, Inc.

Figure 5.5. *Imagine a world without physical activity.*

For More Information on the Philosophy of Sport

Academic Organizations
British Philosophy of Sport Association
European Association for the Philosophy of Sport
International Association for the Philosophy of Sport

Scholarly Journals
Journal of Sport and Social Issues
Journal of the Philosophy of Sport
Quest
Sport, Ethics and Philosophy

REFERENCES

1. Drewe, S., *Why Sport?: An Introduction to the Philosophy of Sport.* Toronto: Thompson Educational Publishing, 2003.

2. Holowchak, M. A., ed., *Philosophy of Sport: Critical Readings, Crucial Issues.* Upper Saddle River, NJ: Pearson Education, 2002.

3. Kretchmar, S., *Practical Philosophy of Sport and Physical Activity* (2nd ed.) Champaign, IL: Human Kinetics, 2005.

4. Morgan, W., *Why Sports Morally Matter.* New York: Routledge, 2006.

5. Simon, R., *Fair Play: Sports, Values, and Society.* Boulder CO: Westview Press, 1991.

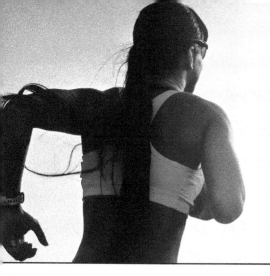

Chapter 6

SPORT HISTORY

OUTLINE

Objectives

What Is Sport History?

The Development of Sport History

Sport History and the Power of Myths

Gender and Sport Participation
   Patterns

A Historical Case Study in
   Globalization and Sports

Summary

References

OBJECTIVES

1. Understand key concepts and research questions in sport history.
2. Understand the development of sport history as an academic field of study.
3. Understand the relevance of sport history to other areas in the field of kinesiology.

WHAT IS SPORT HISTORY?

The purpose of this chapter is to provide kinesiology students with an introduction to the field of sport history. The chapter begins with an explanation of what sport history is, followed by an overview of the development of sport history as an academic field, and concludes with several illustrations of how sport history has particular relevance for students in kinesiology.

Sport history can be regarded as a subdiscipline of the parent discipline of *history* or as one of the disciplines that contribute to *sport studies*, a branch of kinesiology that specifically covers the sociocultural aspects of sport, exercise, and physical activity. These relationships can be confusing, but they illustrate the cross-, trans-, and multidisciplinary aspects discussed in Chapter 1. Given the diversity of approaches within sport history, it is challenging to provide a concise overview of the field. Thus, students should realize that the following summary is only intended as a general introduction, and those wishing to gain further insight about sport history should consult some of the references provided at the end of this chapter.

To provide a definition at the most basic level, sport history involves a study of sport-related events and individuals from the past. Sport historians contribute to our understanding of kinesiology in a broad sense by helping us make sense of how and why movements of human bodies have been organized into what we currently call *sports* and the meanings with which these practices have been imbued. One way to understand the work of sport historians is to make a distinction between descriptive and analytical research (20). Specifically, descriptive history seeks to identify details that help locate events and individuals in the past, while analytical history seeks to make sense of these details. For example, if one was trying to investigate the history of softball, a descriptive question would be "When did the first softball game take place?" An analytical question would be "Why has softball been primarily played by females at the youth level?" See the box for some additional examples of descriptive and analytical research questions. Later, we will return to the discussion of what sport historians do and how they do it by providing some examples that are relevant to students in kinesiology. First, we will provide an overview of the organizational development of sport history as an academic discipline with a specific focus on the growth of the field in North America.

THE DEVELOPMENT OF SPORT HISTORY

While sport history was not organized and institutionalized as an academic field until the second half of the 20th century, people have been researching the history of sport for a longer period of time. This was especially the case in Germany during the late 18th and early 19th centuries, when teachers and scholars rediscovered and reinterpreted physical activities from ancient Greece and other cultures. The work of Vieth, published in 1794 on the history of physical exercises, for example, contributed to the foundation of the development of German gymnastics, known as *Turnen* (24). Subsequently, understanding the history of physical activities

Research Questions in Sport History (adapted from [2])

Descriptive
Where (was softball first played)?
When (did the first softball game take place)?
Who (originated the sport of softball)?
What (is Little League Softball)?
Analytical
How (did softball become popular in the United States)?
Why (has softball been primarily played by females at the youth level)?

and their philosophical foundations became a major part of the training of physical educators. Despite these antecedents, it took until the 1960s and 1970s for the systematic academic study of the development of sport to gather momentum in Europe. Initially, most of the research on the history of sport was conducted in college and university departments that specialized in sports and physical education (18). Only gradually did the study of sport become more acceptable within history departments, as some established scholars regarded sport to be too trivial as a topic.

The development of the field in North America was similar to that which took place in Europe. The next box presents a timeline of some notable events in the development of sport history in North America. Here, among the earliest works helping to lay the foundation for the development of sport history was Frederic Paxson's *The Rise of Sport*, published in 1917 (14). Paxson suggested that as the old, continental American frontier was closed, organized sport constituted a new frontier for Americans. By recognizing sport as an important aspect of American society, Paxson helped usher in a shift in which historians increasingly gave serious scholarly attention to sport, whereas previously they tended to focus primarily on what were seen as the more important topics of war, politics, and "high culture" (21). Despite the increasing attention given to historical research about sport, it was not until after World War II that more organized efforts to promote sport history as an academic field in its own right began to coalesce.

One of the first achievements by individuals working to develop an organization dedicated to the historical study of sport was the creation of a History of Sport subgroup of the College Physical Education Association (CPEA) in 1960 (later renamed the National College Physical Education Association for Men, or NCPEAM). This was a notable step in that it created a forum for historians of sport and physical education to share their research. However, there were significant limitations to having only a subgroup within a broader physical education organization. Notably, women were excluded from the CPEA/NCPEAM meetings, and the History of Sport subsection failed to draw scholars from outside the field of physical education (21). In turn, it became apparent that independent meetings and organizations would be necessary to move the field of sport history forward.

Meetings dedicated specifically to sport history began to emerge in the late 1960s, with the First International Seminar on the History of Physical Education and Sport hosted by the Wingate Institute for Physical Education in Netanya, Israel, in 1968. Shortly thereafter, the First Canadian Symposium on the History of Sport and Physical Education was held in Edmonton, Alberta, in 1970, closely coinciding with the publication of the *Canadian Journal of the History of Sport and Physical Education* (later renamed *Sport History Review*). Perhaps more importantly, however, was the development of the North American Society for Sport History (NASSH), which held its first annual meeting in Columbus, Ohio, in 1973. Equally notable, NASSH also initiated a scholarly journal devoted specifically to sport history, the *Journal of Sport History* (*JSH*), first published in 1974. These developments were particularly meaningful because unlike researchers in laboratory sciences who often work in teams, sport historians labor primarily as individuals (21).

Key Events in the Development of Sport History

1917: *The Rise of Sport* published by Frederick Paxson; helped foster serious academic interest in sport history
1960: College Physical Education Association established a History of Sport section; gave historians of sport a specific forum in which to share research
1970: First Canadian Symposium on the History of Sport and Physical Education (Edmonton, Alberta)
1973: First conference of the North American Society for Sport History (Columbus, OH)
1974: *Journal of Sport History* first published

Table 6.1. Selected Academic Journals in Sport History

Journal Title	Information about Journal
International Journal of the History of Sport	First published in 1984
Journal of Sport History	First published in 1974; official journal of the North American Society for Sport History
Sport History Review	First published in 1970; published as the *Canadian Journal of the History of Sport and Physical Education* from 1970–1980; published as the *Canadian Journal of the History of Sport from 1980–1995*
Sport in History	First published in 1981; published as *The Sports Historian* prior to 2003; official journal of the British Society of Sports History
Sporting Traditions	First published in 1984; official journal of the Australian Society for Sports History

With the initiation of organizations and journals such as NASSH and the *JSH*, sport historians now had their own forums in which to present and exchange ideas. The continued growth of the field since that time is evidenced by the fact that there are now several journals dedicated specifically to publishing sport history research (see Table 6.1 for a summary). There are, however, notable limitations of the organizational development of the field, such as the fact that, as of 2007, the leading professional organization for sport historians in *North America* (NASSH) had no scholar from Mexico among its members and its journal had not published a single article in Spanish (Dyreson, 2007). Further, as of 2013, NASSH has yet to hold a meeting in Mexico.

SPORT HISTORY AND THE POWER OF MYTHS

In 2010, Major League Baseball Commissioner Bud Selig sent the following response to a fan who inquired about the origins of the sport of baseball: "From all of the historians which I have spoken with, I really believe that Abner Doubleday is the 'Father of Baseball.' I know there are some historians who would dispute this though" (1). A problem with Selig's reply, however, is that the story of Abner Doubleday being the father of baseball is a myth. When he suggested that "some historians" would dispute Doubleday's status as the sport's founder, he is wildly distorting the fact that the story of Abner Doubleday inventing the game of baseball is regarded to be untrue by virtually all historians who have investigated it.

Selig's statement speaks to the power of myths. The "Doubleday myth," as it is often referred to, has endured for over a century, despite having been widely refuted by sport historians. The endurance of such myths poses a substantial challenge for sport historians who often must play the role of "myth-busters" seeking to provide more accurate understandings of people and events from the past (2).

The Doubleday myth initially emerged from a commission organized in the early 1900s to investigate the origins of baseball. The commission was backed by Albert Spalding—a former player, baseball executive, and sporting goods magnate—and chaired by former National League President Abraham Mills. Notably, this was a time period in which the United States was still relatively young as a nation and baseball had emerged as the "national pastime." In 1903, a prominent sportswriter named Henry Chadwick had written that baseball was descended from a British game called "rounders" (19). Given the cultural significance that baseball had attained in the United States, however, there was a strong nationalistic interest in having baseball branded as a uniquely American invention. After some investigation, the Mills Commission concluded that baseball was actually invented by a man named Abner Doubleday in Cooperstown, New York, in 1839. Doubleday, who was a well-known Union Army general in the Civil War, was credited with having arranged the bases in a diamond pattern and using the term "base ball." The evidence for this story came from the testimony of a man named Abner Graves, who had met Doubleday while he was a soldier in the Union Army.

Since the commission publicized Doubleday's status as the "Father of Baseball," the story has been challenged by sport historians for numerous reasons. For example, Graves, who claimed to be present on the day in 1839 when Doubleday drew a diagram of the playing field with the bases arranged in a diamond pattern, would have been only 6 or 7 years old at this time (17). When he provided his testimony to the Mills Commission, however, nearly 70 years had passed. The childhood memories of a man in his 70s seem to be a questionable foundation upon which to base any confident conclusions, particularly when this was the only evidence that Doubleday had founded the game. Further, Graves' story contained many apparent inconsistencies, and he was later institutionalized after murdering his wife and being found not guilty by reason of insanity (17). Casting further doubt on Graves' claims are some of the facts about Doubleday's life. For example, in 1839 Doubleday was in his first year as a cadet at the United States Military Academy in West Point, New York, and he would have been unlikely to receive leave to travel to Cooperstown at that point in time (17). Doubleday was also a prolific writer, yet made no mention of having been involved in baseball prior to his death in 1893. Given these inconsistencies, no serious historians accept the story of Doubleday as the "Father of Baseball."

So, who did "invent" the game of baseball? The reality is that it would probably be inappropriate to label any one individual as the inventor of baseball. Rather, the sport evolved incrementally from other bat-and-ball games. While the British games of rounders and cricket likely played a key role in the development of baseball, it is important to note that bat-and-ball games have been played in many societies throughout history. Although it would be inaccurate to identify a single person as the originator of baseball, there were certainly key individuals involved in the sport's development. For example, Alexander Cartwright led the New York Knickerbocker Base Ball Club in the 1840s and played an important role in advancing the game to its modern version. Many other individuals, however, have been important in the development of baseball into the sport we know today.

Despite all this evidence to the contrary, the Doubleday myth still persists to some extent today. One of the primary symbols of the myth's continued relevance is the National Baseball Hall of Fame, which is located in Cooperstown (Figure 6.1). In fact, the Baseball Hall of Fame was originally dedicated in 1939 to commemorate the supposed founding of baseball in Cooperstown 100 years earlier. Today, the Hall of Fame's website contains a page with a headline that proclaims "the Doubleday Myth is Cooperstown's Gain" (13). The site acknowledges that the Doubleday myth has been exposed as false, but proclaims that the myth "has grown so strong that the facts will never deter the spirit of Cooperstown." Thus, in addition to being a representation of the myth's continued relevance, the Hall of Fame simultaneously acts to further perpetuate the myth. This is an example of how, when people become heavily invested in a myth (for example, the construction of a hall of fame and museum building in Cooperstown), it can be particularly difficult to completely dispel. Thus, myth-busting often takes significant effort. However, by doing so and, in turn, helping to provide more accurate accounts of events and people from the past, sport historians provide an important contribution to the field of kinesiology. They help us better understand the historical factors that influence the world of sport and physical activity we observe today.

When we examine historical claims like the origin of baseball, we can write descriptive narratives about the "who, what, and when" of what "really" happened, or we can delve deeper by analyzing why these myths were created and how they have been reproduced. Other sporting myths include the notion that our sense of amateurism goes back to the ancient Olympics and the idea that William Webb Ellis invented rugby in 1823. By going beyond studying individual cases, we can build theories about why myths exist at all and what role they play in human culture. Another area to explore is the role historians themselves play in creating historical accounts as versions of the past (2). This discussion should encourage us to critically examine not only the past, but also what present-day ideas we take for granted and why we assume them to be true. What claims do you think are made today that future generations will regard as myths?

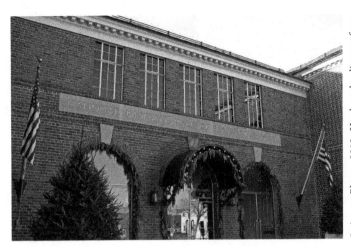

Figure 6.1. *The National Baseball Hall of Fame, located in Cooperstown, NY, is a symbol of the continued persistence of the "Doubleday myth."*

GENDER AND SPORT PARTICIPATION PATTERNS

Another way in which sport history is important to students and professionals in kinesiology is that it can help us understand the historical basis for current participation patterns in sport and physical activity. As many readers may know, there were relatively few sport participation opportunities for women in the United States prior to the 1970s. Since that time, however, there has been massive growth in women's sport participation. Yet, sport and physical activity patterns differ substantially between men and women. As an obvious example, some sports are played primarily by men, while other sports are played more widely by women. Why is this? While some people may be tempted to assume there is a natural order to sport participation patterns, this is not necessarily the case. Rather, there are historical factors involving people struggling to gain access to sport that have shaped the sport participation patterns existing today.

Prior to the 20th century, women's exclusion from sport was rationalized by a belief that women's bodies were physically incapable of enduring strenuous activity. Specifically, there was a widespread notion that, due to the recurring menstrual cycle, women were chronically weak and had only a finite amount of mental and physical energy. This belief was widely held by influential medical practitioners, most of whom were men, and was ostensibly based on scientific evidence. Menstruation was conceived as a pathological condition that necessitated the exclusion of women from competitive sports and any other physical exertion considered to be overly exhausting by experts in the medical community. Sport historian Patricia Vertinsky labeled this belief the idea of the "eternally wounded woman" (23). By propagating this idea, medical practitioners played the role of human engineers, influencing women's perceptions of their own physical capabilities in a negative way. Although mainstream medical practice no longer views menstruation as pathological, we still see evidence of this idea persisting, for example, at some tennis tournaments in which men play best of five sets, while women play best of three.

Even as beliefs such as the "eternally wounded woman" began to be debunked through research, there was still substantial resistance to women's entry into sport. This was particularly true in sports such as baseball. To help us gain insight about why this was the case, it is useful to understand that organized participatory sports were developed during the late 19th century in part as a solution to what scholar Michael Kimmel has called the "crisis of masculinity" in the United States (8). As Kimmel explains, several factors contributed to this "crisis," which was essentially a perceived erosion of traditional middle-class white masculinity that began during the second half of the 19th century (Figure 6.2).

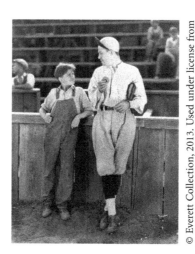

© Everett Collection, 2013. Used under license from Shutterstock, Inc.

Figure 6.2. *During the "crisis of masculinity" in the late 1800s, baseball became a way of revitalizing American masculinity and helping boys learn to become men.*

As westward expansion was coming to an end, the rise of industrialization was dramatically altering men's relationships to their work. Whereas nearly nine of every 10 American men were farmers or self-employed businessmen in the first half of the 19th century, fewer than one of every three men were economically autonomous by the first decade of the 20th century (8). This meant that many men lost control of their labor and were dispossessed of ownership. Accompanying industrialization and urbanization was a tremendous infusion of immigrants into major U.S. cities during this time period, which further threatened traditional white American masculinity. Additionally, women's rights movements become more common at this time and challenged men's domination of politics and business. It was in this context, as a response to the crisis of masculinity, that organized competitive sport in general flourished, and baseball specifically emerged as the "national pastime." In short, sport (baseball in particular) began to be seen as a way of revitalizing American manhood and helping boys learn to become men.

Given that organized competitive sports developed in the United States in part as a way of reviving masculinity during a time of perceived crisis, it should not be surprising that there has been substantial resistance to women's participation in sport. The development of baseball and softball illustrate this point. When baseball emerged as a sport for adults in the mid-19th century, it was organized by men and for men. Softball, on the other hand, developed as an activity for both men and women in the late 19th and early 20th centuries (3). In the context of the depression era, softball's popularity boomed in the 1930s and 1940s. It was relatively inexpensive, required less space and fewer resources than baseball, and benefitted from funding for public works projects as part of the *New Deal* initiated by President Franklin D. Roosevelt. Girls and women flocked to softball, particularly in working-class communities. Here, notions of appropriate femininity were less restrictive since working-class women historically had to be physically active as part of their daily labor. Despite their early entry into softball, women's participation was contested and resisted. Gender and social class ideologies caused many observers to wonder if female softball players were becoming "too manly."

Girls and women interested in baseball, however, faced a greater level of resistance. For example, Little League Baseball (LLB) was founded in the late 1930s and operated with a policy that only boys were eligible to participate. When in the 1960s and early 1970s a few individual teams allowed girls to participate, LLB responded by threatening to revoke the charters of leagues in which girls participated. With this strategy, LLB was able to resist the entry of girls for a few years. However, following a civil rights grievance filed in 1973 by the National Organization for Women on behalf of Maria Pepe (a young baseball player in New Jersey), LLB was forced to allow girls onto its teams (11). Rather than embrace this decision by welcoming girls into Little League Baseball, Little League officials moved quickly to create a softball program in 1974. In other words, once forced by law to include girls, Little League responded by creating a separate niche for girls, channeling boys and girls into different tracks and ensuring that baseball remained a largely sex-segregated institution (12). We can see the legacy of these decisions today, given that baseball is still primarily played by boys and men, while girls and women largely play softball.

While providing a thorough overview of the gendered history of sport and physical activity is beyond the scope of this chapter, our intent was to highlight a few key historical factors that can help us better understand the sport participation patterns we observe today. By understanding how such historical factors continue to act as impediments to women's participation, professionals across the field of kinesiology may be better equipped to create sport and physical activity opportunities that are more inclusive and open to all.

A HISTORICAL CASE STUDY IN GLOBALIZATION AND SPORTS

American football serves as a case study for the globalization of sport, illustrating how sport history can help increase understanding of the current sports landscape on a broader level. "The world is growing smaller," is a familiar statement, but the degree to which this phrase applies depends on where you live, how old you are, and how much money you have. It is difficult to deny that different parts of the world—and the people who live there—have become increasingly connected and interdependent. In part, this is due to advances in communication technology and travel. Today, access to the Internet can make a kid growing up in a small town in Ohio a die-hard fan of the British soccer team, Manchester United. Games can be watched live online while chatting with soccer fans around the world. London's Wembley Stadium became the site of the first NFL exhibition game abroad in 1983. In 2007, the same stadium was the site of the NFL's first regular season game held outside North America (Figure 6.3). Clearly, the world of sport has been changing.

One concept used to describe and analyze these changes is *globalization*, which refers to a "transplanetary process or set of processes involving growing multi-directional flows of increasingly liquid people, objects, places, and information and the structures they encounter and create that are barriers to, or expedite, those flows" (16). This does not mean that the world is necessarily becoming the same everywhere. For example, although sports are seemingly played around the world, important differences, nuances, and local variations still exist. Thus, using the concept of globalization, we can study historical developments that help explain why Americans are most likely to play baseball, basketball, or gridiron football, while the rest of the world tends to play cricket, soccer, or rugby (10, 22).

The migration of American football abroad illustrates possibilities and obstacles in the international flow of sports. As an example, the American football federation in Germany (AFVD) counted over 45,000 members in 2012, including tackle and flag football players as well as cheerleaders of all ages. While this may sound like a lot of participants, the AFVD ranked just 38th among the 62 member federations of the German sport

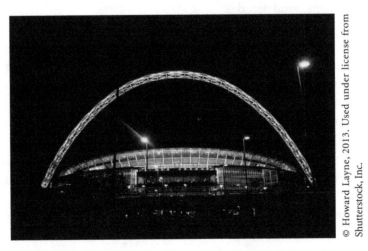

Figure 6.3.   *In 2007, London's Wembley Stadium hosted the first regular-season NFL game played outside of North America.*

federation, just below triathlon and above jujutsu. The German soccer federation, meanwhile, was the largest organization with close to 7 million members (4). Thus, it is fair to say American football is still a minor sport in Germany. Internationally, American football has very limited appeal as a participant sport. Comparatively, however, Germany is a relative success story. Almost half of all organized gridiron players in Europe play in Germany, and it appears that outside of North America, no other country produces more players.

The development of American football in Germany is best understood in a broader sociocultural context. This includes how the influence of foreign cultures (including sports) have been embraced, negotiated, and opposed by different groups of people over the last two centuries. In the early 19th century, *Turnen* (gymnastic exercises) became a means for German men to galvanize nationalistic sentiments to overcome French rule. The formation of clubs for instruction in a variety of balancing and climbing activities was part of a larger political movement with an aim to abolish the old feudal order and the formation of a united nation state (15). In England, the emergence of modern sport resulted in the formation of the Football Association in 1863, which governed the standardization and rationalization of what Americans would end up calling soccer. The influence of the British Empire in trade and military quickly facilitated the international diffusion of the sport. By the end of the 19th century, the kicking game also reached Germany. In one case in 1874, Konrad Koch, a German schoolteacher, returned from a visit in England with a soccer ball and began to teach the game to his students. The introduction of soccer was met with considerable resistance by Germans who favored their *Turnen* to English sports. In an effort to minimize the English origins of the sport, and thus lessen opposition, German soccer enthusiasts translated the game's terminology. Offside became *Abseits*, corner kick turned into *Eckball*, and penalty transformed into *Elfmeter* (literally: eleven meters). The game found a following mainly in those who were considered outsiders, including young people, members of the working class, and especially upstart white-collar workers, who looked to create new social networks (6). By the 1920s, soccer was well on its way to becoming *König Fußball* (king football) in Germany.

When American football arrived in Germany, the country's sporting culture was not only dominated by soccer, but the arrival occurred in a particular historical context (5). After World War II, American soldiers attempted to introduce their version of football in an effort to reach out to German youth. The efforts resulted in the formation of a few, short-lived clubs in the American-occupied zone of West Germany. It appears the Americans would have had more success in reaching and influencing young Germans had they been more experienced in the game of soccer. In post-War West Germany, the complicated game of American football did not have the same appeal as other American products (for example, chocolate, cigarettes, and chewing gum)— all of which were immensely popular and valuable. For many Germans, these consumer goods promised a new beginning and perhaps their version of "the American dream." American football was not able to tap into these symbolic meanings for another several decades.

At the grassroots level, American football gained its first down in the late 1970s in West Germany. At this time, the young Federal Republic was becoming less politically and economically dependent on the United States. Some protesters even demanded the withdrawal of the several hundred thousand American troops still stationed in Cold War West Germany. Despite these animosities, many West Germans had developed a taste for American popular culture and many personal friendships had developed between American soldiers and German civilians. It is important to understand the presence of Americans in Germany in order to make sense of the emergence of American football. Between 1950 and 2000, Germany hosted over 10 million U.S. military members (7), most of whom were concentrated in the southwest of the country, which is also where most of the first football teams started. One of these encounters resulted in the founding of the first long-term American football club in 1977 (5). Two years later, there were enough clubs to form a league and a federation. Instead of simply being a foreign export, the sport was now organized by Germans for Germans and integrated into the traditional structure of clubs, leagues, and federations. Although the proximity of American military bases was instrumental for the emergence of the first clubs, Germans took active measures to limit dependence on Americans. On the field, the rules changed from requiring a minimum amount of Germans per team to eventually setting a limit of two American players on the field for each team.

As Germans "Germanized" the organizational structure of the sport, they embraced the American cultural iconography. Whereas German soccer enthusiasts a hundred years earlier had changed the game's terminology to make it appear less English, this time the organizers made it a point to use American team nicknames and words like "quarterback" or "touchdown." This, they argued, made the game sound "cool" and less old fashioned than soccer. Football promoters presented their games as a stereotypical American event, including music, barbeque, and cheerleaders. This "party atmosphere" appealed to those who had grown up with American pop music, movies, and TV shows.

In 1991, the NFL built on this concept when it introduced the World League of American Football as the first intercontinental league in professional team sports. The league started ambitiously with teams in Canada, England, Germany, Spain, and the United States. This move by the NFL coincided with several historical developments. The breakup of the Soviet Union and the fall of the Iron Curtain opened new markets in East Europe, causing a gold-rush mentality among Western entrepreneurs. This added further impetus to what LaFeber referred to as the new global capitalism dominated by multinational corporations (9). Although companies had operated internationally for some time, LaFeber pointed to a number of characteristics that indicated a considerable shift in the late twentieth century. By the 1980s and 1990s, American-based multinational corporations like Nike produced the majority of their goods abroad and depended on foreign labor markets. Thus, they transcended and escaped the control of single governments and nations. In the case of the NFL's operation of a professional league in Europe, this meant that its teams did not have to become part of the traditional governance structure of clubs and federations. The league played by its own rules, literally and figuratively.

Further, these multinational companies not only produced, but also sold products abroad, as they increasingly targeted and depended on the world market. Coca-Cola, for example, sold four of every five bottles outside the United States in 1996. Figures like this made NFL owners wonder how much more merchandize they could sell outside the United States. To reach these markets, these companies employed massive advertising campaigns on a global scale. And like Coca-Cola and Nike, the NFL sold not only products, but also lifestyles based on American culture. Recent technological advancements made it possible to broadcast these messages instantly across the globe. In the 1980s, the development of fiber-optic cables, along with direct broadcast satellites and personal computers, had catalyzed the revolution in the global telecommunications market. Whereas a European football enthusiast in the 1970s had to custom order VHS recordings of his or her favorite NFL teams that would arrive by mail two weeks after the game, worldwide audiences were now able to watch live NFL games from the comfort of their homes in Paris, Tokyo, and Sydney. Maintaining an international league, however, was challenging for the NFL.

At the end of the league's tenure in 2007, now called NFL Europa, all teams but one were located in Germany, which proved to be the most viable market for professional football. But an average attendance of about 20,000 spectators per game was not enough to overcome the costs of operating a league that required almost all players, coaches, and staff to be flown in from the United States. The league was also not able to land major TV contracts in Europe. Although a discussion of the complex reasons for the demise of NFL Europa is beyond the scope of this chapter, future professionals in sport business would do well to consider potential lessons from this historical case study. First, supporting a steady, organic growth from a participant sport to a spectator sport might be vital for those interested in promoting a new professional sport. Second, understanding local culture and history is essential for producing and selling in a global market.

Marketing sports as an explicitly American spectacle can turn out to be a double-edged sword in foreign markets, as a distinct American image might be a selling point for some and a turn-off for others. For some, American football's military-like armor and drill, combined with violent collisions on the field, might confirm negative stereotypes of the United States as a violent country, riddled with drugs and crime, and overly commercialized. This potential ambivalence toward America helps to explain both the relative success and relative failure of American football in Germany. At the risk of simplifying complex processes, this brief historical sketch illustrates the multidirectional flow of sport in a globalized world and the importance of cultural competence and a historical perspective for students aspiring to work in sport.

SUMMARY

Sport history is a field that involves the study of sport-related events and individuals from the past. It began to develop as a distinct field of academic study in the mid-20th century, and today there are numerous academic journals, organizations, and conferences dedicated to sport history. This chapter provided several specific illustrations of how understating sport history can be useful to aspiring kinesiology professionals. First, we discussed how sport historians often face the challenge of myth-busting when seeking to provide accurate accounts of people and events from the past. Next, we highlighted some key historical factors related to differing sport participation patterns between women and men. Finally, we provided a historical case study related to globalization and sport.

In closing, we wish to emphasize that this chapter is only intended to provide an initial introduction to the field of sport history. There are likely to be a number of history courses offered at your university, perhaps some of which may focus on historical aspects of sport. We encourage students who wish to gain further insight into sport history to investigate such courses or to consult some of the references provided at the end of this chapter for further reading. Ultimately, understanding sport history can be of great benefit to professionals throughout the field of kinesiology.

REFERENCES

1. Arango, T., "Myth of baseball's creation endures, with a prominent fan." *The New York Times* (November 12, 2010). Retrieved from http://www.nytimes.com

2. Booth, D., *The field: Truth and fiction in sport history*. New York: Routledge, 2005.

3. Cahn, S. K., *Coming on strong: Gender and sexuality in twentieth-century women's sport*. New York: Free Press, 1994.

4. Deutscher Olympischer Sportbund, DOSB Bestanderhebung, 2012. Frankfurt/Main.

5. Dzikus, L., "American football in West Germany: Cultural transformation, adaptation, and resistance." In A. Hofmann, ed., *Turnen and sport: Transatlantic transfers*. Münster: Waxman, 2004, pp. 221–239.

6. Eisenberg, C., "The middle class and competition: Some considerations of the beginnings of modern sport in England and Germany." *The International Journal of the History of Sport 7*: 265–287.

7. Kane, T., *Global U.S. troop development, 1950–2003*. Washington DC: The Heritage Foundation, 2004.

8. Kimmel, M. S., "Baseball and the reconstitution of American masculinity, 1880–1920." In M. A. Messner & D. F. Sabo, eds., *Sport, men, and the gender order*. Champaign, IL: Human Kinetics, 1990, pp. 55–65.

9. LaFeber, W., *Michael Jordan and the new global capitalism*, 2nd ed. New York: W. W. Norton, 2002.

10. Markovits, A., and S. Hellerman, *Offside: Soccer and American exceptionalism*. Princeton, NJ: Princeton University Press, 2001.

11. McDonagh, E., and L. Pappano, *Playing with the boys: Why separate is not equal in sports*. New York: Oxford University Press, 2008.

12. Messner, M. A., *It's all for the kids: Gender, families, and youth sports*. Berkeley: University of California Press, 2009.

13. National Baseball Hall of Fame and Museum, "The Doubleday myth is Cooperstown's gain." Retrieved from http://baseballhall.org/museum/experience/history

14. Paxson, F. L., "The rise of sport." *Mississippi Valley Historical Review 4*: 143–168.

15. Pfister, G., "Cultural confrontations: German Turnen, Swedish gymnastics and English sport—European diversity in physical activities from a historical perspective." *Culture, Sport, Society 6*(1)(2003): 61–91.

16. Ritzer, G., *Contemporary sociological theory and its classical roots: The basics,* 3rd ed. Boston: McGraw-Hill, 2010.

17. Ryczek, W. J., *Baseball's first inning: A history of the national pastime through the Civil War.* Jefferson, NC: McFarland & Company, 2009.

18. Schiller, K., and C. Young, "The history and historiography of sport in Germany: Social, cultural and political perspectives." *German History* 27(3)(2009).

19. Seymour, H., *Baseball: The early years.* Oxford, UK: Oxford University Press, 1989.

20. Struna, N., "Historical research in physical activity." In J. Thomas & J. Nelson, eds., *Research methods in physical activity.* Champaign, IL: Human Kinetics, 1996, pp. 251–275.

21. Struna, N., "Sport history." In J. D. Massengale & R. A. Swanson, eds., *The history of exercise and sport science .* Champaign, IL: Human Kinetics, 1997, pp. 143–179.

22. Szymanski, S., and A. S. Zimbalist, *National pastime: How Americans play baseball and the rest of the world plays soccer.* Washington, DC: Brookings Institution Press, 2005.

23. Vertinsky, P., "Exercise, physical capability, and the eternally wounded woman in late nineteenth century North America." *Journal of Sport History* 14(1)(1987): 7–27.

24. Vieth, G. U. A., *Beiträge zur Geschichte der Leibesübungen.* Berlin, 1794.

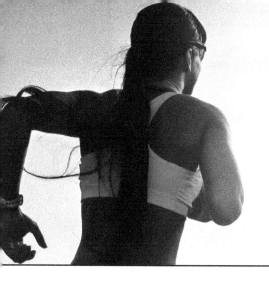

Chapter 7

SPORT SOCIOLOGY

OUTLINE

Objectives

Development of Sport Sociology

Doping and Overconformity to the "Sport Ethic"

The Social Construction of Obesity

Control, Freedom, and Change in Coaching Discourses

You've Got to Look and Act the Part

Learning to Do Your Job

Summary

References

OBJECTIVES

1. Understand key concepts and research questions in sport sociology.
2. Understand the historical development of sport sociology as an academic field.
3. Understand the relevance of sport sociology to other areas in the field of kinesiology.

This chapter provides an overview of sport sociology as an academic field of study and notes several key areas in which the work of sport sociologists is particularly relevant to students and professionals in kinesiology. As an academic discipline, the term *sport sociology* implies a field in which sociological analysis is applied to sport. However, while sport sociology certainly has important roots in both kinesiology and sociology, scholars in the field have also drawn inspiration from such disciplines as anthropology, cultural studies, geography, history, media studies, and political economy, to name a few. Such a diverse theoretical background makes it challenging to provide a succinct overview of the field. Thus, students should realize that this chapter is only intended to provide a general introduction to the field. Those wishing to gain further insight about sport sociology should consult some of the references provided at the end of the chapter.

Sociology involves the study of human society, social interactions, organizations, and institutions. Specifically, many sociologists seek to examine *social structure* in an effort to understand the established patterns of social relations that shape society. A focus on social structure entails identifying recurrent and enduring characteristics of social interactions, relationships, and networks rather than individual qualities of the persons involved in these relationships (17). In turn, sport sociologists commonly conduct research to help us understand patterns of social interaction and organization in sport. For example, a sport sociologist might study how interactions in the context of sport and physical activity are patterned along the lines of gender, race, or social class. Sport sociologists may use both empirical research and theory to develop knowledge about sports as a part of our cultural life and social worlds.

In this chapter, we use the term *sport* broadly to refer to a wide range of activities involving various levels of human movement in order to reflect the breadth of the field of sport sociology. The breadth of the field is sometimes very wide indeed, ranging from research about masculinity in the context of American football to the culture of risk taking associated with mountain climbing.

Two key concepts for understanding a sociological approach to studying sport are the ideas that sports are *social constructions* and *contested activities*. Viewing sports as social constructions emphasizes the fact that sports are created by individuals as they interact with one another under a particular set of social structural conditions. As social constructions, sports have continually changed throughout the past, and they will continue to change in the future.

Sports are also contested activities. Saying that sports are contested has two distinct meanings: (a) the outcomes of sporting events are literally decided on the field of play and (b) that people struggle over the ways in which sports are organized and carried out in society (1). From a sociological perspective, we are most interested in the second definition. In a youth sport setting, for example, individuals may disagree about the extent to which competitiveness should be emphasized: Should all children on a team be given playing time, or should only the most skilled athletes by rewarded with time on the field? Further, should youth sport programs be supported by public money, making them more accessible to people with fewer financial resources, or is it acceptable to restrict sport opportunities to those with the ability to pay club dues and other participation costs?

At all levels of competition, there have been struggles about such issues as whether women should be allowed to play sports, whether people from different racial backgrounds should play together, and how people with disabilities should be included in sports programs. Some examples of questions that often shape the research of sport sociologists are provided in the following box.

THE DEVELOPMENT OF SPORT SOCIOLOGY

In order to better understand the current state of sport sociology, this section discusses some of the key events in the development of the field. The second box presents a timeline of notable events in the development of sport sociology. Recognition of physical activity and physical education within the parent discipline of sociology dates back prior to the beginning of the 20th century (14). However, sport sociology first emerged as a specific, named endeavor with the publication of Heinz Risse's 1921 book-length study, *Soziologie des Sports* [Sociology of Sports] (5).

Prominent Research Questions in Sport Sociology (adapted from [1])

- Why are certain activities selected and designated as sports in particular groups and societies?
- Why are sports created and organized in different ways at different times and in different places?
- How do people include sports in their lives, and does participating in sports affect individual development and social relationships?
- How do sports and sport participation affect our ideas about bodies, human movement, masculinity and femininity, social class, race and ethnicity, work, fun, ability and disability, achievement and competition, pleasure and pain, deviance and conformity, and aggression and violence?
- How do various sports compare with other physical activities in producing positive health and fitness outcomes?
- How are the meaning, purpose, and organization of sports related to the culture, social structure, and resources of a society?
- How are sports related to important spheres of social life such as family, education, politics, the economy, the media, and religion?
- How do people use their sport experiences and knowledge about sports as they interact with others and explain what occurs in their lives and the world around them?
- How can people use sociological knowledge about sports to understand and participate more actively and effectively in society, especially as agents of progressive change?

The first programmatic call for a sociology of sport appears to have been issued by Ulrich Popplow in his paper, "Zu einer Soziologie des Sports" [Toward a Sociology of Sports], published in the journal *Sport und Leibeserziehung* [Sport and Physical Education] in 1951. Further growth of the field is illustrated by the formation of the International Committee for the Sociology of Sport (ICSS), which was the first academic organization devoted specifically to sport sociology. In 1966, the ICSS held its first international symposium in Cologne, Germany, and also began publishing the *International Review of Sport Sociology* (renamed the *International Review for the Sociology of Sport* in 1984), which was the first academic journal specifically devoted to the field. Notably, the development of sport sociology was quite international in nature, exemplified by the first executive board of the ICSS, which included scholars from Cuba, Finland, France, the German Democratic Republic (East Germany), the Federal Republic of Germany (West Germany), Great Britain, Japan, Poland, the Soviet Union, Switzerland, and the United States (13).

In the context of North America, John Loy and Gerald Kenyon's *Sport, Culture and Society*, published in 1969, was the first English-language edited collection focused on the sociology of sport (5). Harry Edwards' 1973 book, *The Sociology of Sport*, meanwhile, was the first American textbook to appear in the field (2). As further evidence of the development of the field, the North American Society for the Sociology of Sport (NASSS) held its first conference in 1980, in Denver, Colorado. Four years later, the first issue of the *Sociology of Sport Journal* (*SSJ*), which is the official journal of NASSS, was published. Today, there are multiple academic journals dedicated specifically to the field of sport sociology as well as numerous others that commonly publish research on sociocultural issues in sport (see box for a summary).

In the following sections, we provide several examples to better illustrate how sport sociology research is relevant to students and practitioners throughout the field of kinesiology. As you read these sections, we encourage you to think about how the ideas presented might be relevant in your particular area of interest.

Key Events in the Development of Sport Sociology

1921: Heinz Risse's book-length study, *Soziologie des Sports* [Sociology of Sports], marked the point at which the sociology of sport first emerged as a specific, named endeavor.

1951: The first programmatic call for a sociology of sport was issued by Ulrich Popplow in his paper, "Zu einer Soziologie des Sports" [Toward a Sociology of Sports], published in the journal *Sport und Leibeserziehung* [Sport and Physical Education].

1966: The International Committee for the Sociology of Sport held its first international symposium in Cologne, Germany.

1966: *International Review of Sport Sociology* became the first journal primarily focused on publishing sport sociology research.

1969: John Loy and Gerald Kenyon's *Sport, Culture and Society* was the first English-language edited collection published in the field.

1973: Harry Edwards' *The Sociology of Sport* was the first American textbook to appear in the field.

1980: The North American Society for the Sociology of Sport (NASSS) held its first conference in Denver, Colorado.

1984: *Sociology of Sport Journal* (*SSJ*), which is the official journal of NASSS, was first published.

DOPING AND OVERCONFORMITY TO THE "SPORT ETHIC"

Doping, a term that refers to the use of banned performance-enhancing substances and methods, is an issue that receives substantial attention in the world of sport. Its relevance in fields such as sport medicine, coaching, sport administration, fitness, and strength training is apparent.

Doping is a frequent topic of discussion in the sports media. Sport organizations contribute millions of dollars each year in an effort to control doping. However, the success of such anti-doping efforts appears to be limited, as reports continue to proliferate that doping is widespread in many sporting contexts. For example, prior to his admission to using a host of performance-enhancing drugs, including erythropoietin and human growth hormone, Lance Armstrong repeatedly emphasized that of the approximately 600 drug tests he had taken throughout his career, he had not failed a single one. If there is to be any hope of successfully controlling doping in sport, it is important to understand why athletes use banned performance-enhancing substances and methods.

As doping is debated among public figures and media personalities, individualistic explanations that view doping as being the result of poor decisions by athletes who lack moral character and integrity are often presented to the public. However, while individual characteristics certainly are relevant, a sociological perspective can help us understand the broader structural forces in sports that lead many athletes to use banned substances. In fact, research suggests that doping generally does not result from a lack of moral character; rather, it is often the most dedicated and hardest working athletes that engage in doping.

The work of sociologists Robert Hughes (10) and Jay Coakley (1) on overconformity to the sport ethic helps us better understand the prevalence of doping in sport (Figure 7.1). The sport ethic refers to a set of norms that commonly exist in sport settings and are used to guide athletes' ideas and actions. Specifically, four norms that comprise the sport ethic have been identified: (a) making sacrifices for the game—the idea that athletes must subordinate other interests for the sake of an exclusive commitment to their sport, (b) striving for distinction—the idea that athletes must constantly seek to push limits, dominate others, and be the best they can be, (c) accepting risks and playing through pain—the idea that athletes are expected to endure pressure,

Sport Sociology Journals

Journals devoted primarily to sport sociology
International Review for the Sociology of Sport
Journal of Sport and Social Issues
Sociology of Sport Journal
Sport in Society

Other sport studies journals in which sport sociology research is commonly published
European Sport Management Quarterly
International Journal of Sport Communication
International Journal of Sport Science and Coaching
Journal of Intercollegiate Sport
Journal of Issues in Intercollegiate Athletics
Journal of Sport Management
Physical Education and Sport Pedagogy
Qualitative Research in Sport, Exercise and Health
Quest
Research Quarterly for Exercise and Sport
Soccer and Society
Sport Coaching Review
Sport, Education and Society
Sport Management Review
Women in Sport and Physical Activity Journal

pain, and risk without backing down, and (d) refusing to accept limits—the idea that athletes have an obligation to overcome all obstacles in the pursuit of competitive success (10).

If one wants to successfully claim an identity as an athlete, it is likely one must adhere to the norms of the sport ethic. Due to such factors as the need to compete for playing time and receive positive assessments from

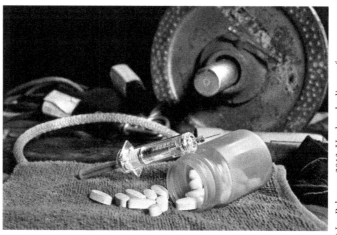

© Joe Belanger, 2013. Used under license from Shutterstock, Inc.

Figure 7.1. *Thinking about doping as a result of overconformity to the sport ethic helps us understand the broader structural forces in sports that can lead athletes to use performance-enhancing drugs.*

coaches, many athletes engage in overconformity to the norms of the sport ethic. For example, an athlete who takes repeated doses of painkillers to continue competing while suffering from a severe injury is demonstrating an uncritical adherence to norms such as making sacrifices for the game and playing through pain. Similarly, the use of banned performance-enhancing substances is also frequently a result of athletes overconforming to the norms of the sport ethic.

To better understand how doping results from overconformity to the sport ethic, it is useful to compare performance-enhancing drug use in sport to recreational drug use in general. When people use a drug like heroin to get high, they are generally demonstrating underconformity—a rejection of societal norms. However, when an athlete uses human growth hormone in an attempt to regain his or her starting position on a team after suffering a potentially career-threatening injury, this athlete is not rejecting the norms of sport ethic. Rather, the athlete is demonstrating overconformity to such norms as accepting risk, making sacrifices, and refusing to back down to obstacles in the pursuit of success. In other words, the athlete using a performance-enhancing drug is generally doing so for much different reasons than a person using an illicit drug. In turn, the methods used to address recreational drug use are not particularly relevant or helpful in efforts to control doping in sport.

In their efforts to control recreational drug use, authorities may use such methods as harsh penalties and aggressive testing. While the effectiveness of such approaches toward recreational drug use is questionable, these types of methods are even less likely to be successful in preventing athletes from using substances they feel are necessary to continue their sport participation. Effective control of doping likely requires structural changes in sport. Coakley has offered suggestions on where to begin the process (1). Several of these are summarized here.

First, sport organizations might critically examine the hypocrisy involved in a sport culture that seeks to ban doping while simultaneously encouraging overconformity to the sport ethic in a variety of other ways. For example, when athletes are compelled to take whatever means necessary to play through injury, including the extensive use of painkilling drugs, this works to foster a culture in which doping is seen as another logical way to push one's body in the pursuit of competitive success.

Second, organizations should more clearly establish rules indicating that certain health risks are undesirable in sport. When athletes who risk their long-term health by playing through injury are treated as heroes, we promote the same type of overconformity that contributes to performance-enhancing drug use. Taking this point a step further, it would be beneficial if athletes do not return to competition until they have been evaluated and cleared by independent medical personnel. The structural pressure to win at all costs that can exist within sport may place pressure on team physicians and trainers (who are employed and paid by the team) to rush athletes back to competition before they are ready.

Third, health and injury education programs can serve a beneficial role in helping athletes be more in tune with their bodies rather than learning to deny pain and injury. This can play an important role in changing a sports culture that encourages athletes to ignore pain in a way that poses risks to long term health. Importantly, critical questions about how the norms of the sport ethic work to encourage doping and drug use should be a key aspect of these education programs. Effecting structural changes in sport is certainly difficult, but the suggestions discussed in this section may serve as important starting points for addressing the broader forces contributing to doping in sport.

Overall, the issue of doping in sport is complex. The information discussed in this section is intended to help you think about how the social norms associated with sport can impact the seemingly individual choice of an athlete to use performance enhancing drugs. Because doping is consistent with many norms of the sport ethic, we suggest it is important to consider these factors if successful methods of addressing doping are to be developed. How do you think the issue of doping in sport might be effectively addressed?

THE SOCIAL CONSTRUCTION OF OBESITY

In recent years, obesity has come to be a "hot" topic for researchers in fields such as medicine, epidemiology, and physiology. Public attention to the issue of obesity is further fueled by the proliferation of "reality" weight-loss shows around the world, such as *The Biggest Loser* in the United States. The World Health Organization has even gone so far as to declare that there is a "global obesity epidemic." However, research by some scholars, such as sport sociologist Geneviève Rail, has challenged the use of the term "epidemic" and the notion of obesity as a disease (19). The sociological insights presented in this section can help provide a fuller understanding about the nature of the so-called "obesity epidemic."

Perhaps a good starting point by which to understand obesity from a sociological perspective is to realize that the concept of obesity is socially constructed. One way in which ideas about obesity are constructed is through *discursive practices*. Discursive practices refer to the processes and techniques through which meanings and definitions are produced. In other words, obesity is not a simple scientific "fact," but rather a process through which regulatory norms, such as the Body Mass Index (BMI), are created and employed to place people into such categories as "obese" or "overweight" (19). In this case, certain groups have created the measure of BMI as a technique to define some people as obese and, in turn, propose specific solutions to address the issue. Further, because of its socially constructed nature, obesity can be transformed over time (definitions may change as to who qualifies as obese) and place (different countries may have different definitions of obesity).

For example, in 1998 the National Institutes of Health and Centers for Disease Control and Prevention in the United States lowered the BMI cutoff point for defining people as "overweight," which resulted in more than 25 million individuals in the "healthy" weight category being suddenly reclassified as overweight. Understanding the socially constructed nature of obesity is a good starting point from which to understand obesity in relation to broader social forces in society.

Earlier in this chapter, we introduced the idea of sports as contested activities. Similarly, because of its socially constructed nature, the ways in which an issue such as obesity is framed (and the solutions that might result from a particular framing) may be quite contested, involving power struggles among parties with competing interests (Figure 7.2). In turn, it is important to consider who benefits from the ways in which obesity is constructed, which may include parties in such industries as pharmaceuticals, agribusiness, and insurance providers. By thinking about the influence of these factors on how obesity is framed, we may better understand why certain definitions of obesity become favored over others.

As groups struggle over how to define and frame the topic of obesity, a prominent area contested in this process involves the ways in which individual or societal factors contributing to obesity are either highlighted or obscured. When the topic of obesity is discussed in the media, for example, it is often framed as an individual "lifestyle" choice—the idea that people simply choose a lifestyle that leads to obesity. The reason such a view is problematic, however, is that individual choices are enabled and constrained in important ways by social structural forces. If we ignore broader social factors contributing to obesity, we limit our ability to understand and address the issue. For example, a focus only on individual choice ignores the finding that socioeconomic status is more related to BMI than any lifestyle factor (19). Further, fatness itself may have an impoverishing effect, resulting from stigmatization, discrimination, and negative impacts on such areas as education,

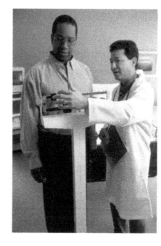

Figure 7.2. *Obesity is socially constructed in that it involves a process by which regulatory norms such as the Body Mass Index (BMI) are created and employed to place people into such categories as "obese," "overweight," and "healthy."*

© Getty Images.

employment, salary, and medical care. Another structural factor to consider in this area is the health impact of poor neighborhoods, resulting from pollution, noise, and lack of access to such things as fresh food and free, safe outdoor activities.

The extent to which obesity is framed as either an individual or societal problem is important, because it has significant implications for the courses of action that become favored to address the issue. For instance, when the cause of obesity is perceived to be unhealthy individual lifestyle choices, then the favored solutions likely involve regulating lifestyle choices in such areas as diet and physical activity. On the other hand, when the social and economic conditions contributing to obesity are highlighted, policy solutions may favor addressing the broader structural conditions (lack of access to education, employment, health care) that tend to promote unhealthy lifestyles. Notably, the obesity "crisis" and the accompanying focus on individual-centered explanations have emerged at a time when some key policy makers are pushing for austerity and cutbacks to areas such as education, health care, and the social safety net.

While the information discussed in this section may challenge some common-sense understandings of obesity and the way it is commonly presented, this discussion is not intended to represent the single, correct way to view obesity. Rather, the intent is to show how considering a topic in multiple ways, specifically using sociological insights, may help achieve a more complete understanding of an issue as complex and contested as obesity. How will you approach the issue of obesity as a kinesiology professional?

CONTROL, FREEDOM, AND CHANGE IN COACHING DISCOURSES

Social theorist Michel Foucault, who labeled himself a "historian of systems of thought," took a socio-historical approach to research and examined the relationship between *power, knowledge,* and *self* (identity) (15). His theories help us understand the ways in which control and power work in the context of coaching and strength training.

In his research, Foucault would choose a topic such as madness (insanity), discipline, or ethics, and conduct a "history of the present" (6). In doing so, he would show how people came to know (theory) and to act (practice) in a particular field. Foucault used the word *discourse* or *discursive formation* to refer to the socially dominant knowledge and practices (ways of thinking, feeling, and behaving) in a field. He also examined how power and knowledge (often simplified to *power-knowledge*) operated together as a relational force to influence our identities and how we live—hence, the triad listed above: power, knowledge, and self. Foucault did not believe the discourse of a given field (such as coaching) was created in a fully rational or linear way. Rather, he suggested that discourses are produced by numerous forces, which often remain unknown or hidden.

For Foucault, and contrary to popular (Marxist) belief at the time, power was not a possession, and the ability to exercise power was not limited to select individuals. That is, one does not wield power like one possesses and wields a sword, and power is not limited to people on the top of an organizational hierarchy, such as the head coach or athletic director. If someone were to state "he has a lot of power over people," this would be inaccurate from Foucault's perspective. Rather, Foucault viewed power-knowledge as a relational force used to achieve a goal by influencing the possible actions of people (Figure 7.3). Every person can exercise some degree of power, although power relations will often be quite unequal.

Think of it this way. One of your professor's goals was to get you to read this chapter. If you read it, you may be rewarded with praise, a good grade on a quiz, and the respect of your professor for engaging in a lively class discussion. For your peers who didn't read this chapter—bad news—they may be scolded or labeled as abnormal. You could have refused, but as you are currently reading this sentence, you complied with the professor's request. Both the professor and the student can exercise power, but the professor normally selects the textbooks and assignments, and is thus in a position to exercise greater power.

For Foucault, a necessary condition for power to operate is freedom. Students, faced with multiple options (drop a class, read the whole chapter, read only parts, or do not read at all), are essentially "free" to choose what to do. However, can you see how things have been structured in a way that controls students' behavior? We will return to this in our discussion of discipline and control.

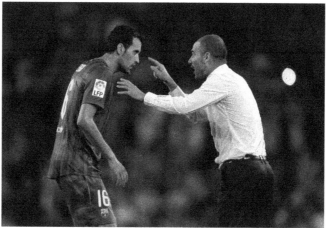

© Maxisport, 2013. Used under license from Shutterstock, Inc.

Figure 7.3. *Foucault used the term power-knowledge to describe how complex relations of power are exercised through knowledge and practice to influence the actions of others. Coaches use a variety of means (control of time, space, and movement) to influence the actions of players on a team.*

With respect to the relationship between knowledge and power, consider that in the field of strength and conditioning, it was once widely believed that resistance training would make athletes slower and become "muscle bound." Because this was accepted as the norm, many athletes did not engage in resistance training, especially with heavy weights. Over the years, multiple research studies showed that resistance training could enhance speed without reducing flexibility, and now this knowledge has become the norm. Regardless of whether this knowledge is true, the dominant discourse has changed over the years, and this change has subsequently affected how people exercise and train.

Foucault did not believe one could necessarily prove knowledge to be true or false. Rather, Foucault was more interested in showing how knowledge was accepted as the "Truth"—a Truth that is universal—and how this limited our ways of thinking, feeling, and behaving. For example, just because multiple set weight training is effective does not mean we should stop using single set training. Quite literally, we are able to select from any number of ways of engaging in exercise or fitness. Also, in the field of strength and conditioning, the "best" knowledge is purportedly produced through the use of experimental research designs, control groups, and statistical tests of probability. To understand the human body, students are required to take courses in anatomy, kinesiology, and biomechanics. By breaking down the body into its physical components and possibilities, we are told this way of knowing—that is scientific and objective—is the best way to understand the human body and ourselves. Those that are able to produce this knowledge naturally have PhDs, usually in exercise physiology or chemistry, and are often employed in university laboratories. Of interest to Foucault was who gets labeled as an expert and how they are able to influence the actions of others.

Other research in areas such as motor learning and sport psychology also informs our coaching practices. This research, for example, tells coaches and physical educators how to organize a practice, manage a large group of athletes, reinforce desired behavior, and punish "bad" behavior. Researchers conduct studies on so-called "expert" coaches and share this research as "The Way" to plan for success, motivate athletes, and provide the most efficient instruction and feedback to reach a (coach's) desired effect. This knowledge becomes popularized through the media (TV, documentaries, sport movies), books (biographies of winning coaches, how-to manuals), and educational programs (college courses, coaching clinics). If this all sounds very natural and good—that's exactly the point from a Foucaultian perspective.

By using a historical approach, Foucault showed how people assumed certain knowledge and practices as the *Truth* because they've become normalized or an accepted way of knowing. Foucault's point was to disrupt accepted truths and to "think otherwise." He would encourage us to look for negative effects, contradictions, gaps in our logic, and develop different, perhaps better, but certainly more ethical (less controlling) ways of practicing.

Within the field of kinesiology, Gearity and Mills used parts of Foucault's work to take a critical look at "normal" strength and conditioning coaching practices (7). It's worth pointing out that many of these practices are commonly used throughout fitness programs (CrossFit, spinning, small groups) and personal training. Borrowing from Foucault's work on the penal system, Gearity and Mills showed how coaches (un)consciously controlled the time, space, and movement of athletes through highly organized and minutely detailed practice plans in an effort to maximize athletic performance and to win. Athletes were continually observed and often treated like objects to be corrected and tested to determine who was abnormal or deficient. These practices, understood by the strength and conditioning coach as normal and effective, led to positive effects (gains in strength), but also negative effects, such as coach-athlete conflict, injuries, and ultimately underperformance. An important point of this research is to show coaches how to think critically and to challenge taken for granted, "normal" ways of coaching.

At this point you may reply, "But that's just what coaches do." It is, however, as illustrated in the cases above, the point is to go further by realizing that what coaches do is not based on some natural order or neutral evidence (4). Rather, what coaches do is influenced by their athletic experiences, mentors, formal education, clinics and conferences, observations of other coaches, to name just a few. Naturally, we are tempted to conclude that what we're doing is effective and ethical, but a socio-historical approach demonstrates human fallibility and changes in ways of practicing. If we want coaches to think critically about their development and to be creative in developing new, and hopefully more effective and ethical, ways of coaching, then we believe thinking with Foucault could help. So—how might you coach with less discipline and punishment (control) of athletes, or promote diverse and creative ways of coaching and being an athlete? How about in the classroom?

YOU'VE GOT TO LOOK AND ACT THE PART

Another highly influential sociological thinker was Erving Goffman (1922–1982). In his well-known work, *The Presentation of Self in Everyday Life,* Goffman presents a way of looking at human interaction from what he called the *dramaturgical* perspective (8). Developed from *ethnographic research*, the dramaturgical perspective is a metaphor that views *life as a stage.*

On stage, actors deliver a compelling performance to show the audience what the story is about. Goffman argued that, like the stage, people throughout society engage in this sort of behavior in everyday life. Goffman presented evidence to support his argument by showing how individuals encounter each other through *impression management.* He argued that within a particular society's social norms or *social roles*, humans engage in impression management in order to control the image presented to others, and ultimately influence others' behavior. Individuals generally play their part by fulfilling pre-established patterns of action, rather than consciously choosing a creative or untested action.

Goffman identified the characters in this sort of performance as an individual, team, or audience. An individual is the one giving the performance. A team is the cooperation of many individuals involved in staging a performance. And the audience is the receiver of the performance. The location where the performance is given is like a stage, divided into two parts. There is a *front region*, which is where the actor delivers the performance. He or she controls the impression given to others through the *setting* (furniture, décor), *appearance* (social status), and *manner* (interaction role). There is also a *back region* where the actor kind of relaxes from his or her role and prepares for giving the performance.

A good example of seeing impression management in coaching can be found in the movie, *The Express: The Ernie Davis Story*. After winning a game, the Syracuse football team has the option of playing top-ranked Texas in the Cotton Bowl for the national championship or a lesser opponent in a different bowl game. Then head coach Ben Schwartzwalder goes to the team in the locker room and asks them to decide whom to play. Looking them all in the eye, he sternly tells them it's their decision and he supports them either way. As he turns away from the team to let them "choose," he smiles, which appears to giveaway the forgone conclusion that they'll play Texas. In this example, we see Schwartzwalder put forth the front of a stern coach who is truly concerned with the opinions of the team, but back stage (as he turns away), he knows he has given a good performance that will guide the players' decision.

Another key concept from Goffman is the idea of *dramatic realization*, which refers to "playing up" one's part in an attempt to ensure the audience understands and is confident in the individual's portrayal. Goffman even uses a baseball umpire as an example to illustrate this point. In an effort to let the audience (managers, baseball players, and fans) know that they are absolutely certain of a decision, umpires may give a dramatic performance by doing a strikeout dance, a forceful first pump, and a loud bark of "STRIKE THREE" (Figure 7.4).

A last concept explored here, although there are many more points to be drawn from Goffman, is *idealization*. In accordance with leading societal values and social expectations, performers try to live up to these values and expectations when giving a certain impression. For example, because American culture often highly values discipline, accountability, and a hard-nosed approach, many youth sport coaches try to enact these behaviors in practice. Observers of youth sport lament that too many of these coaches think of themselves as disciples of former Green Bay Packers coach Vince Lombardi or Alabama football coach "Bear" Bryant. Regardless of its desirability, many performers (coaches) pick an idealized model to guide their coaching behavior.

There are numerous ways that the dramaturgical perspective can help us better understand a field such as sport coaching. For example, depending on the time (before, during, after practices or games) and location, coaches need to interact with the media, owners, athletic directors, athletes, family members, officials, boosters, recruits, fans—and the list goes on. As theorized by Goffman and briefly outlined above, we may consider each of these interactions to be governed by different rules of engagement. To fulfill the role of the coach involves not only giving athletes instruction on how to kick a ball, for example, but interacting with numerous audiences. If a coach fails to play the proper role, he or she may be lose credibility, become embarrassed, or suffer from shame or

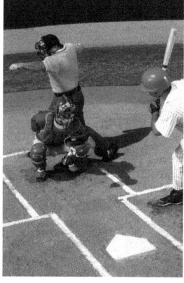

© JupiterImages, Inc.

Figure 7.4. *An umpire makes a dramatic call of "strike three!" Goffman's dramaturgical perspective helps us understand why umpires often make calls with great emotion in order to convince the audience that they are certain of a decision.*

stigma, a concept Goffman elaborated upon (9). At times, a coach's physical appearance is so important that he or she may do things like lifting weights to gain muscle mass, growing facial hair, or dressing "professionally" in order to convey a proper coaching image. Several years ago a former head coach in the Southeastern Conference said that his athletic director once quipped, "You don't even look like a football coach."

There are a few scholarly examples in kinesiology that have drawn upon Goffman's work. In the area of sport coaching, Jones drew upon his own coaching experiences to present a fictionalized story of himself as a high-performing soccer coach (11). In interacting with his athletes, Jones presented a front that was to be received as confident and all-knowing. Notably, he had long been managing a speech impediment, which is often viewed as a sign of weakness or unintelligence. For a coach, anything outside the social norm (i.e., coaches are expected to know what they're doing at all times, state clearly what athletes are to do, and lead the team onward to victory) could be fatal. Although in reality he was doubtful and uncertain of what to do as a coach, he worked hard to maintain a particular image in order to keep the athletes' respect. Jones hoped that his more authentic story would help coaches and coach educators address typically ignored issues. By drawing upon Goffman, he showed how we might better understand why coaches do what they do and the ensuing negative effects.

There are ample opportunities to extend the use of Goffman's dramaturgical perspective in the field of kinesiology. For example, think of the assistant coach who presents the image of a "yes-man" to the head coach in an attempt to garner support, the female coach who acts like "one of the guys" in order to fit in, the coach who presents a united and loyal front in order to possibly hide what really goes on or unethical acts of other coaches, and, of course, the collegiate coach who paints a particular picture of his or her university in order to sign a top recruit. How else do you see coaches putting on a good front? How does this differ from what things are *really* like?

LEARNING TO DO YOUR JOB

We often think of learning as something that occurs inside our heads. That is, our brains or minds perceive, attend to, and process some sort of stimuli to make sense of it and act. This type of approach, which focuses on the individual, is usually categorized as a cognitive learning theory. Different, but not unrelated to cognitive approaches, are sociocultural learning theories. These theories look at how individuals learn, make sense of, and act within the context of social structural forces in society.

By this point in the chapter, it should make sense that a sociological approach would focus on individuals within society and how knowledge and practices change over time. Like Foucault and Goffman, we can again see how sociological approaches are interested in the changing nature of knowledge and practice.

One sociocultural learning theory that has gained popularity in kinesiology is *situated learning*. Situated learning was a term used by Jean Lave and Etienne Wenger that highlighted the importance of how people learn by doing in a specific context (12). In their research, Lave and Wenger, scholars in artificial intelligence and learning theories, present rich descriptions of people's actual experiences of mentoring. By analyzing mentor-mentee relations, they developed the concept of *legitimate peripheral participation* to denote how novices begin authentic learning by taking on fewer and lesser responsibilities, which eventually gives way to becoming a *full participant* with greater and more central responsibilities. In this view, knowledge is not seen as being in the hands of just one person, but rather it is a historical product created and accepted within a particular community. Through collaboration, interaction, and engagement within the specific environment, the beginner or novice learns the beliefs, values, actions (knowledge) of how a task or job is done. This learning by doing, learning from others, and learning in context is *authentic learning* because the knowledge gained is genuine to the job, rather than abstract knowledge gained from an inauthentic environment as is often the case with the classroom.

In many kinesiology jobs, we can see the importance of having a quality mentor and the need for authentic learning. A new personal trainer or fitness specialist would likely benefit from having an experienced health club owner or a successful personal trainer mentor him or her about leading a business or developing a clientele. Most athletic trainers or physical therapists likely would be initially unprepared to start their own practices and wary about the "ins and outs" of what really works in practice, such as how to manage multiple patients simultaneously or which modalities and therapeutic exercises are most efficient and effective. A novice physical education teacher or coach, meanwhile, would need to learn how to fill out paperwork, structure the curriculum, motivate multiple and diverse students, and when and how much instruction and feedback to offer.

Universities have the goal (among others) to educate and prepare students for careers, but with limited time and resources, and often the unavailability of a realistic context to do the actual work, we can see why many kinesiology students may be, to a degree, unprepared for day one on a job. We could also look at kinesiology curriculums for knowledge gaps in preparing future practitioners. Many programs tend not to emphasize the development of interpersonal skills, issues related to disabilities, and counseling for athlete or client drug and alcohol abuse. This gap seems to imply that practitioners would either need to learn this knowledge from others in the field, on their own, or perhaps not at all. In order to address their limitations, many university programs require internship or practicum experiences as a means to apply what was learned in the classroom, and hopefully, to learn situation specific, authentic knowledge from a quality mentor.

In a follow-up text, *Communities of Practice: Learning, Meaning and Identity*, Wenger expanded on situated learning by detailing the notion of *communities of practice*, which refers to groups of people who share a concern or passion about a topic, and who deepen their knowledge and expertise about the topic by interacting on an ongoing basis (20). He also elaborated upon the three essential structures of a community of practice. The simplest to understand is what he called the domain or the *joint enterprise*, which refers to the field (athletic training, fitness) or specific problem (best treatment, insurance billing) community members are addressing. Within the domain, people are *mutually engaged*, which speaks to the type and depth of relationships fostered. Last, people are engaged in a *shared repertoire*, which is the practice of creating knowledge, skills, and tools to solve problems. Communities of practice exist, quite literally, everywhere these three structures exist, and multiple communities may exist within the same workplace. Individuals within the community learn new things and may forget past knowledge, while people come and go and the unequal use of power affects what is known and what is done. While we may assume that communities are well-oiled, high-functioning machines, it is important to realize this is not inherently the case. For example, a mentor may not be a good ethical model, may not properly engage with the mentee, or may be ineffective in modeling how to complete tasks.

Because authentic learning is sought within a community of practice, scholars across many fields such as sports coaching (3), physical education (16), and athletic training (18) have noted its potential use to improve practitioner education and effectiveness. For example, Nash drew upon communities of practice theory to develop a program to assist pre-service physical education teachers in Australia (16). The program partnered pre-service teachers with university mentors and practicing physical education teachers within area schools. The results of the program showed that most of the 118 pre-service teachers thought their knowledge and skills, as well as confidence, were improved by the support and mentoring provided.

What do you think you'll need to learn on the job? In what ways can you better prepare yourself to become a master within your domain?

SUMMARY

Sport sociology is a field that examines how patterns of social relations, interactions, organizations, and institutions impact how we understand and experience sport and physical activity in society. It began to develop as a distinct field of academic study in the mid-20th century, and today there are numerous academic journals, organizations, and conferences dedicated to sport sociology. This chapter provided several specific illustrations of how sociological research and theory can be useful to aspiring kinesiology professionals. First discussed was how doping in sport can be understood as a form of overconformity to the "sport ethic." Second, the socially constructed nature of obesity was examined. Next, we illustrated how the work of social theorist Michel Foucault helps us understand the ways in which relations of power and control work in the context of coaching and strength training. We then explored how the work of sociologist Erving Goffman helps us understand the multiple roles kinesiology professionals have to play in different aspects of their careers. Finally, we discussed the concept of situated learning in order to illustrate the social nature of the process through which people acquire the knowledge and skills necessary to become professionals in their chosen field.

REFERENCES

1. Coakley, J., *Sports in Society,* 10th ed. New York: McGraw-Hill, 2009.

2. Coakley, J., "Sociology of sport in the United States." *International Review for the Sociology of Sport* 22(1987): 63–77.

3. Culver, D. M., P. Trudel, and P. Werthner, "A sport leader's attempt to foster a coaches' community of practice." *International Journal of Sports Science & Coaching* 4(3)(2009): 365–383.

4. Denison, J., "Michel Foucault: Power and discourse: The 'loaded' language of coaching." In R. L. Jones, P. Potrac, C. Cushion, and L. T. Ronglan, eds., *The Sociology of Sports Coaching.* New York: Routledge, 2011, pp 27–39.

5. Dunning, E., "Sociology of sport in the balance: Critical reflections on some recent and more enduring trends." *Sport in Society 7* (2004): 1–24.

6. Foucault, M., *Discipline and Punish: The Birth of the Prison* (A. Sheridan, Trans.). New York: Random House, 1977.

7. Gearity, B. T., and J. Mills, "Discipline and punish in the weight room." *Sport Coaching Review* (2013). *http://dx.doi.org/10.1080/21640629.2012.746049*

8. Goffman, E., *The Presentation of Self in Everyday Life.* New York: Doubleday, 1959.

9. Goffman, E., *Stigma: Notes on the Management of Spoiled Identity.* New York: Simon & Schuster, 1963.

10. Hughes, R., and J. Coakley, "Positive deviance among athletes: The implications of overconformity to the sport ethic." *Sociology of Sport Journal* 8 (1991): 307–325.

11. Jones, R., "Dilemmas, maintaining 'face,' and paranoia: An average coaching life." *Qualitative Inquiry* 12(5) (2006): 1012–2021.

12. Lave, J., and E. Wenger, E., *Situated Learning: Legitimate Peri–heral Participation.* Cambridge, UK: Cambridge University Press, 1991.

13. Loy, J. W., B. D. McPherson, and G. S. Kenyon, *The Sociology of Sport as an Academic Specialty: An Episodic Essay on the Development and Emergence of an Hybrid Subfield in North America.* Ottawa, Ontario: Canadian Association for Health, Physical Education, and Recreation, 1978.

14. Lüschen, G., "Sociology of sport: Development, present state, and prospects." *Annual Review of Sociology* 6(1980): 315–347.

15. Markula, P., and R. Pringle, *Foucault, Sport and Exercise: Power, Knowledge and Transforming the Self.* London: Routledge, 2006.

16. Nash, M., "Using the idea of 'communities of practice' and TGFU to develop physical education pedagogy among primary generalist pre-service teachers." *Asian Journal of Exercise & Sport Science* 6(1)(2009): 1–7.

17. Nixon, H., *Sport in a Changing World.* Boulder, CO: Paradigm Publishers, 2008.

18. Peer, K. S., and R. C. McClendon, "Sociocultural learning theory in practice: Implications for athletic training educators." *Journal of Athletic Training* 37(4 suppl)(2002): S136–S140.

19. Rail, G., "The birth of the obesity clinic: Confessions of the flesh, biopedagogies and physical culture." *Sociology of Sport Journal* 29(2012): 227–253.

20. Wenger, E., *Communities of Practice: Learning, Meaning and Identity.* Cambridge, UK: Cambridge University Press, 1998.

Section 2

APPLIED PHYSIOLOGICAL KNOWLEDGE BASE

Section 2 of the text introduces the three disciplines of kinesiology that have been heavily influenced by the physiological sciences. Exercise physiology is introduced first not only because it is the oldest discipline of kinesiology, but because its content is basic to the understanding of sport nutrition and physical activity epidemiology. The central theme of Chapter 8 is that exercise, sports performance, and general physical activities can be explained by bioenergetic processes in the contracting muscle cell. Chapter 9 concentrates on nutritional ergogenics, optimal dietary needs of athletes, and how nutrition affects performance. Chapter 10 describes the science of epidemiology and focuses on physical inactivity as a major determinant of disease risk. Students are cautioned at the outset to view these chapters as incomplete works of each field. Individual textbooks have been devoted to these three disciplines. In the case of exercise physiology, entire books covering some of its subfield content have even been written. Rather, the chapters are meant to present a brief snapshot of the discipline with enough content to communicate the basic scope and range of the science. There is no doubt that within the confines of the course for which this book is being used instructors will expand or constrict what is written here in exploring these fields with their students.

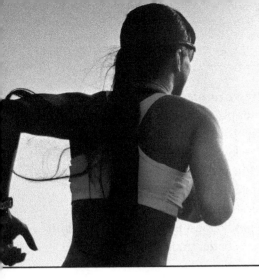

 Chapter 8 ///

EXERCISE PHYSIOLOGY

☑ OUTLINE

☑ OBJECTIVES

1. Explore exercise physiology as a discipline of kinesiology.
2. Distinguish activities based on metabolic considerations.
3. Understand basic principles related to anaerobic and aerobic production of energy.
4. Understand how the cardiovascular and pulmonary systems are integrated with aerobic metabolic processes.
5. Understand the importance of thermoregulation during exercise.

Exercise physiology is the study of the function of the body under the stress of *acute* and *chronic* exercise. It is equally concerned with how the body responds to the intense demands placed on it by physical activity and the changes that occur in the body as individuals regularly participate in exercise training (1).

Physical activity takes many forms. Activities as diverse as a slow stroll, raking leaves, a mile run at a fast pace, a dock worker's day-long labor, an Olympic weightlifter's 200 kg snatch lift, an elite bodybuilder's grueling three-hour workout, and a marathoner's 26.2-mile run are but a few examples of the activities to which the principles of exercise physiology can be applied. These diverse forms of physical activities require our bodies to make varying degrees of physiological adjustments. The role of the exercise physiologist is to examine specific responses in an attempt to delineate the alterations made with acute exercise to better understand the chronic adaptations that occur with exercise training.

The term *acute* refers to the performance of a single bout of exercise. This may take a few seconds (running a 40-yard dash) or many hours (competing in an ultramarathon race). Exercise physiologists investigate how the body makes internal adjustments in the face of massive disruptions to homeostasis occurring with exercise stress.

The study of acute responses represents only half of what is of interest in exercise physiology. Of concern also are the adaptive processes to chronic exercise stress. The term *chronic* refers to a length of time over which changes take place in different physiological systems during exercise training. These changes, or adaptations, generally can be interpreted as an improvement in the body's function at rest and during submaximal and maximal exercise.

Using the framework of acute responses and chronic adaptations, the exercise physiologist applies the knowledge gained from the basic sciences to problems in exercise physiology, thereby gaining insights into how the body functions during the stress of exercise. This can then be used as a basis for developing the best training practices to enhance athletic performance or improve health, two areas of special interest to the exercise physiologist.

METABOLIC AND HEMODYNAMIC CONTINUA

The differences in the acute responses and chronic adaptations among physical activities are often astounding. For example, it is possible to classify all exercises, athletic activities, and general physical activities on continua based on the two key physiological perturbations to exercise—*metabolic* and *hemodynamic* responses. In terms of metabolic responses, exercises can range from those that require the anaerobic production of energy in the cell to those that require the aerobic production of energy. In terms of hemodynamic responses, exercises can range from those that impose a volume load on the heart to those that impose a pressure load.

The metabolic continuum illustrates physical activities as energetic events (Figure 8.1). Activities are placed in a time frame that depicts the duration of the maximal effort during the event. The descriptors power, speed, and endurance are intensity factors with the greatest intensity (and shortage duration) being on the power end of the continuum and the lowest intensity (and longest duration) on the endurance end. Power and speed events are anaerobic, that is, they do not require the production of adenosine triphosphate (ATP) via oxygen metabolism to fuel the event. The further an event moves along the continuum toward the right, the more it relies on oxygen metabolism and the longer will be the duration of the event or exercise. Therefore, endurance events are aerobic, requiring oxygen for the production of ATP.

Track and field events are ideal examples of the use of these descriptors. For instance, the shotput requires all-out effort from the first instance of movement to displace the shot with as much force and distance as possible.

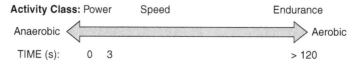

Figure 8.1. *Metabolic continuum.*

The event is over in less than 3 seconds. Other examples of power activities are Olympic weightlifting (single, maximal lifts) and running up a short flight of stairs. From an energetics standpoint, the fuel used for events classed in the power category is resting stores of phosphagens, particularly ATP and creatine phosphate (CP).

Speed events require a slightly longer time period. Examples of speed events are sprints (100 and 200 meters) and longer runs (400 meters). Weightlifting performed as a bodybuilding routine involving many repetitions per bout also qualifies as a speed event since the time frame during which the performer lifts is longer, but not approaching the endurance end of the continuum. Events and exercises of this nature rely on glycogen stores in the muscles to fuel maximal performance of the activity, which results in the production of lactic acid. Lactic acid buildup is what sets the boundary for duration of the maximal effort during speed events.

Endurance events are at the extreme right end of the continuum and are of much longer duration than both power and speed events. However, endurance activities are not very intense, allowing the production of ATP largely through aerobic metabolism. The 1500-meter run and runs of much longer duration are in this category. It must be noted that activities are not mutually exclusive in a metabolic sense; no one activity relies solely on a single energy system.

Sometimes placing an event or activity or sport on the metabolic continuum to determine the main way ATP is supplied to the contracting muscle can be tricky. For example, is soccer play aerobic or anaerobic? What about basketball? The answer to those questions depends on the action of the performer. If the play is of low intensity, as is sometimes the case, aerobic production of ATP predominates. If, however, an athlete steals the ball and there is a fast break to the goal, the anaerobic production of ATP predominates. So how would such an athlete train? The answer is that training should employ a combination of methods to ready the athlete for the various rigors of the sport.

It can be seen then that some activities fall in a "gray" zone with the energy output dependent on both anaerobic and aerobic sources. Generally, the shorter the activity, the greater is the contribution of anaerobic energy production. Conversely, the longer the activity, the greater is the contribution of aerobic energy production. The type of training program adopted to improve performance in an activity or sport event depends heavily on where the activity falls on the continuum.

An important concept related to the metabolic continuum and the type of exercise training employed is *specificity*. To maximize benefits, training should be carefully matched to an athlete's specific performance needs. Physiological adaptations produced from exercise training are highly specific to the nature of the training activity. Because of this principle, athletes should avoid certain kinds of training regimens, since the adaptations they receive from them may run counter to their performance requirements. For example, a power performer would not want to train with long distance jogging because the physiological adaptations gained from that form of exercise would tend to weaken his performance in the power event or sport.

Another example is the classic misconception that weight training will produce aerobic or cardiovascular benefits. The reasons why this is false are physiological and biochemical in nature and relate to the fact that specific kinds of adaptations (i.e., the aerobic benefits supposedly produced by weight training) follow only if there is a demand made on the bioenergetic processes and the physiological systems thought to be adapting. Cardiovascular benefits do not follow weight training because weightlifting does not sufficiently engage aerobic bioenergetic pathways.

Exercise can also be classified on a hemodynamic continuum (Figure 8.2). The degree to which an activity promotes blood movement (volume load) and the amount of blood pressure produced (pressure load) by the activity are important considerations when attempting to understand acute responses.

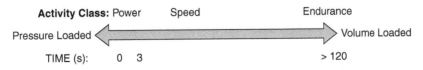

Figure 8.2.   *Hemodynamic continuum.*

Hemodynamic refers to the circulation of blood and encompass the forces restricting or promoting its circulation. Exercises that promote a great deal of blood movement are the endurance forms. These exercises are also associated with moderate elevations in blood pressure and are classified under the volume load heading. In typical aerobic or endurance exercise, the heart is loaded or stressed by pumping a great deal of blood volume through the circulation. There is a necessary link between aerobic metabolism (the metabolic continuum) and blood flow (the hemodynamic continuum). When an exercise is primarily aerobic, the hemodynamic response is largely one that promotes large blood flow. In contrast, those exercises that restrict blood movement, as in resistance forms (weightlifting), are also the ones that lead to a sharp increase in blood pressure. The heart is said to be pressure loaded in this class of exercise. While resistance exercise promotes moderate increases in blood movement, the amount of blood flow during resistance exercise is still very limited in comparison to volume load exercise. Therefore, pressure load exercises also are said to be largely anaerobic. Weightlifting is a perfect example of a pressure load exercise.

Activities, exercises, and sports events will fall at some point along the continua, but a few can be placed at either extreme. The concept of metabolic and hemodynamic continua is extremely useful in helping the coach or personal trainer design the best exercise training programs for clients. With knowledge of where a sport event or exercise falls on the continua, it becomes a matter of designing an exercise program that stresses training in the time frame of the event. For those sports events that are somewhere in the middle of the metabolic continuum, a mixed training program is needed.

ENERGY

Understanding energy conversion in the cell is vital for a sound understanding of muscular activity. The most rudimentary understanding of movement can be reduced to the study of the biochemical processes that release bound energy, converting it to free energy that is involved at any moment in all biological processes. Energy is the ability to perform work. Work and energy are directly related; as work increases, so does the transfer of energy from one form to another.

Different forms of energy are important in biological processes. The following are a few examples:

- Skeletal and heart muscle contraction, metabolic processes: chemical energy
- Nerve conduction: electrical energy
- Maintenance of body temperature: thermal energy

The laws of thermodynamics dictate energy conversions. The first law states that energy conversions result in no lost energy. This is the law of conservation of energy—energy is neither created nor destroyed, but is converted from one form to another.

The body's bioenergetic systems are part of the thermal processes that govern life on the entire planet, the sun being the ultimate source of energy for life. The massive amount of thermonuclear energy on the sun is released during fusion reactions, which then irradiates the earth where it drives the reactions of photosynthesis, the process that makes carbohydrates in plants (Figure 8.3).

The energy from one reaction (energy releasing—*exergonic*) is transformed to another form (energy absorbing—*endergonic*). Exergonic and endergonic reactions are coupled. In the example of photosynthesis radiant energy from fusion reactions (exergonic) on the sun is transformed to chemical energy in the form of carbohydrates (endergonic) on earth. The same coupling of energy-releasing and energy-conserving reactions takes place in our cells with muscle contraction (an endergonic process) being the ultimate outcome.

Energy for movement comes from energy-rich nutrients in the form of carbohydrates, fats, and proteins. These three energy nutrients are broken down during digestion to their constituent building-block molecules that enter the body from the digestive tract and are processed by the liver for storage and usage. These building-block molecules are rich in potential energy that is available to be converted to free energy for future muscular work. The energy bound in the building-block molecules, however, cannot be directly used by the

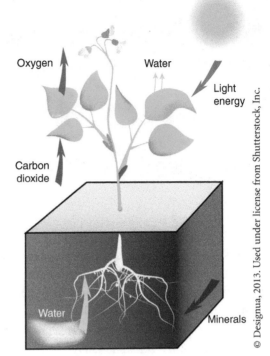

Figure 8.3. *The exergonic process on in the sun is nuclear fusion, which gives off energy in the form of the light and heat. Plants capture this energy and use it to build carbohydrates and other chemical compounds. Since the sun is releasing energy, its reaction is exergonic, and since plants are storing this energy, their reaction is endergonic.*

contracting muscle. It must first be converted to another chemical form that can then become the direct source of energy for muscle contraction.

Metabolism is the sum of the chemical processes that convert energy from indirect sources (the energy nutrients) to the source that can be used directly to do muscular activity. Another way to state this is that metabolism is the sum of all catabolic and anabolic reactions. Catabolism is the process of breaking down large energy nutrient molecules to their smaller constituent building blocks. In this process a transfer of energy takes place.

Anabolism is the process whereby smaller biomolecules are built up to larger biomolecules (glucose to glycogen, for example). An input of free energy is necessary to produce these kinds of reactions, making them energy-requiring reactions. For movement to occur, catabolic (energy releasing—exergonic) processes are linked with anabolic (energy trapping—endergonic) processes for the purpose of producing another high-energy product that then becomes the direct donor of free energy for muscular activity. This high-energy compound is ATP.

The subsequent breakdown of ATP releases its bound energy, converting it to free energy, which is then used for all of the energy-requiring processes in our cells, including muscle contraction. How ATP is created in the cell to power muscular activity is one of the major topics in the study of exercise physiology. As we have seen, the processes that produce ATP can proceed by anaerobic or aerobic means. These metabolic pathways are controlled by mechanisms inside the cell that regulate energy storage. All of this activity is precisely integrated for the most efficient production of ATP for a given sport activity or exercise.

Anaerobic Production of ATP

ATP can be produced without involving the cellular mechanisms that involve oxygen. The anaerobic production of ATP is a very important means of powering movement and makes possible a greatly expanded repertoire of activities. Table 8.1 provides examples of activities that are powered by the anaerobic production of ATP divided into power and speed activities. Without the anaerobic production of ATP, activities such as a sprinting or heavy weightlifting would not be possible. What makes power and speed activities possible is the rapid production of ATP in the cell by means of anaerobic metabolic pathways.

Table 8.1. Examples of the Time Course of Anaerobic Sport Events and Bodybuilding Training

Activity	Power	Speed	Duration (s)
Weight Training (Olympic Style)	X		< 5
Track and Field Throwing Events	X		< 10
100 m sprint	X		
200 m sprint		X	< 20
Weight Training (Bodybuilding)		X	> 30
400 m run		X	< 45

The phosphagen system is the first and simplest anaerobic metabolic pathway, so named because it uses two important high energy phosphate compounds stored in muscles in small quantities. The release of energy from ATP upon its breakdown causes muscle fibers to shorten (contraction). Every cell in the body contains a quantity of ATP and other high-energy phosphates. These quantities are very small, and because the high energy phosphates cannot be supplied from other areas of the body to the muscle, ATP must be continuously remade in muscle and every other cell. The *energy charge* of the cell, therefore, is directly related to ATP concentration—low ATP concentration means low energy charge and vice versa. A central role of metabolism is to guarantee that the cell is properly charged by the transfer of bound energy in the form of the energy nutrients to ATP, a process called *phosphorylation*.

Because anaerobic activities are highly intense, they require a very rapid re-supply of ATP for the rate of muscle contraction, and therefore the activity, to be sustained. Aerobic activities are much less intense, which means ATP production can proceed slowly through the coordinated integration of both cellular and cardiopulmonary system interactions.

To understand these differences more fully, it is important to introduce the concept of metabolic power versus metabolic capacity. A metabolic pathway is powerful if it has the ability to rapidly supply ATP during highly intense activity. Therefore, power relates to the rapidity of the pathway to produce ATP. Capacity, however, refers to the ability to make large quantities of ATP. Power and capacity are inversely related. Metabolic pathways that are the most powerful also have the least capacity, and vice versa. The anaerobic pathways are far more powerful than the aerobic pathways, but have a very limited capacity for ATP production.

ATP is referred to as the *energy currency* of the cell, because the free energy released from its breakdown powers cellular functions, including muscular contraction. However, since the concentration of ATP is very low in muscle, it is possible to deplete it rapidly in highly intense exercise. The depletion rate of ATP during intense activity would be much greater if it were not for creatine phosphate (CP) serving as a reservoir of phosphate units. The breakdown CP sustains ATP concentrations by the donation of the phosphate group from CP to ADP during the simultaneous breakdown of ATP. The breakdown of CP serves to sustain ATP levels in the muscle until the CP reservoir is itself depleted. When the reservoir is depleted, ATP concentration decreases precipitously, and so does the power output of the activity. In essence, the runner in a 200-meter run cannot complete the event at 40-meter sprint velocities, because of rapidly declining ATP concentrations. Muscle cells, in effect, run out of energy (ready ATP supply) and sprint velocity necessarily falls off. Without the presence of the next anaerobic metabolic pathway a 200-meter run could not be completed with much intensity of effort at all, and neither could anaerobic activities of longer duration such as the 400-meter run.

Two hundred meter sprints and races of longer distances can be completed in a very intense fashion due to the fact that our muscles have the capability to break down glucose to produce ATP in intense activity. The breakdown of glucose is termed *glycolysis*. During intense activity, longer than 10 to 15 seconds, exercising muscles rely more and more on glycolysis to pick up where the phosphagen system left off. This has very important implications, because without glucose breakdown during intense activity we would have to severely curtail our running velocity before we finished our 200-meter sprint. In effect, our range of anaerobic activities would be limited to those activities that could be completed with a very high intensity of effort before our reservoir of creatine phosphate ran out, which is only a few seconds. We would not be able to engage in the speed activities (intense activities that are more enduring than the power activities, but of much shorter duration than the endurance activities). Fortunately, the glycolytic pathway provides an adequate backup.

According to the concept of power versus capacity, glycolysis, while capable of supplying ATP very rapidly, is less powerful than the phosphagen system. One reason for this is that glycolysis is a far more complicated metabolic pathway. It involves the use of eleven enzymes, whereas the phosphagen system needs only two to produce ATP.

Remember that when power is low, capacity is high. This means that the capacity of glycolysis to produce ATP is much greater than the phosphagen system. The reason for this is that there is a lot more energy reserve stored as glucose, so much so that its storage quantity is not a limiting factor for intense activity. This means that glycolysis will be limited or forced to cease during intense activity prior to glucose being depleted in the cell. Recall that the reason ATP production via creatine phosphate breakdown stopped was that creatine phosphate exists in very limited quantities in muscle. These concepts make glycolysis an ideal backup to the phosphagen system in producing ATP anaerobically, greatly increasing our range of anaerobic activities.

The cell's capacity for glycolysis is crucial beyond the initial 10 to 15 seconds of very intense activity and up to approximately 90 seconds. However, there is a limit to the ability of glycolysis to sustain ATP production in intense activity. This limitation is brought about by the end product of glycolysis during intense activities, lactic acid. When glucose is metabolized in muscle during intense activity, lactic acid, formed in the last of 11 reactions, increases in concentration in the muscle and spills over in the blood circulating through the muscle. Since this is an acid buildup, the pH of the cell significantly decreases to the point at which muscle contraction begins to be compromised due to at least two reasons. First, the buildup of acid in the muscle cell causes any further chemical breakdown of glucose to be hampered by decreasing the activity of the enzymes responsible for glucose breakdown. Second, as the watery medium of the muscle cell (the sarcoplasm) becomes more acidic, the ability of the muscle to continue to contract forcibly is reduced. The net result of this is that exercise intensity (i.e., running speed) must be reduced.

Lactic acid is a fatiguing substance and in this respect its buildup is detrimental. However, the ability of the cell to form lactic acid early in intense activity is actually what provides the cell with the capability to continue to make ATP rapidly. Therefore, lactic acid can be seen as necessary initially and detrimental later in intense activity.

Aerobic Production of ATP

When exercise is at an intensity level that can be maintained continuously for long periods of time, ATP is produced in muscles through cellular respiration, a process that uses oxygen. In terms of power versus capacity, the aerobic production of ATP has by far the least power. It is not capable of providing ATP rapidly. In turn, the capacity of this system far exceeds the anaerobic systems. Glycolysis releases only approximately 5% of the energy in the glucose molecule when its final product is lactic acid. When the exercise intensity is lower, the rest of this energy is liberated by cellular processes that are located in the mitochondria. Glucose breakdown continues in the mitochondria during activity that can be extended for long periods of time.

The processes of cellular respiration are very complex, involving the integration of cellular aerobic metabolism with several organ systems designed to coordinate fuel (energy nutrient) and oxygen delivery to the working muscles. Cellular respiration involves five separate metabolic pathways in the breakdown of the two main energy nutrients (triglyceride and glucose) used during steady-state (endurance) exercise.

The breakdown of triglycerides is termed *lipolysis*, a process that liberates fatty acids from the triglyceride molecule. This takes place primarily in adipose tissue. The fatty acids are released to the blood and transported to muscle cells where they are metabolized. The breakdown of fatty acids is termed *beta-oxidation*. In this process acetyl-CoA is formed. Other pathways involved in the aerobic production of ATP are the Krebs cycle and the electron transport chain.

Beta oxidation and glycolysis are coordinated in that both funnel their end products to the respiratory mechanisms inside the mitochondria. Beta-oxidation ends in the formation of acetyl-CoA. Unlike the form of glycolysis that runs during intense activity, ending in lactic acid buildup, the form of glycolysis that proceeds during endurance activity ends in the formation of pyruvate. Pyruvate is placed into the mitochondria where it is also converted to acetyl-CoA. Therefore, acetyl-CoA is referred to as the *common degradation product*, because it is derived from both carbohydrate and fat catabolism. In the aerobic production of ATP during endurance-types of activities, both glucose and fats are metabolized simultaneously with common end products entering cellular respiration in the mitochondria.

The aerobic production of ATP is far more complicated, because these reactions involve many separate metabolic pathways each with many enzyme steps that are located in different parts of the cell and the body. For instance, fatty acids are mobilized from fat cells during lipolysis and are catalyzed via beta oxidation in muscle during exercise. Muscle stores of triglycerides are also used. Recall that both anaerobic pathways were located in the sarcoplasm of the muscle fiber and had relatively few steps. This allowed ATP to be produced very rapidly for quick muscular activity. Thus, power was increased at the expense of capacity. In the aerobic system this is turned around, with the advantage now toward capacity. Also, now that fat is being utilized as a fuel substrate, the energy source is almost unlimited. This great increase in capacity, however, comes at the expense of decreases in power.

In many ways the Krebs cycle can be considered the beginning of the aerobic system, since it is the point of entry for all metabolic intermediate compounds that serve as fuel substrate to be completely broken down in cellular respiration. Starting in the Krebs cycle these compounds are further broken down to form additional energy-rich carrier molecules—nicotinamide adenine dinucleotide (NADH) and flavin adenine dinucleotide (FADH). These high-energy carrier molecules funnel hydrogen ions to the inner mitochondrial wall where the electron transport chain makes large quantities of ATP molecules in a process called *oxidative phosphorylation* (as opposed to substrate level phosphorylation when ATP was formed during glycolysis).

The Krebs cycle is also significant because it is the process whereby carbon dioxide is produced. The aerobic system is aptly named since a regular supply of oxygen is needed in the mitochondria to serve as a final repository for the hydrogen atoms that are stripped off of the energy nutrients during metabolism. With enough oxygen, NADH, and FADH present, oxygen serves as the final acceptor of hydrogen atoms as these atoms are passed along a series of intermediate acceptors. Throughout this process ATP is generated, and metabolic water is produced. This process, therefore, utilizes the oxygen that we breathe in and deliver to the working muscles. In this process oxygen is said to be consumed. In the next section the physiological systems that deliver oxygen to the muscles where it is extracted from blood and used in aerobic metabolism are examined. The ATP supplied to the muscles provides the energy for contraction to occur.

THE CARDIORESPIRATORY SYSTEM

Major organ systems must provide an adequate supply of oxygen to meet the demand contracting muscles have for oxygen during endurance exercise. The organ system that absorbs oxygen from the atmosphere and into blood is the pulmonary system. The cardiovascular system then delivers oxygen carried by the blood to the working muscles and all other organ systems. The heart and lungs are controlled to precisely match the increased metabolic demand for oxygen that occurs with exercise. These systems work as a unit to maintain oxygen and carbon dioxide homeostasis in the body.

The integration of the pulmonary and cardiovascular systems in the delivery, extraction, and utilization of oxygen can be depicted by an equation that expresses the relationship between three important variables: oxygen consumption, cardiac output, and the arteriovenous oxygen difference. The blood delivered depends on the size of the cardiac output (the volume of blood circulated per minute). The amount of oxygen extracted depends in large part by the ability of the muscles to absorb and utilize oxygen. The three variables are shown in the equation below.

Oxygen Consumption = Cardiac Output   Arteriovenous Oxygen Difference
(Utilization) = (Amount Delivered)   ×   (Amount Extracted)
Central Factor (Heart)   Peripheral Factor (Tissues)

There is an immediate need to meet the increased demand for oxygen with an adequate supply during endurance exercise. Heart rate and strength of cardiac contractions increase so that the cardiac output closely matches any level of oxygen consumption. The increased strength of cardiac contractions produces a greater cardiac stroke volume. Cardiac output is the product of heart rate and stroke volume. These factors result in an increase in the delivery of blood to the working muscles, and constitute the central factor (pertaining to the heart itself) for the increase in oxygen consumption that occurs with exercise. The increased delivery of blood is accomplished not only by an increase in blood flow (cardiac output), but by the massive redistribution of blood away from areas that do not participate in producing movement (the gastrointestinal tract, bone, skin) and toward the working muscles (where the greatest demand is). The increase in cardiac output, heart rate, and oxygen consumption during endurance activities is proportional to exercise intensity. For instance, both cardiac output and oxygen consumption increase in a step-by-step fashion as walking or running rate increases. However, during weightlifting, a resistance exercise that requires the anaerobic production of ATP, oxygen consumption is much lower for a given level of heart rate.

Second, as exercise intensity increases more oxygen is extracted from the blood as the blood passes through the capillaries of the working muscles. This can be measured as a larger difference between the oxygen content of the arteries feeding the muscles and oxygen content of the veins leaving the muscles. This greater difference in the oxygen content of arteries versus veins constitutes the peripheral (away from the heart) factor for the increase in oxygen consumption that occurs with exercise.

Third, the increase in oxygen consumption with exercise results from an increase in pulmonary ventilation. Pulmonary ventilation is the bulk flow of air into and out of the lungs. Upon the initiation of exercise the rate and depth of breathing increase, which results in an increase in pulmonary ventilation. As the exercise intensity during endurance activity increases, more air is passed in and out of the lungs. The increased rate at which the lungs are ventilated allows more oxygen to be delivered to the working muscles.

Thermoregulation

Mammals are classified as homeothermic, meaning that regardless of the state of the external environment, they must maintain internal body temperatures within narrow limits for survival. This is often quite challenging when faced with extremes of temperatures. One of the functions of the cardiovascular system is to remove heat from the body. This function is especially important during aerobic exercise, because of the large amount of heat produced and subsequently trapped in the body.

Part of the energy liberated during aerobic exercise is used to perform useful work. However, this portion of the energy expenditure is relative small (only about 20%–30%). This means that the remaining part of the energy produced is stored as heat and must be eliminated to maintain core temperature within reasonable levels. If this is not done adequately, the result may be some form of heat illness or possibly even death.

When aerobic exercise is performed in environmental conditions that are favorable (low to moderate air temperature and relative humidity), the body's ability to thermoregulate is sufficient to keep core temperature increases to a minimum. The increase in core temperature is linked to exercise intensity (as the percentage of maximal oxygen consumption). Exercise at 50% maximal oxygen consumption would mean a core temperature increase of only 1°C. This represents a successful thermoregulatory effort.

If environmental conditions are at the extremes of temperature, relative humidity, or both, thermoregulation is much harder to accomplish. The result of exercising in environmental extremes is an increased core temperature and a reduced work output. The reduced work output is a direct result of the extra burden placed on the cardiovascular system, which must not only supply oxygen to the working muscles to sustain the work output, but now it has an even more important role in delivering heat to the superficial regions of the body to dissipate the heat. This would have the direct effect of reducing maximal oxygen consumption and reducing exercise performance. In this case two areas of the body are competing for same cardiac output: the muscles to sustain the exercise intensity and the skin to dissipate the heat being carried by the blood. As the skin region receives more of the cardiac output, there is of necessity a reduction in endurance performance.

The ability to adequately dissipate the extra heat produced during aerobic exercise depends on the evaporative transfer of heat to the environment as water is vaporized from the respiratory passages and from the surface of the skin. Evaporation of water (sweat) off the skin is especially important since it represents the major way heat is removed from the body during exercise, except in hot, humid environments. Anything that retards this process will hinder exercise performance and carries a certain amount of risk to the exercising subject.

Evaporation is aided when the vapor pressure gradient from the skin surface to the air is large. This occurs when the relative humidity of the air is low. In this condition sweat easily evaporates to air that is relatively more dry than the skin. As water evaporates from the skin, heat is also transferred to the surroundings, and the body is cooled. Exercising in conditions of low relative humidity is, therefore, desirable. This problem is also independent of environmental temperatures since deaths have occurred in high humidity conditions even when temperatures have been moderate.

Inappropriate clothing greatly retards the evaporation of sweat from the skin. Different types of clothing are more effective in setting up a microenvironment around the skin than others, resulting in evaporation being retarded even when the outside environmental conditions are favorable. Certain types of athletic wear are specifically designed to provide a vapor barrier that completely stops the evaporative cooling process.

One of the most important things that can be done when exercising in a hot environment is to drink enough water. Studies have shown that water replacement is very effective in keeping the increase in core temperature seen with aerobic exercise to a minimum. When water balance (water intake that matched water loss) is maintained core body temperature increases are minimal.

SUMMARY

Exercise physiology is the science of how the body functions during exercise and sports activities and how the body adapts to chronic exercise training. The scope of exercise physiology covers both acute and chronic exercise responses and adaptations and includes the study of activities that can be placed on metabolic and hemodynamic continua. Exercise physiology is the study of how the body utilizes energy from the standpoint of cellular mechanisms to a systems approach. In this chapter the major organ systems supporting energy-transferring processes were briefly featured to show the integration of these systems with cellular mechanisms in the production of energy.

REFERENCE

1. Brown, S.P., Miller, W.C., Eason J.M. *Exercise Physiology: Basis of Human Movement in Health and Disease*, Baltimore: Lippincott Williams & Wilkins, 2006.

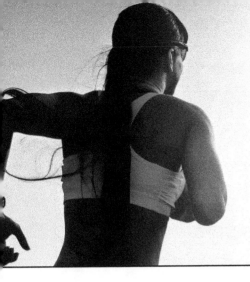

Chapter 9

SPORT NUTRITION

OUTLINE

OBJECTIVES

1. Describe the six classes of nutrients.
2. Learn the nutrients that can be used to produce energy in the body.
3. Identify the fat and water soluble vitamins and list their main functions.
4. Identify main minerals required by athletes and describe their main functions.
5. Learn the proper hydration techniques.
6. Learn the ideal body fat percentage of physically active adults.
7. Describe the different methods used to assess body composition.
8. Discuss the role that dietary supplements have on exercise performance.

The science of nutrition is the study of metabolic and physiological responses that occur in the body as a result of what we eat (i.e., our diet). Sport nutrition, a subdiscipline of the multidisciplinary field of nutrition, is the study and application of nutritional principles to people that exercise. Proper and balanced nutrition is not only important to professional athletes, but also to people who exercise for recreation and even to others whose daily activities require high energy expenditures. In the arena of high-level collegiate and professional sports, it is important for athletes to maintain the competitive edge that proper nutrition can give them. It is also important to note at the outset that sound nutrition is not only essential for competitive success, but is vital for overall health.

This chapter briefly describes major components of sport nutrition. First, the six classes of nutrients (i.e., carbohydrate, fat, protein, vitamins, minerals, and water) are described. Each nutrient is defined, and information on the quality and quantity a healthy individual must consume is provided. Also discussed is whether athletes require higher quantities of each of the six classes of nutrients. The chapter then moves to a discussion of the interaction of exercise and nutrition and the influence of these two components on body composition. Factors that influence body composition are also discussed. In general our body weight and body composition change as a result of caloric intake (e.g., food consumption) and calories expended (e.g., exercise). A comparison of the methods available to determine body composition is given along with the healthy range of body fat percentage for active adults. Finally, dietary supplements are discussed and evidence provided for and against the use of each by athletes.

The trend in increased leisure time physical activity requires that the general public understand the role nutrition plays in the lives of people pursuing an active lifestyle. Unfortunately, the danger of exploitation still exists in the area of nutritional supplementation. Oftentimes, our sports-conscious culture and media-driven society help perpetuate fads and misconceptions. The public is usually ill equipped to decipher the good from the bad, which leads to a proliferation of quackery, or the promotion of unproven or fraudulent practices. Even weekend athletes want to perform better, but few are able to decide whether it is prudent to take a nutritional supplement in the face of media reports even when the science is known to be lacking. It is therefore paramount in this day of record-breaking performances by athletes who have soiled the purity of sport by the use of questionable ergogenic aids for individuals to be discerning consumers. The field of sport nutrition can play a central role in helping elite and recreational athletes make healthful choices. Students of kinesiology have a solid foundation in sport nutrition to help individuals avoid the pitfalls of those who propagate faddism and quackery.

THE SIX CLASSES OF NUTRIENTS

Carbohydrates

Carbohydrates and fats (described below) are the main sources of energy in the diet. There are two main classes of carbohydrates. The first class of carbohydrates, sugars and starches, can be digested and metabolized for energy. Sugars are mainly found in soft drinks, syrups, jellies, and cookies, whereas starches are found in potatoes and other vegetables. The second class of carbohydrates is known as dietary fiber and is of plant origin. This form of carbohydrate is resistant to digestion and absorption by the human small intestine. Despite the fact that humans cannot digest dietary fiber, it is now well established that dietary fiber promotes beneficial physiologic effects, such as maintaining gastrointestinal health (5).

Carbohydrates are divided into three groups: monosaccharides, disaccharides, and polysaccharides. Monosaccharides are the simplest form of carbohydrates and contain only one sugar (derived from the Greek word *sákkharon*, meaning sugar). Examples of monosaccharides include glucose (also referred to as blood sugar), fructose, and galactose. Disaccharides contain two monosaccharides and include sucrose (e.g., table sugar) that is composed of the monosaccharides glucose and fructose. Another disaccharide is lactose (e.g., milk sugar) that is composed of the monosaccharides galactose and glucose. Polysaccharides are composed of numerous (e.g., three or more) monosaccharides and include glycogen, starch, and cellulose. Glycogen is the storage form of carbohydrates in humans, and it is mainly found in the liver and skeletal muscles. Starch and cellulose are the storage forms of carbohydrate in plants. As discussed above, humans can digest and absorb starch, but cannot digest cellulose, the main component of plant fiber.

Carbohydrate Ingestion before and during Exercise and Its Effect on Exercise Performance

During low intensity exercise the primary fuel for energy production is fat. As exercise intensity increases, carbohydrate utilization increases and during high intensity exercise most of the energy is supplied by carbohydrate metabolism (3). Years of sport nutrition research has shown that carbohydrate consumption during long-term exercise (i.e., more than 90 minutes) can maintain and/or improve exercise performance. During the early stages of exercise, the body breaks down glycogen stored in skeletal muscles into glucose, and this glucose is subsequently used for energy production. As the exercise duration increases, glycogen stores and even those of the liver can be depleted. If a person continues to exercise, hypoglycemia (i.e., low blood glucose concentration) can occur when liver glycogen is depleted. If blood glucose levels decrease to very low levels, numerous central nervous system symptoms can ensue (e.g., fainting). Therefore, consuming carbohydrates (exogenous or out of the body source) during long-term exercise activities is recommended to replenish the glucose used for energy consumption. The typical recommendation is to consume about 30 to 60 grams of carbohydrate every hour during prolonged exercise activities.

An additional important topic in sport nutrition has been the role of carbohydrate consumption before exercise. This practice is known as carbohydrate loading or glycogen supercompensation. Specifically, research has shown that if a person intending to perform a long-term exercise activity (e.g., running a marathon) modifies his or her diet for a few days before the event, exercise performance can be improved. The rationale behind this practice is that the body can store additional glycogen before the event, and thus depletion of glycogen stores can be delayed. There are two ways of achieving this goal—the "classic method" and the "modified method." To learn more on this topic please, refer to the following references (7, 12).

Carbohydrates are metabolized in the body to produce adenosine triphosphate (ATP), which is the cell's energy currency. It is used to support energy demands, including skeletal muscle contractions (e.g., exercise). At rest, carbohydrate metabolism accounts for about 30% of bodily energy needs, but as exercise intensity increases, the percentage of energy produced in the body from carbohydrate metabolism increases (13). Consumption of carbohydrates before and during exercise can improve exercise performance (see box on carbohydrate ingestion).

One gram of carbohydrate yields 4 kilocalories (kcal) of energy. Typically, about 60% of an athlete's total kcal intake should come from carbohydrates. Most of the carbohydrate intake should be in the form complex carbohydrates (e.g., rice, whole grain breads, potatoes) rather than simple carbohydrates (e.g., cookies, pastries, candy). The main reason consumption of complex carbohydrates is recommended over simple carbohydrates is based on the glycemic index. Complex carbohydrates have a low glycemic index, indicating slower rates of digestion and absorption of carbohydrates (16). A lower glycemic response usually equates to a lower insulin demand and may improve long-term blood glucose control and decreases the risk of developing diabetes.

Fats

The body requires a dietary supply of fats (lipids) to function properly. For example, fats are used for energy production (stored in adipose tissue) and hormone production. Fats are also involved in cell membrane structure and during the absorption of fat-soluble vitamins from the gastrointestinal tract. Thus, it is currently recommended that about 20% to 30% of the total calorie intake should come from dietary fats.

Fats are more energy dense than carbohydrates. Specifically, one gram of fats yields 9 kcal of energy. This property of fats may be viewed both as a benefit and a detriment. The benefit is that we can store reserved energy in the body in a "packed" form. However, since fats have a very high caloric density, it requires a long period of time to reduce the mass of adipose tissue when on a diet.

Fats can be divided into different forms (e.g., saturated fats, monounsaturated fats, and polyunsaturated fats). As Figure 9.1 illustrates, saturated fats (i.e., no double bonds between carbon atoms of the fatty acids) are found in high concentration in animal products (e.g., butter, ice cream, lard). The consumption of such fats has been linked to increased risk of cardiovascular disease (e.g., atherosclerosis). Therefore, it is currently recommended that saturated fats should make up only about 7% of the total fat intake. Monounsaturated fats (i.e., one double bond between carbon atoms of the fatty acids) should cover about 13% of the total fat intake. Food sources high in monounsaturated fats include olive oil, avocadoes, and peanut oil. Finally, the consumption of polyunsaturated fats (i.e., more than one double bond between carbon atoms of the fatty acids) should be about 10% of the total fat consumption. Food sources high in polyunsaturated fats include sunflower oil, nuts, seeds, and fish. Importantly, recent evidence indicates that the consumption of dietary polyunsaturated fats can reduce the risk of developing cardiovascular disease and cancer (4).

In summary, the dietary source of fats does not necessarily affect exercise performance, but since certain types of fats (e.g., saturated fats) have been linked with increased risk of chronic disease, an athlete should be aware of these issues and the consumption of fats should be closely regulated according to the current dietary recommendations.

Protein

The third class of nutrients is protein. Protein metabolism yields the same amount of energy as carbohydrates (4 kcal per gram protein). However, protein is not considered a primary energy source, and under normal conditions it only supplies less than 2% of the energy used by the body (13).

Protein is composed of amino acids chemically linked to each other; these amino acids are the building block of skeletal muscle. There are 20 amino acids divided into those that are essential (sometimes refer to as indispensable) and nonessential. The nine essential amino acids cannot be synthesized in the body and therefore must be consumed in the diet. The 11 nonessential amino acids can be synthesized in the body from other substrates. Table 9.1 lists the essential and nonessential amino acids for adult humans. It is important

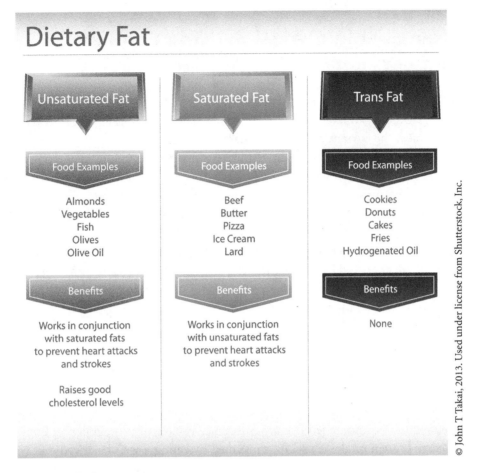

© John T Takai, 2013. Used under license from Shutterstock, Inc.

Figure 9.1.   *Different forms of dietary fat.*

Table 9.1.   The Essential and Nonessential Amino Acids for Adult Humans.

Essential	Nonessential
Histidine	Alanine
Isoleucine	Arginine
Leucine	Asparagine
Lysine	Aspartate
Methionine	Cysteine
Phenylalanine	Glutamate
Threonine	Glutamine
Tryptophan	Glycine
Valine	Proline
	Serine
	Tyrosine

Is Protein Supplementation Using Commercial Supplements Required in Athletes?

The use of protein supplements has increased exponentially over the past several years by both recreational and professional athletes. However, as we have discussed earlier, most people consuming a well-balanced diet meet the current adult Recommended Dietary Allowance for protein. Therefore, in most cases the use of commercial protein supplements is not warranted. Even if an athlete does require a higher protein intake, it is recommended that the extra protein intake comes from dietary sources since this is less expensive. Also, when the athlete increases his or her protein intake by consuming food items high in quality protein (e.g., milk, eggs, tuna,) the athlete also consumes additional nutrients (e.g., vitamins, minerals).

It is also important to note that consumption of excessive and unnecessary amounts of protein may have a harmful effect on the body (e.g., increased loss of calcium). In summary, it appears that most individuals that exercise consume adequate amounts of protein in their diet, and supplementation with commercial protein supplements is unnecessary.

to note that some of the amino acids listed as nonessential are required by infants and growing children (e.g., histidine). Also, some other nonessential amino acids may be essential in certain situations (e.g., arginine and cysteine.).

The current adult Recommended Dietary Allowance is 0.8 g of protein per kg body weight per day. This amount of dietary protein intake is usually consumed by eating a well-balanced diet (Figure 9.2). However, certain groups of people (e.g., vegetarians) may require a protein supplement to meet this requirement. It is also important to note that the protein requirement for athletes has been and continuous to be an unresolved issue (see box on protein supplementation). Several studies have investigated this issue, but still no clear answer remains.

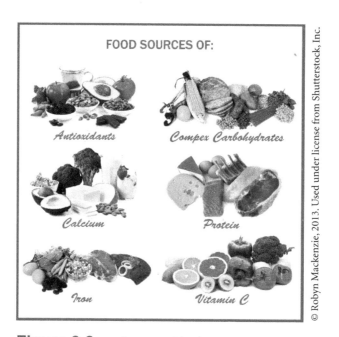

Figure 9.2. *Sources of food items to be included in a well-balanced diet.*

Athletes appear to require more protein in their diets than sedentary individuals because of tissue damage during exercise and the higher turnover of skeletal muscle (e.g., recovery and repair of tissue after exercise). The current recommendation by the American College of Sports Medicine is that elite athletes performing high-intensity endurance exercise may require 1.2 to 1.4 g of protein per kg body weight per day. Also, the current recommendation by the American College of Sports Medicine is that strength-training elite athletes that are adding muscle mass may require 1.2 to 1.7 g of protein per kg body weight per day (15).

Vitamins

Vitamins are required by the body in smaller amounts than carbohydrates, fats, and proteins. Vitamins do not produce energy, but they do play a major role in numerous energy-producing metabolic reactions. Vitamins can be divided into two categories: fat-soluble vitamins and water-soluble vitamins.

The four fat-soluble vitamins are listed in Table 9.2. Vitamin A is essential for proper vision and growth. Some food items high in vitamin A include liver, carrots, and broccoli. Vitamin D is required for calcium and phosphorous absorption and optimal bone development. Food items high in vitamin D include milk, fish oils, and salmon. Vitamin E is a potent antioxidant and its deficiency can lead to hemolysis of red blood cells. Vitamin E food sources include vegetable oils, sunflower seeds, and peanuts. Finally, vitamin K is required during blood clotting and bone metabolism. Green vegetables and liver contain high amounts of vitamin K.

The water-soluble vitamins include vitamin C and the B vitamin complex (Table 9.2). All of the B vitamins are involved in energy-producing reactions. Additional functions of the B vitamins are nerve function (thiamin), hemoglobin synthesis (pyridoxine), and DNA synthesis (folic acid). Food items rich in thiamin include peas and brewers' yeast. Mushrooms contain high levels of riboflavin, niacin, and pantothenic acid. Cheese and eggs yolks contain a high concentration of biotin. Fortified grain products (e.g., pasta, cereal, bread) are high in folic acid. Animal protein foods are high in pyridoxine and B12.

Vitamins are required in small quantities in the body, and inadequate consumption of these vitamins can lead to deficiency. However, excess consumption of vitamins can lead to vitamin toxicity. Fat-soluble vitamins are stored in adipose tissue; therefore, excess consumption of any of the four fat-soluble vitamins can lead to vitamin toxicity (8). Vitamin toxicity of the water-soluble vitamins is not common since these vitamins are readily metabolized and excreted from the body.

Table 9.2. The Fat- and Water-Soluble Vitamins.

Fat soluble	Water soluble
vitamin A	vitamin C
vitamin D	thiamin (B1)
vitamin E	riboflavin (B2)
vitamin K	niacin (B3)
	pantothenic acid (B5)
	pyridoxine (B6)
	biotin (B7)
	folic acid (B9)
	cobalamin (B12)

Vitamin and Mineral Supplementation for Athletes—Is It Necessary?

Sport nutritionists have been trying for years to identify whether vitamin and/or mineral supplementation is needed for athletes compared to sedentary individuals. Unfortunately, to this date the results of numerous studies remain equivocal and thus no consensus answer is available. There may be instances where certain individuals do require supplemental vitamins/minerals. For example, female athletes must pay close attention in the amount of calcium and iron consumed. Inadequate consumption of calcium and iron minerals can lead to reductions in bone mineral density and anemia, respectively. Unfortunately, both of these conditions are commonly seen in female athletes, and under these circumstances supplementation may be warranted.

Consumption of excess (i.e., over the Recommended Dietary Allowances) vitamins and/or minerals does not appear to increase exercise performance. On the other hand, excess consumption of vitamins/minerals can lead to toxicities. Specifically, excess fat-soluble vitamins are stored in the adipose tissue and can lead to side effects (muscle weakness, fatigue, etc). Consuming high doses of minerals can also lead to toxicities and negatively influence the metabolism of other minerals. Specifically, excess iron consumption can interfere with copper and zinc metabolism.

In summary, vitamins and minerals are required by the body in relatively small amounts. The preferred way of meeting vitamin and mineral dietary intake recommendations is by consuming a well-balanced diet. However, certain individuals (e.g., vegetarians) may require a multivitamin/mineral supplement to meet their daily requirements. However, a person taking a multivitamin/mineral supplement must be careful not to exceed the dietary requirements of each of these nutrients.

Minerals

Just like vitamins, minerals do not produce energy, but are required by the body for numerous functions. Minerals can be broken into two categories. Macrominerals (major minerals) are required in larger amounts (0.3 – 5.0 g per day) than microminerals (trace elements) that are required in milligrams or smaller quantities.

There are seven macrominerals: calcium, phosphorus, potassium, sulfur, sodium, chloride, and magnesium. Calcium and phosphorus play a critical role in bone and teeth development, and dairy products contain high levels of these two macrominerals. Sodium, potassium, and chloride function as major ions in intracellular and extracellular fluids. Table salt is made of sodium and chloride, and bananas contain high levels of potassium. Finally, magnesium is a critical cofactor (i.e., aids enzyme function) and can be found in green vegetables and nuts.

There are numerous microminerals required by the body (Figure 9.3), but in this chapter we will only discuss several key ones: iron, copper, zinc, iodide, selenium, chromium, and fluoride. Iron is part of hemoglobin, and copper functions in iron metabolism. Zinc plays a role in growth and sexual development, and iodide is required for proper thyroid function. Selenium is an antioxidant, and chromium functions in carbohydrate metabolism. Finally, fluoride is essential for maintaining the tooth enamel and prevents dental caries. Food sources that contain high levels of these minerals are iron (meat and spinach), copper (cocoa and beans), zinc (seafood), iodide (saltwater fish and iodized table salt), selenium (eggs and fish), chromium (egg yolks), and fluoride (fluoridated water and toothpaste).

Finally, there is a continuous debate whether athletes require higher intakes of vitamins and minerals than sedentary individuals. This topic is addressed in the box on vitamin and mineral supplementation.

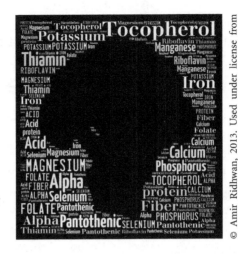

© Amir Ridhwan, 2013. Used under license from Shutterstock, Inc.

Figure 9.3. *Numerous vitamins and minerals are required for health and maximal exercise performance.*

Water

Water, the last class of nutrient to be discussed, is as important as the previous five nutrients. Our bodies are about two-thirds water, and losing 3 to 4% of body water can lead to decreased exercise performance. A sedentary adult loses about 2.5 liters of water daily. Usually, this water loss is replenished by beverages and food. Some water is also produced in our bodies through metabolic processes. On the other hand, an athlete who exercises at a high intensity and for long periods of time can lose up to 6 liters of water per day. This water loss must be replenished to avoid detrimental side effects (e.g., fatigue, dizziness) and even death.

The current recommendation for athletes is to drink liquids before, during, and after exercise. It is very important to note that if an athlete waits to become thirsty before drinking, it may be too late since the body may have already become hypohydrated. Usually athletes drink water or sport drinks to replenish the water loss during exercise (Figure 9.4). Water consumption is usually sufficient to prevent exercise-induced hypohydration. However, sport drinks are excellent alternatives to water since they usually contain other nutrients (e.g., carbohydrates and electrolytes) that may offer additional benefits to the exercising body.

As previously mentioned, athletes should not wait to become hypohydrated before they start consuming liquids. The color of the urine can serve as an excellent marker to check hydration status. Dark-colored urine is an indication of hypohydration. Hydration status can also be monitored by fluctuations in body weight before and after exercise. To avoid hypohydration, the following general guidelines should be followed. Several hours before exercise an athlete should consume about 0.5 liters of liquids, and a few minutes before exercise he or she should consume an additional 0.25 liters of liquids. Also, during exercise an athlete should consume about

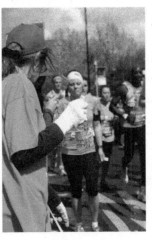

© Michaelpuche, 2013. Used under license from Shutterstock, Inc.

Figure 9.4. *Adequate hydration is required for optimal exercise performance.*

0.25 liters of liquids every 15 minutes of exercise. Also, at the cessation of exercise, an athlete should consume about 1 liter of water for each kilogram body weight lost during exercise.

NUTRITION AND BODY COMPOSITION

The United States and other industrialized countries face an obesity epidemic. Obesity can be due to consumption of excess calories or lack of exercise and has been linked to numerous diseases (i.e., hypertension, diabetes). Although the obesity epidemic is of great concern, it is also important to note that significant health problems may be present in an individual who is underweight.

In today's society there is a push to look good and have the "perfect" body. In some instances, the "perfect" body is someone who is underweight. This is especially true in young female athletes. Female athletes are often faced with three common health problems that are interrelated and are known as the female athlete triad. These health concerns are described in the box of the same name.

The Female Athlete Triad

The female athlete triad is composed of three interrelated conditions: eating disorders, amenorrhea, and bone mineral loss.

Eating Disorders

Bulimia is portrayed by overeating that is followed by vomiting. This is also known as binge eating (i.e., excessive food intake) and purging (i.e., vomiting). People who suffer from this condition practice purging to lose or maintain their weight, and most of them actually have a normal weight. Bulimia is believed to have a psychological origin. People who suffer from bulimia have negative emotions (e.g., guilt). Most of these individuals are females.

People suffering from bulimia require professional treatment, because the condition can lead to severe health issues. For example, frequent vomiting may damage the teeth and the esophagus because of the high acidity of the stomach contents. Common signs that may indicate that a person is suffering from bulimia include excessive concern about caloric intake, continuous trips to the bathroom especially after a meal, depression, low self-esteem, and fixation on body weight.

Anorexia nervosa is another eating disorder that is more common in females than males. Anorexia nervosa is depicted by limiting food intake to a state of starvation. This can lead to emaciation. People suffering from this condition are in a high risk of dying from starvation. Similar to bulimia, anorexia nervosa is also linked to psychological problems. Anorexia nervosa may be induced by family and/or peer pressure to be thin in order to "fit" in today's society. People suffering from anorexia nervosa have a constant fear of gaining weight. They take all preventive measures (e.g., not eating) to avoid any weight gain. Common signs of anorexia nervosa include rapid and extreme weight loss, constant obsession with food and calorie intake, mood swings, avoiding family and friends during food-related activities, and fatigue.

Amenorrhea

Amenorrhea is characterized by the lack of menstrual period in females during their normal reproductive years. The incidence of amenorrhea is higher in female athletes compared to the general population, but the exact cause of amenorrhea is not known. Female distance athletes have the highest incidence of amenorrhea, and data indicate that the amount of training is related to the development of amenorrhea.

The large amount of training can influence several hormones in the female body, which in turn have an influence in the hypothalamus. This homeostatic disturbance can have a negative influence on the female reproductive hormones and thus alter normal menstruation. Also, females who engage in long-distance training each week may suffer from psychological stress, which can also influence several hormones (e.g., catecholamines, endogenous opioid peptides) that can in turn disrupt the reproductive physiology of the female athlete.

Bone Mineral Loss

Exercise training has a beneficial effect on the bone mineral content of both males and females. However, females are at a higher risk of having reduced bone mineral content because of their hormonal physiology. Female athletes sometimes suffer from an eating disorder (e.g., bulimia, anorexia nervosa) that can result in inadequate nutrient intake (e.g., calcium, vitamin D). Importantly, an eating disorder can also cause amenorrhea (i.e., absence of a menstrual period) that can lead to a disruption of estrogen homeostasis. Collectively, the inadequate intake of calcium and vitamin D and disruption in estrogen homeostasis can lead to loss of bone mass. Exercise can reduce bone mineral loss in females, but exercise alone cannot completely prevent the loss. Therefore, in order to prevent the bone mineral loss, the underlying conditions (e.g., amenorrhea, eating disorder) must be treated by a trained professional.

Body mass index (BMI), an easy way to estimate body composition, is calculated as body weight (kg)/height^2 (m^2). Once BMI is determined the value is compared to a universally accepted table so that a classification is made. Specifically, a BMI of less than 18.5 indicates that the individual is underweight, a BMI between 18.5 and 24.9 indicates a normal weight, a BMI of 25.0 to 29.9 indicates that the person is overweight, and a BMI of greater than 30.0 indicates that the person is obese. The BMI is used because it is easy to calculate, but it is paramount to note that it does not measure the percentage of body fat in an individual. For example, a heavily muscled person (e.g., bodybuilder) can be classified as overweight or obese, even though his or her body fat percentage is in the normal range. Therefore, being able to evaluate the body composition of the general population and athletes and monitor changes in body composition is essential.

For this reason, several other techniques exist that offer a more direct measure of the body fat percentage. The most commonly used techniques to estimate percentage body fat are briefly described below. Once percentage of body fat has been obtained, its value should be compared (Table 9.3) since the healthy range of percentage of body fat depends on factors such as age, sex, and activity level. The percentage of body fat of an individual can be reduced by several factors including exercise and calorie intake (Figure 9.5).

Skinfold Thickness

This technique incorporates several skinfold measurements of subcutaneous (just beneath the skin) fat by using skinfold calipers. Once obtained, the skinfold measurements are inserted into an equation and an estimation of body fat is determined. Different prediction equations exist, each requiring a different number of skinfold measurements. Typical sites used to estimate body fat percentage by this technique include triceps, biceps, chest, subscapula, abdomen, suprailiac, thigh, and calf. This technique is also easy to use, but determining body fat percentage via skinfold measures has several drawbacks (10). Measurement of subcutaneous fat has a high rate of error due to instrument (e.g., improper calibration of calipers) or human error (e.g., not properly trained). Also, numerous equations exist that were developed by using a certain population, and thus one must be careful to use the most appropriate equation for each individual.

Table 9.3. Recommended Body Fat Percentage for Physically Active Individuals.

	Low	Middle	Upper
18–34 years			
Male	5	10	15
Female	16	23	28
35–55 years			
Male	7	11	18
Female	20	27	33
55+ years			
Male	9	12	18
Female	20	27	33

Adapted from (9).

Hydrostatic Weighing

This technique is also known as underwater weighing. The technique is based on the principle described by Archimedes (a Greek mathematician). This principle states that the upward buoyant force exerted on a body immersed in a fluid is equal to the weight of the fluid the body displaces. This information can be used to estimate body density, and then percentage body fat can be calculated by various equations. This technique produces fairly accurate results and for many years it has been considered the gold standard in measuring body composition.

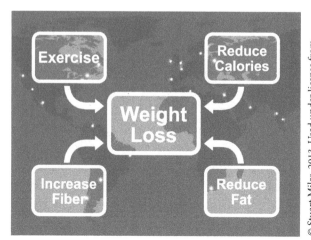

Figure 9.5. *Factors that can influence body composition.*

© Stuart Miles, 2013. Used under license from Shutterstock, Inc.

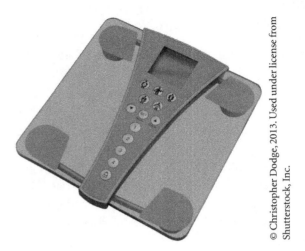

Figure 9.6. *An example of the equipment needed to determine body composition by using the bioelectrical impedance analysis (BIA) technique.*

Air Displacement Plethysmography

Another technique to estimate body composition is air displacement plethysmography, which is also known as the Bod Pod method. The principle behind this method is similar to hydrostatic weighing, but air displacement is used to estimate body density instead of water displacement. Once body density has been obtained, it is used in an identical way as described in the underwater weighing method, and body fat percentage can be calculated. The hydrostatic weighing and air displacement plethysmography methods give very similar results, but an advantage of the Bod Pod is its ease of use (10).

Bioelectrical Impedance Analysis

The bioelectrical impedance analysis (BIA) technique is used to estimate percentage of body fat, and its principle is based on the observation that fat is not as good a conductor of electricity as is muscle. A small current is sent through the body and the electrical impedance (i.e., opposition to the current) is determined. From this information, total body water can be estimated, and then percentage of body fat can be calculated from various established equations. The bioelectrical impedance analysis method is not considered to be a very accurate method of determining percentage body fat, but its use has grown over the years because of the simple equipment required and ease of use (Figure 9.6). An additional note is that hydration levels of an individual can greatly confound the results obtained by using this technique (11).

Dual Energy X-ray Absorptiometry

The dual energy X-ray absorptiometry (DEXA or DXA) method was originally developed to measure bone density. This technique incorporates the use of x-rays. The amount of x-ray energy absorbed in the body is analyzed by computer software and subsequently used to calculate body composition (e.g., percentage of body fat). It is now established that dual energy X-ray absorptiometry method gives accurate results in regards to body composition, but it requires very expensive equipment (2).

USE OF SUPPLEMENTS TO IMPROVE EXERCISE PERFORMANCE

The use of ergogenic aids to boost sport performance has been growing in recent years. This section presents several key methods used, brief explanations as to why athletes use them, and whether any of the supplements can actually improve physical performance.

Supplemental Oxygen

Oxygen is required for the production of adenosine triphosphate (ATP) through aerobic metabolism. Under physiological conditions, blood is about 97% saturated with oxygen. Therefore, the possibility exists that breathing pure oxygen (i.e., 100% oxygen) can increase the amount of oxygen in the blood, and this extra oxygen can be used to produce more ATP and thus improve endurance exercise performance. However, research has shown that while it is possible to increase the amount of oxygen in the blood before exercise by breathing pure oxygen, this extra oxygen will be lost if the athlete breaths normal air several times before exercise (Wilmore, 1972). Therefore, breathing pure oxygen before competition does not offer any advantage to the athlete. In contrast to this, if an athlete was able to breathe air that contained more than 21% oxygen while exercising, the exercise performance would be improved. However, during competition, that is not allowed and would be practically impossible to achieve. Also, a lot of athletes (e.g., football players) breathe a gas mixture that is higher than 21% oxygen shortly after an exercise bout in order to recover quicker. However, this practice does not offer any improvement in subsequent exercise performance (18).

Creatine Monohydrate

Since the early 1990s, athletes have been using creatine monohydrate to improve exercise performance. Creatine monohydrate is used to regenerate ATP via the creatine phosphate pathway. Typically, our creatine supply is obtained through the diet (e.g., meat and fish), and this creatine is stored in the muscles to be used later. However, the amount of creatine in the muscles can be increased by consuming extra amount of creatine (e.g., creatine monohydrate supplement). Importantly, several studies indicate that this extra creatine in the muscles can improve muscular force and power output during high-intensity, short-term, and repetitive exercise events (e.g., sprinting, weightlifting). However, creatine supplementation has no effect on long-duration exercise activities. Finally, it is important to note that several side effects (nausea and gastrointestinal distress) have been linked with creatine monohydrate supplementation.

Blood Doping

Red blood cells contain hemoglobin that binds oxygen and transports it to the exercising muscles. Increasing red blood cells would increase the capacity of an individual to deliver oxygen to the muscles where it can be used to produce ATP by aerobic metabolism. There are different ways that the red blood cell count can be increased in an athlete. The first method is where an individual removes and stores his or her own red blood cells a few weeks before competition. A few days before the competition the athlete infuses the red blood cells back into the circulation. The result is an increased oxygen-carrying capacity that can improve aerobic exercise performance. Another way to increase the amount of red blood cells in the body is by using the drug erythropoietin (6). Erythropoietin stimulates the generation of new red blood cells in the body. However, both of these techniques to increase red blood cells are banned in many sports. Several sport agencies are currently disqualifying and taking sanctions against athletes who have a higher than 50% hematocrit (i.e., red blood cell concentration in blood) level.

Buffers

During high-intensity exercise, most of the energy in the body is produced by anaerobic metabolism, and lactic acid production increases. Lactic acid dissociates to lactate and hydrogen ions, and the accumulation of hydrogen ions can interfere with muscle contraction and exercise performance overall. The body contains several substances that can act as buffers (i.e., chemicals that prevent changes in pH by maintaining hydrogen ion homeostasis). However, the amount of naturally occurring buffers in the body might not be enough to counteract the increased hydrogen ions produced during exercise. Therefore, consumption of exogenous buffers has been practiced by athletes to improve exercise performance. The majority of the research studies have shown that consumption of a buffer (e.g., sodium bicarbonate) before high-intensity exercise can improve time to exhaustion; perhaps by maintaining pH homeostasis for a longer time. However, the use of exogenous buffers is banned by numerous sport agencies.

Caffeine

Caffeine is a natural product that can be found in numerous food items consumed daily. For example, coffee, carbonated cola drinks, and chocolate contain relatively high amounts of caffeine. Caffeine is a central nervous system stimulant and can play a role in improving exercise performance (17). Specifically, athletes who consume caffeine have a lower rate of perceived exertion and reduced perception of fatigue. Caffeine can also increase the mobilization of free fatty acids to be used for energy production; at the same time, this provides a glucose/glycogen sparing effect. Currently, the International Olympic Committee lists caffeine as a restricted drug where up to 12 μg/L (i.e., about eight cups of coffee) are allowed. Caffeine ingestion can also be associated with side effects that include high heart rate and blood pressure (Figure 9.7). Caffeine can also produce hypohydration since it is a potent diuretic (1).

Nitric Oxide Stimulators

In the past few years, several supplements have become available that are marketed as nitric oxide stimulators. Most of these supplements contain L-arginine, which can be the rate-limiting step for nitric oxide production in the body. Nitric oxide is a potent vasodilator and thus high levels can increase blood flow. The elevated blood flow can result in improved exercise performance since the delivery of oxygen and nutrients to the contracting skeletal muscles can be increased. However, the ergogenic benefits of such supplements have not been consistently proven in the current literature. Also, consuming supplements that contain L-arginine can result in adverse effects (e.g., palpitations, dizziness, syncope) requiring hospital admission. Therefore, the use of such supplements is not recommended as an ergogenic aid for healthy individuals.

Dietary Antioxidants

Numerous dietary antioxidants are consumed by athletes in an effort to improve exercise performance. The rationale for ingesting antioxidants stems from the notion that exercise can induce an increased level of reactive oxygen and nitrogen species production leading to increased oxidative stress. It has been shown that increased oxidative stress can be detrimental to exercise performance (14). However, it is also important to note that low and physiological levels of reactive oxygen and nitrogen species are required for maximal force production by

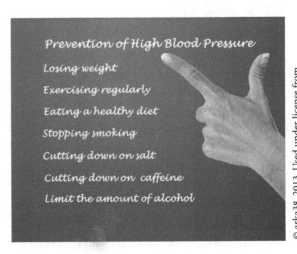

Figure 9.7. *Factors that can influence blood pressure.*

the contracting skeletal muscles. Therefore, consuming vast amounts of antioxidants can also result in reduced exercise performance.

N-acetylcysteine is a dietary antioxidant that prevents oxidative stress induced by skeletal muscle contractions. N-acetylcysteine increases the force generation of skeletal muscle; however, the ergogenic benefits of N-acetylcysteine in athletes have not been consistently shown. Also, N-acetylcysteine supplementation causes severe side effects (e.g., nausea and gastrointestinal distress), and therefore its practical use by athletes is limited.

Vitamin E is a lipid soluble dietary antioxidant that is commonly consumed by athletes in an effort to improve exercise performance. Vitamin E can prevent lipid oxidation and converts potent oxidants to less-harmful compounds. Although vitamin E supplementation can offer beneficial effects to certain groups of people, the use of high doses of vitamin E is currently not recommended. Even people with chronic vitamin E deficiency do not show reduced exercise performance.

Vitamin C is a water-soluble antioxidant and a very powerful scavenger of reactive oxygen species. Thus, physiological levels of vitamin C are paramount in maintaining overall health. However, when individuals consume large doses of vitamin C, harmful events can occur. Specifically, vitamin C can interact with the minerals iron and copper and actually promote increased oxidative stress. Therefore, athletes should avoid megadoses of vitamin C supplementation.

SUMMARY

Carbohydrates yield 4 kilocalories per gram, fat yield 9 kilocalories per gram, and protein yields 4 kilocalories per gram. About 60% of an athlete's diet should be from carbohydrates, 30% from fat, and 10% from protein.

There are two classes of vitamins: fat soluble and water soluble. Insufficient intake of any one of these vitamins can lead to deficiencies. Excessive intake of mainly fat-soluble vitamins can lead to vitamin toxicity.

There are two classes of minerals: macrominerals and microminerals. Athletes should consume the recommended dietary allowances of these minerals by eating a well-balanced diet.

Water is a vital nutrient, and it is required for optimal exercise performance. Athletes should always remember to adequately hydrate before, during, and after exercise.

Body composition of athletes should be monitored closely since it relates to exercise performance and overall health. There are different techniques available to determine body composition, but each offers advantages and disadvantages.

Numerous dietary supplements exist on the market. Some of them may offer an ergogenic benefit, but most of them do not.

REVIEW QUESTIONS

1. What are the six classes of nutrients?
2. Which nutrients can be used to produce energy? How much energy does each one of them produce?
3. What is the simplest form of carbohydrate?
4. What are the different forms of dietary fats?
5. What do the terms *essential* and *nonessential amino acids* mean?
6. Which are the essential and nonessential amino acids?
7. What are the two groups of vitamins?
8. What are the two groups of minerals?
9. Describe the proper hydration practices.
10. Compare and contrast the different techniques used to determine body composition.
11. What are ergogenic aids?
12. Discuss the effectiveness of the dietary supplements listed in this chapter.

REFERENCES

1. Armstrong, L. E., D. J. Casa, C. M. Maresh, and M. S. Ganio, "Caffeine, fluid-electrolyte balance, temperature regulation, and exercise-heat tolerance." *Exerc Sport Sci Rev* 35(3)(2007): 135–140.

2. Bonnick, S. L., and L. A. Lewis, *Bone Densitometry for Technologists.* Springer, 2013.

3. Brown, S. P,, W. C. Miller, and J. N. Eason, *Exercise Physiology. Basis of Human Movement in Health and Disease:* Lippincott Williams & Wilkins, 2006.

4. de Oliveira Otto, M. C., D. Mozaffarian, D. Kromhout, A. G. Bertoni, C. T. Sibley, D. R. Jacobs, Jr., and J. A. Nettleton, "Dietary intake of saturated fat by food source and incident cardiovascular disease: The Multi-Ethnic Study of Atherosclerosis." *American Journal of Clinical Nutrition* 96(2)(2012): 397–404.

5. Duke Medical Health News, "The considerable health benefits of fiber. Fiber helps prevent weight gain and disease, and enhances cardiovascular and gastrointestinal function." *Duke Medical Health News* 16(6) (2010): 6.

6. Eichner, E. R., "Blood doping: Infusions, erythropoietin and artificial blood." *Sports Medicine* 37(4–5) (2007): 389–391.

7. Fairchild, T. J., S. Fletcher, P. Steele, C. Goodman, B. Dawson, and P. A. Fournier, "Rapid carbohydrate loading after a short bout of near maximal-intensity exercise." *Med Sci Sports Exerc* 34(6)(2002): 980–986.

8. Hayman, R. M., and S. R. Dalziel, "Acute vitamin A toxicity: A report of three paediatric cases." *Journal of Paediatric and Child Health* 48(3)(2012): E98–100.

9. Heyward, V., *Advanced Fitness Assessment and Exercise Prescription.* Human Kinetics, 2010.

10. Heyward, V., and D. Wagner, *Applied Body Composition Assessment:* Human Kinetics, 2004.

11. Kyle, U. G., I. Bosaeus, A. D. De Lorenzo, P. Deurenberg, M. Elia, J. Manuel Gomez, . . . Espen, "Bioelectrical impedance analysis-part II: utilization in clinical practice." *Clinical Nutrition* 23(6)(2004): 1430–1453.

12. Pizza, F. X., M. G. Flynn, B. D. Duscha, J. Holden, and E. R. Kubitz, "A carbohydrate loading regimen improves high intensity, short duration exercise performance." *Internatioal Journal of Sport Nutrition* 5(2) (1995): 110–116.

13. Powers, S. K., and E. T. Howley, *Exercise Physiology. Theory and Application to Fitness and Performance.* New York: McGraw Hill, 2012.

14. Radak, Z., *Free Radicals in Exercise and Aging.* Human Kinetics, 2000.

15. Rodriguez, N. R., N. M. Di Marco, and S. Langley, "American College of Sports Medicine position stand. Nutrition and athletic performance." *Med Sci Sports Exerc* 41(3)(2009): 709–731.

16. Sun, F. H., S. H. Wong, Y. J. Huang, Y. J. Chen, and K. F. Tsang, "Substrate utilization during brisk walking is affected by glycemic index and fructose content of a pre-exercise meal." *European Journal of Applied Physiology* 112(7)(2012): 2565–2574.

17. Weinberg, B. A., and B. K. Bealer, *World of Caffeine: The Science and Culture of the World's Most Popular Drug.* New York: Routledge, 2002.

18. Wilmore, J., *Ergogenic Aids and Muscular Performance Oxygen.* Academic Press, 1972.

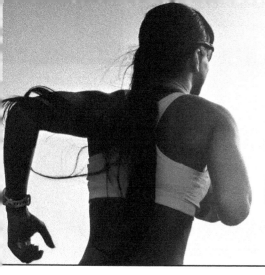

Chapter 10

PHYSICAL ACTIVITY EPIDEMIOLOGY

 OUTLINE

 OBJECTIVES

1. Appreciate the historical foundations of physical activity epidemiology.
2. Understand basic epidemiological terminology.
3. Understand basic epidemiological study designs.
4. Know current physical activity guidelines and how they were developed.

"If we could give every individual the right amount of nourishment and exercise, not too little and not too much, we would have found the safest way to health." ~Hippocrates

The term *epidemiology* is comprised of *epi–*, meaning upon, *–demos–*, meaning people, and *–ology* meaning the study of. Epidemiology is literally the study of what falls upon the people. Epidemiology is more commonly understood to mean the study of the distribution and determinants of health-related states or events in speci-fied populations (1). The field of epidemiology is rooted in the study of infectious diseases, most notably by the work of Dr. John Snow (1813–1858) during the cholera outbreak in London in 1854 (2). Snow combined (at the time) ground-breaking observational scientific data with logical reasoning techniques to determine how cholera spread throughout a community. The importance of this accomplishment is better realized when we consider that the bacteria that causes cholera was not discovered for another year, a vaccine was not developed for another 45 years, and antibiotics were not discovered until 1928! Snow observed that more cases occurred with closer proximity to the community water pump and only among people who drank the water from that pump. These conclusions led to the removal of the pump handle to prevent further consumption of the con-taminated water and, ultimately, ended the outbreak (2). The statistical mapping (Figure 10.1) of the disease and observational tools that Snow used in this landmark study are still used in present-day epidemiological investigations and unquestionably shaped the public health practices all over the world.

As treatment and prevention strategies for infectious diseases improved, morbidity (illness) and mortality (death) due to these diseases decreased. Epidemiologists turned their focus toward morbidity and mortality due to chronic diseases, such as heart disease. *Morbidity* refers to the illness or sickness associated with disease, and *mortality* refers to death (1). This shift in focus is the segue that eventually led to the inception of physi-cal activity epidemiology. Physical activity epidemiology is a subdiscipline of epidemiology that examines the role of physical activity in the development or prevention of various diseases. Dr. Jeremy Morris is credited with the first study to examine the influence of physical activity on health in his 1953 study of London munici-pal workers (3, 4). Morris examined drivers and conductors of the city's double-decker bus transportation

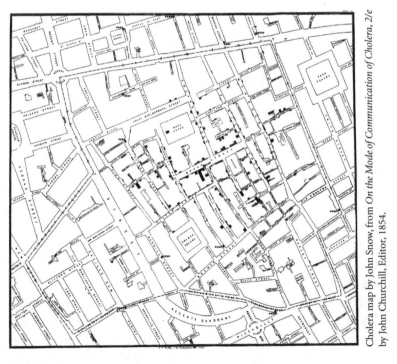

Cholera map by John Snow, from *On the Mode of Communication of Cholera, 2/e* by John Churchill, Editor, 1854.

Figure 10.1. *Original dot map, made by John Snow, illustrating cases of cholera in proximity to the community water pump (2).*

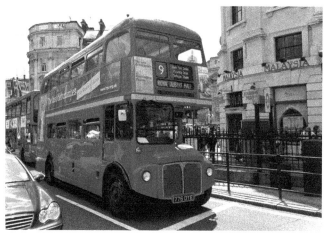

Figure 10.2. *Double-decker bus conductors walked the length of the bus and climbed up and down the stairs the stairs many times each day to collect passenger fares. This physical activity reduced their risk for CHD compared to the drivers who remained seated most of the day.*

system (Figure 10.2). The conductors' job responsibilities required them to walk the length of the bus and traverse the stairs many times each day to collect passenger fares. By comparison, conductors were much more active than the drivers, whose job required them to remain in the driver's seat. Incidence of coronary heart disease (CHD) among conductors was half that of the drivers. The concept of incidence and its utility in descriptive epidemiology is discussed later in the chapter, but the difference in health between the conductors and drivers is clear. Likewise this initial physical activity epidemiological study also showed that in addition to occupational physical activity levels, other factors may also be involved with the development of CHD. Because all of the workers got their uniforms at the same place, Dr. Morris was able to conclude that body size also played a role in the development of CHD, as evidenced by the smaller uniforms worn by the conductors (3, 4). Since this first study in 1953, physical activity epidemiologists have been working to better understand how physical activity act as both a preventive and treatment measure for improving health, all the while using the epidemiological principles stemming from Dr. Snow's work with cholera in the mid-19th century.

BASIC PRINCIPLES OF EPIDEMIOLOGY

As previously mentioned, epidemiology is the study of the distribution and determinants of health-related states or events in specified populations (1). Everything about epidemiology is very clearly defined and delimited. This emphasis on specificity allows epidemiologists a great deal of confidence when relating the findings of a study to the general population.

Epidemiology research is categorized in two major ways, either *descriptive* or *analytical* (5). As the name implies, the purpose of descriptive epidemiology is to describe. Descriptions are about the group being studied, and the sole purpose is to examine the distribution of variables of interest (1). The only research question being answered is, "What does the data look like?" This type of research is important to assess current health status of the group being studied. Two valuable pieces of information we gain from descriptive epidemiology are prevalence and incidence. When we assess *prevalence*, we are looking at the total number of individuals in the group being studied who exhibit a certain characteristic at a given point in time. For example, imagine you are interested in studying individuals in your *Fundamentals of Kinesiology* class. Your class is effectively a *cohort*, or study group of interest defined based on the defining criteria of being enrolled in the course. For the sake of this example, let's say you are interested in knowing the prevalence of flip-flop wearers. If there are 100 students in the class and 55 students are wearing flip-flops on the day you decide to do you prevalence study, then the prevalence of flip-flop wearers is 55%. *Incidence*, on the other hand, is an indicator of the number of new cases during a specified period of time. Using that same flip-flop example, imagine you assess the number of flip-flop wearers a week later and this time 75 of the 100 students are wearing flip-flops. The incidence of flip-flop wearers is 20% and the prevalence is now 75%. If flip-flop wearing was an adverse health condition, we might be concerned that the number of people wearing flip-flops is increasing so rapidly. However, since this was only an example to illustrate the concepts of prevalence and incidence, we need only be concerned that your classmates have adhered to proper sandal-wearing etiquette.

Analytical epidemiology allows us to determine relationships among variables and differences between groups. Ultimately, analytical epidemiology is used to explain *causality*. That is, does exposure to a certain variable cause a specific health outcome? We cannot experimentally make someone sick just to test if an exposure will act as an effective treatment. Likewise, in the case of prevention, if a person never develops a disease, we must have a way of determining if exposure to some specific variable actually helped prevent the disease or was it merely a coincidence that a person was exposed and did not develop the disease. To remedy this issue, researchers employ a set of criteria, commonly referred to as causal criteria. A few variations of causal criteria have been postulated, but the one most frequently used in physical activity epidemiology literature are those from the work of John Stuart Mill from work in 1875 (6). Contemporary adaptation of this work, referred to as Mill's Canons, suggest five causal criteria: (a) temporal sequence, (b) strength of association, (c) consistency, (d) dose response, and (e) biological plausibility (7) (Box 10.1). Every research study conducted examining the influence of physical activity on health addresses one or more of these criteria. In a sense, you can think of it as gathering the evidence to make the case that physical activity is beneficial to health. In fact, epidemiologists use the term *evidence-based medicine* and *evidence-based public health* to describe the application of the best available evidence when setting patient care and public health policies and practices (1).

Analytical epidemiology employs a variety of study designs to address causal criteria. When discussing study designs, it is important to establish the concepts of independent and dependent variables first. Independent variables, sometimes called exposure variables, are the variables that are being examined for their potential influence on the outcome. Dependent variables, also called outcome variables, are the variables in the study for which the value is influenced by the independent variables.

In addition to independent and dependent variables, epidemiologists are also concerned with *third variables*. When we consider the relationship between the independent and dependent variables, rare is the case when the independent variable causes the effect observed in the dependent variable without any influence from any other variable. Third variables are those other variables of interest in a study. There are three types of third variables: mediating, moderating, and confounding variables. *Mediating variables* are variables that occur in the causal pathway between the independent and dependent variables. *Moderating variables* are variables the presence or absence of which results in variation in the relationship between the independent and dependent variables. *Confounding variables* are variables that, because of their common relationship with both the independent and dependent variables, cause an artificial relationship between the independent and dependent variables.

BOX 10.1   Causal Criteria Using Mill's Canons

Temporal sequence: Exposure to the variable of interest must precede the development of the disease with enough for the disease to develop.

Strength of association: A large and clinically meaningful difference must exist when comparing the risk of developing the disease between those exposed and those not exposed to the variable of interest.

Consistency: The observed association between the variable of interest and the disease is always observed if the variable of interest is present; repeated in the literature in people of different age, gender, ethnicity, and race.

Dose response: The risk of developing the disease increases proportionately with greater exposure to the variable of interest.

Biological plausibility: The observed association between the variable of interest and the disease is explainable by existing knowledge about possible biological mechanisms.

The way in which the independent, dependent, and third variables are examined determines the research question. Each study design is able to answer a specific research question and is applied accordingly.

Cross-Sectional Study Design

Cross-sectional studies are like taking a snapshot of the individuals being studied. The independent and dependent variables are measured at the same time. This study design is ideal for determining prevalence and incidence and is effectively used in descriptive epidemiology. Because the time-order of variables cannot be determined in this design, when applied to analytical epidemiology, a cross-sectional study can only show relationships, there is no way to infer cause and effect.

Case-Control Study Design

Case-control studies compare the probability of developing a disease in participants who were exposed to a risk factor relative to participants who were not exposed. A *risk factor* is any variable known to increase the probability of developing a disease (1). Typically, participants are selected into a study based on the presence of a disease and then compared to non-diseased controls according to the odds of past exposure to a risk factor (5). Case-control studies can be retrospective, present time, or prospective. Because of the nature of the participant selection in this study, only one disease can be studied at a time.

Prospective Cohort Study Design

As suggested by the flip-flop example earlier in the chapter, participants in this type of study are identified as a member of a group based on some defining characteristic. The term *prospective* infers that this cohort of participants will be followed in to the future. Prospective cohort studies can be analyzed as a series of cross-sectional studies or longitudinally. This type of study design has issues with maintaining the all of the original cohort members through additional follow-ups, particularly in studies that span several decades.

Randomized Controlled Trial Study Design

Randomized controlled trials are truly experimental in design. Potential participants are thoroughly screened to determine their eligibility. Eligibility criteria are specific to each study, but very strictly monitored and adherence is required. Participants who are selected to be in the study are randomly assigned to groups that either receive an experimental manipulation or control condition. Baseline and follow-up assessments of all of the variables of interest are conducted and used to determine magnitude of the change due to the experimental manipulation. Randomized controlled trials tend to be expensive because all of the independent variables being studied must be closely monitored in the experimental and control groups to ensure that any differences in dependent variables are actually due to the prescribed dose of the experimental group. Because this type of study design is so stringently restricted to certain participation eligibility criteria and experimental manipulation, the findings from these studies are sometimes difficult to generalize to the average population.

PHYSICAL ACTIVITY ASSESSMENT, GUIDELINES, AND SURVEILLANCE

Regardless of the study design, researchers must be very deliberate in the methods they choose to assess the variables of interests in each study. Perhaps the most important variable to a physical activity epidemiologist is *physical activity*. Physical activity is defined as any bodily movement produced by skeletal muscles that results in an increase in energy expenditure above resting rate (8). This broad definition allows the researcher a considerable amount of latitude in the description and categorization of physical activity. Physical activity can be weight-bearing, non-weight-bearing, occupational, leisure-time, continuous, intermittent, organized or nonorganized. Physical activity can also be (and is most commonly) categorized by the type, frequency, duration, and intensity of the activity. When describing and measuring physical activity, it is important not to confuse the term with similar and related variables such exercise and fitness. *Exercise* is described as planned, structured, and repetitive bodily movement done to improve or maintain one or more components of physical fitness (9). By definition, exercise is physical activity, but physical activity does not have to be exercise.

While physical activity and exercise refer to behaviors, *physical fitness* refers to a set of physiological attributes and is categorized as either health- or skill-related. Skill-related fitness is comprised of agility, balance, coordination, power, reaction time, and speed and is related to performance of motor skills associated with athletic ability. Health-related fitness consists of body composition, aerobic fitness, flexibility, muscular endurance, and strength. (See Chapter 22 for an expansion of this concept.)

Given the well-established connection with health outcomes, aerobic fitness receives considerable attention relative to the other components. Aerobic fitness is a physiological characteristic that reflects the maximal amount of oxygen utilized (8). The multifactorial nature of physical activity and its distinct difference from related terms can make assessment challenging.

Several techniques (surveys and questionnaires, pedometers, accelerometers) are commonly used to assess physical activity. However, a detailed account of each of these methods is beyond the scope of this chapter (see *Medicine and Science in Sports and Exercise, vol. 29, Supplement 6*). Likewise, several excellent reviews are available that examine the relative precision and practicality of the available assessment tools (10–14). In general, physical activity assessments can be thought of as using a continuum of those instruments that are high practicality/lower accuracy (surveys, questionnaires) to low practicality/higher accuracy (direct observation, accelerometer). Large studies or limited funding may motivate a researcher to sacrifice some accuracy for a more feasible method of assessing physical activity. Nonetheless, several excellent tools are available at all locations along the continuum and selection of the most appropriate one should be considered early on in the design of the study.

The intensity of physical activity receives a great deal of attention in physical activity epidemiological research, as it is most applicable to health-related research. The descriptive terms "very light," "light," "moderate," "hard," "very hard," and "maximal" have been matched to relative percentages of maximal aerobic capacity or assigned metabolic equivalent (MET) values as a means of standardizing the classification of physical activity (15). This classification system is used as the basis for recommendations designed to improve or maintain health and cardiorespiratory fitness.

The U.S. Department of Health and Human Services published the *2008 Physical Activity Guidelines for Americans*, which provides detailed recommendations for all age groups (16). Any physical activity epidemiologist would agree that this is one of the most significant advances in the field of physical activity epidemiology as it is the first comprehensive guidelines on physical activity to be issued by the federal government. Until these federal guidelines we relied on the recommendations of leading organizations like the American College of Sports Medicine and the American Heart Association (17), or consensus statements from experts in the field (18). The *2008 Physical Activity Guidelines for Americans* have age-appropriate recommendations for children (aged 6–17 years), adults (aged 18–64 years), and older adults (aged 65 and older) (Table 10.1).

Current recommendations for children and adolescents require school-aged youth to participate in at least 60 minutes of physical activity daily. It is recommended that the majority of that 60 minutes be spent participating in activities that are of moderate-to-vigorous intensity and aerobic. Furthermore, the recommendations suggest that at least three of the days should be at a vigorous intensity. Muscle- and bone-strengthening activities should also be incorporated as part of the 60 minutes of activity at least three days each week (16).

Current recommendations for adults (aged 18–64 years) suggest that they should avoid inactivity and reinforces the notion that some physical activity is better than none, and adults who participate in any amount of physical activity gain some health benefits. Additionally, the Guidelines suggest that substantial health benefits can be gained if adults do at least 150 minutes a week of moderate-intensity, or 75 minutes a week

Table 10.1. 2008 Physical Activity Guidelines for Americans.

Age	Recommendation
Children & Adolescents (6–17)	60 minutes or more of physical activity every day (moderate- or vigorous-intensity aerobic physical activity). Vigorous-intensity activity at least three days per week. Muscle-strengthening and bone-strengthening activity at least three days per week.
Adults (18–64)	150 minutes a week of moderate-intensity, or 75 minutes a week of vigorous-intensity aerobic physical activity Muscle-strengthening activities that involve all major muscle groups performed on two or more days per week.
Older Adults (65+)	Follow the adult guidelines, or be as physically active as possible. Avoid inactivity. Exercises that maintain or improve balance if at risk of falling.

of vigorous-intensity, aerobic physical activity, or an equivalent combination of moderate- and vigorous intensity aerobic activity. It is recommended that the aerobic activity should be performed in episodes of at least 10 minutes, and preferably, it should be spread throughout the week. Further, adults may enjoy additional and more extensive health benefits should they increase their aerobic physical activity to 300 minutes a week of moderate intensity, or 150 minutes a week of vigorous intensity aerobic physical activity, or an equivalent combination of moderate- and vigorous-intensity activity and additional health benefits are gained by engaging in physical activity beyond this amount. Adults should also do muscle-strengthening activities that are moderate or high intensity and involve all major muscle groups on two or more days a week, as these activities provide additional health benefits (16).

The guidelines for adults also apply to older adults (aged 65 and older). Additionally, older adults should be as physically active as their abilities and conditions allow when they cannot do the recommended 150 minutes of moderate-intensity aerobic activity a week because of chronic conditions. Likewise, older adults should do exercises that maintain or improve balance and determine their level of effort for physical activity relative to their level of fitness. Older adults with chronic conditions should understand whether and how their conditions affect their ability to do regular physical activity safely (16).

PHYSICAL ACTIVITY EPIDEMIOLOGY IN TRANSLATIONAL MEDICINE

Recent data suggest that approximately 65% of U.S. adults are overweight or obese, which represents an increase of 16% from previous estimates (19). A similar trend is also observed in the pediatric population, where the prevalence of overweight and obesity among 6- to 19-year-olds is approximately 32% (20). This trend is not limited to the United States, as obesity rates are increasing globally, particularly in developed countries (21). Approximately 1.1 billion adults are estimated to be overweight or obese worldwide (21). Given that obesity is a global public health concern, it is a condition that holds considerable promise in the realm of *translational medicine*. Translational medicine is the integration of research from multiple disciplines (basic sciences and social sciences) for the purposes of improving patient care and health outcomes. The potential for a multidisciplinary approach to addressing obesity is intensified when we consider the co-morbidities that tend to cluster with obesity.

The constellation of abdominal obesity, insulin resistance, elevated triglycerides and blood pressure, and low high-density lipoprotein cholesterol (HDL-C) constitute a condition that is referred to as *metabolic syndrome*. Persons with metabolic syndrome are at greater risk for CVD (22–25), with a recent meta-analysis (26) suggesting the risk to be almost twofold. In addition to CVD, metabolic syndrome is also associated with a number of other adverse health conditions, such as polycystic ovary syndrome, non-alcoholic fatty liver disease, gallbladder disease, sleep disorders, impotence, endothelial dysfunction, osteoarthritis, psychosocial dysfunction, and some types of cancer (23, 27).

The evidence for the beneficial relationship between physical activity and obesity and/or metabolic syndrome is clear (28–31). The challenge is in translating that evidence into practice. As we progress in the field of physical activity epidemiology, researchers must consider a comprehensive, multidimensional approach in determining the causal pathways involved in the development of obesity and metabolic syndrome. As human behavior and the activity (or inactivity) of individuals is constantly fluctuating, the field of epidemiology is an ever-changing and dynamic field with plenty of opportunities for research and employment.

SUMMARY

This chapter examined the fundamental historical perspective of physical activity epidemiology and its influence on present-day research in the field. This chapter also provided an overview of basic epidemiological principles and terminology. Additionally, the federal guidelines for physical activity are discussed as well as their significance to the field of physical activity epidemiology.

REFERENCES

1. Last, J.M., International Epidemiological Association. *A dictionary of epidemiology*, 4th ed. New York: Oxford University Press, 2001, xx.

2. Snow, J., *On the mode of communication of cholera*, 2nd ed. London: J. Churchill, 1855, vii, 1.

3. Morris, J. N., J. A. Heady, P. A. Raffle, C. G. Roberts, and J. W. Parks, "Coronary heart-disease and physical activity of work." *Lancet* 265(6796)(1953): 1111–1120; concl. Epub 1953/11/28.

4. Morris, J. N., J. A. Heady, P. A. Raffle, C. G. Roberts, and J. W. Parks, "Coronary heart-disease and physical activity of work." *Lancet* 265(6795)(1953): 1053–1057; contd. Epub 1953/11/21.

5. Szklo, M., Nieto FJ. Epidemiology: beyond the basics. Sudbury, Mass.: Jones and Bartlett; 2004. xvi, 495 p. p.

6. Mill JS. The logic of the moral sciences. La Salle, IL: Open Court Pub. Co.; 1988. 144 p. p.

7. Dishman RK, Heath G, Lee IM. Physical activity epidemiology. 2nd ed. Champaign, IL: Human Kinetics; 2013. xxii, 585 p. p.

8. Casperson CJ, Powell KE, Christenson GM. Physical activity, exercise, and physical fitness: definitions and distinctions for health-related reserch. Public Health Rep. 1985; 100: 126–30.

9. American College of Sports Medicine., Thompson WR, Gordon NF, Pescatello LS. ACSM's guidelines for exercise testing and prescription. 8th ed. Philadelphia: Lippincott Williams & Wilkins; 2010. xxi, 380 p. p.

10. Ainsworth BE, Montoye HJ, Leon AS. Methods of assessing physical activity during leisure and work. Bouchard C, Shephard RJ, Stephens T, Sutton JR, McPherson BD, editors. Champaign, IL: Human Kinetics; 1994. 146–59 p.

11. Melanson EL Jr, Freedson P. Physical activity assessment: A review of methods. Critical Reviews in Food Science and Nutrition. 1996; 36: 385–96.

12. Wareham NJ, Riennie KL. The assessment of physical activity in individuals and populations: Why try to be more precise about how physical activity is assessed? Int J Obes Relat Metab Disord. 1998; 22: S30–S8.

13. Baranowski T, Simmons-Morton BG. Children's physical activity and dietary assessments: Measurement issues. Journal of School Health. 1991; 61: 195–7.

14. Pate RR. Physical activity assessment in children and adolescents. Crit Rev Food Sci Nutr. 1993; 33: 321–6.

15. Howley ET. Type of activity: Resistance, aerobic and leisure versus occupational physical activity. Med Sci Sports Exerc. 2001; 31: S364–S9.

16. Physical Activity Guidelines Advisory Committee. Physical activity guidelines advisory committee report, 2008. Washington, DC: 2008.

17. Haskell WL, Lee I, Pate RR, Powell KE, Blair SN, Franklin BA, et al. Physical activity and public health: Updated recommendation for adults from the American College of Sport Medicine and the American Heart Association. Med Sci Sports Exerc. 2007; 39: 1423–34.

18. Strong WB, Malina RM, Blimkie CJR, Daniels SR, Dishman RK, Gutin B, et al. Evidence Based Physical Activity for School-age Youth. J Pediatr. 2005; 146(6): 732–7.

19. Flegal KM, Carroll M, Ogden C, Johnson C. Prevalence and trends in obesity among US adults, 1999-2000. JAMA. 2002; 288: 1723–7.

20. Hedley A, Ogden C, Johnson C, Carroll M, Curtin L, K F. Prevalence of overweight and obesity among US children, adolescents, and adults, 199-2002. JAMA. 2004; 291: 2847–50.

21. Haslam DW, James WP. Obesity. Lancet. 2005; 366: 1197–209.

22. Tillin T, Forouhi N, Johnston DG, McKeigue PM, Chaturvedi N, Godsland IF. Metabolic syndrome and coronary heart disease in South Asians, African-Caribbeans and white Europeans: a UK population-based cross-sectional study. Diabetalogia. 2005; 48: 649–56.

23. Grundy SM, Cleeman J, Daniels SR, et al. Diagnosis and management of the metabolic syndrome: an American Heart Association/National Heart, Lung and Blood Institute scientific statement. Circulation. 2005; 112: 2735–52.

24. McNeil AM, Rosamond WD, Girman CJ, Heiss G, Golden SH, Duncan BB, et al. Prevalence of coronary heart disease and carotid atrerial thickening in patients with the metabolic syndrome (The ARIC study). Am J Cardiol. 2004; 94: 1249–54.

25. Lakka HM, Laaksonen DE, Lakka TA, Niskanen LK, Kumpusalo E, Tuomilehto J, et al. The metabolic syndrome and total and cardiovascular mortality in middle-aged men. JAMA. 2002; 288: 2709–16.

26. Gami AS, Witt BJ, Howard DE, et al. Metabolic syndrome and risk of incident cardiovascular events and death: a systematic review and meta-analysis of longitudinal studies. J Am Coll Cardiol. 2007;49:403–14.

27. Bray GA, Bellanger T. Epidemiology, trends, and morbidities of obesity and the metabolic syndrome. Endocrine. 2006; 29: 109–17.

28. Despres J-P, Bouchard C, Malina RM. Physical activity and coronary heart disease risk factors during childhood and adolescents. Exerc Sport Sci Rev. 1990; 18: 243–61.

29. Blair SN, Clark DG, Cureton KJ, Powell KE. Exercise and fitness in childhood: implications for a lifetime of health. In: Gisolfi CV, Lamb DR, editors. Perspectives in Exercise Science and Sports Medicine. Indianapolis, IN: Benchmark; 1989. p. 401–31.

30. Riddoch C. Relationships between physical activity and physical health in young people. In: Biddle S, Sallis J, Cavill N, editors. Young and Active? Young People and Health-enhancing Physical Activity—Evidence and Implications. London: Health Education Authority; 1998. p. 17–48.

31. Sallis JF. Epidemiology of physical activity and fitness in children and adolescents. Crit Rev Food Sci Nutr. 1993; 33: 403–8.

Section 3

STRUCTURAL/MECHANICAL KNOWLEDGE BASE

To understand human movement requires a grasp of the body beyond that of the physiological and chemical. Historically, the study of kinesiology coupled anatomy with principles and concepts from physics, the marriage of which created what we know today as biomechanics. This section focuses on concepts important to anyone interested in how the body moves. Regarding health care, this has obvious application to the medical profession and fields such as occupational and physical therapy, ergonomics, athletic training, along with others falling under the kinesiology umbrella.

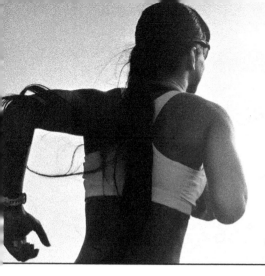

Chapter 11

APPLIED ANATOMY

OUTLINE

Objectives

Reference Terminology

    Terms of Relationship and Comparison

    Terms of Laterality

    Terms of Movement

Osteology

    Skeletal Functions

    Bone Markings and Formations

Structure of Bone

Types of Bones

    Articulations (Joints)

Roles of Muscles

    Actions of Muscles

Summary

References

OBJECTIVES

1. Gain a better understanding of anatomical terminology.
2. Describe and name fundamental movement patterns.
3. Examine factors that contribute to joint stability and range of motion.
4. Define the planes of the body and axes of motion.
5. Investigate bone function, bone markings, and types of bone.
6. Identify the roles and types of contractions of muscles.

Applied anatomy is defined as that aspect of the discipline of anatomy important for a sound understanding of basic structure and how these structures produce movement. Applied anatomy integrates the components of skeletal structure and function in the practice of medicine, dentistry, and allied health. From the standpoint of gross movement, applied anatomy is a foundational science for kinesiology students.

There are a number of approaches to studying anatomy (Greek—dissection). The three main ways are regional anatomy, systemic anatomy, and applied anatomy. *Regional anatomy* is the method of studying body structures by investigating a specific part (thigh, knee) with its associated structures (nerves, muscles, and bones). *Systemic anatomy* is the method of studying anatomy that investigates each body system and its associated structures (muscular system, nervous system). *Applied anatomy* (clinical anatomy) centers on movement and from that standpoint is a foundational discipline to kinesiology. It incorporates the regional and systemic approaches, but unlike these previous two systems, applied anatomy stresses the clinical application (7). A good analogy would be to compare a physician with a police detective. They both have a certain amount of information, now they must determine what has happened and the appropriate course of action. In a physician's case a patient may be experiencing decreased muscular activity in a certain limb, which could indicate a problem in the nervous system or muscular system. The physician then must prescribe the appropriate tests in order to make a final diagnosis. Applied anatomy may also provide a teacher, coach, researcher, or therapist with valuable information on how a movement is produced to guide training and conditioning techniques.

REFERENCE TERMINOLOGY

It is important for anyone studying anatomy to begin with a reference point. This reference point is generally referred to as the *anatomical position*. The anatomical position has been a standard of reference for many years for anatomists, biomechanists, and the medical professions. In this position, the body is upright, with the head facing forward, arms at the side of the trunk with the palms facing forward, and the legs together with the feet pointing forward. Instead of this reference position, some anatomists prefer to utilize the fundamental starting position, which is similar to the anatomical position except that the palms are at the sides facing in toward the trunk (a more natural position than the anatomical position). However, no matter which starting position is used, all movement analyses are made according to a standard starting position (Figure 11.1) (4).

Anatomy, like other disciplines, has a language that is unique and can be initially intimidating. The Greeks and Romans were the first civilizations to allow the human body to be studied through dissection. Therefore, many anatomical terms have names with Greek or Latin origins and reflect information about the shape, size, function, and location of a structure. For instance, the term *condyle*, which is the Latin word for knuckle, refers to an articulating surface of a joint because to the early anatomist, it resembled the knuckles on the hand. The deltoid muscle of the shoulder received its name because it resembled the Greek letter delta to the early anatomist (8).

Terms of Relationship and Comparison

The term *anterior* refers to the front of the body. The term *ventral* can be used interchangeably with anterior and is often used when referring to the front of the spinal cord. Structures located on the anterior side of the body include the sternum, the nose, and the patella. An anterior view of the body can be seen in Figure 11.1. The opposite of anterior is *posterior*, which refers to the back of the body. The term *dorsal* can be used interchangeably with posterior. Structures on the posterior side of the body include the vertebrae, scapula, and calcaneus. These terms can also be used to compare different anatomical structures. The biceps femoris is posterior to the quadriceps, and the quadriceps is anterior to the biceps femoris. A posterior view of the body can be seen in Figure 11.2.

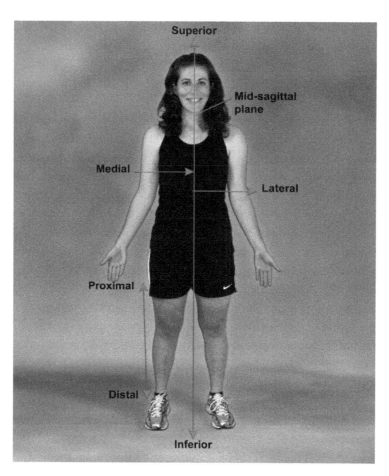

Figure 11.1. *Anterior view of the body.*

Superior refers to the top of the body (near the head), while inferior refers to the bottom of the body (near the feet). The heart would be superior to the liver, while the ankle would be inferior to the knee. *Medial* refers to a structure that is close to the midline of the body. The midline is an imaginary line that divides the body into equal left and right halves. The nose and sternum are medial structures. *Lateral* refers to a structure that is away from the midline, such as the ears. Medial and lateral are often used to define different sides of a joint. The medial side of the knee is closest to the midline, and this is where the medial collateral ligament is located, while the lateral side of the knee is the side farthest away from the midline, and this is where the lateral collateral ligament is located.

Proximal is a term that refers to a structure being near the trunk or to the point of origin. *Distal* refers to a structure being farther away from the trunk or the point of origin. For example, when looking at the joints of the upper extremity, the shoulder is proximal to both the elbow and wrist, because it is closest to the point of origin of the arm. The elbow and wrist would both be distal to the shoulder, because they are farther away from the point of origin. The hip would be proximal to the knee and ankle, and the ankle would be distal to both the knee and hip. Proximal and distal are also used to describe the attachments of tendons. The proximal attachment of the rectus femoris muscle is on the pelvis (anterior inferior iliac spine), while the distal attachment of the rectus femoris is on the tibia (tibial tuberosity).

Palmar refers to the palm of the hand, while *plantar* refers to the sole or undersurface of the foot. *Volar* can be used to refer to both the palm of the hand and the sole of the foot. *Supine* refers to a position where the person is lying on his or her back, facing upward, while *prone* refers to a position where the person is lying on his or her stomach, facing downward. *Superficial* refers to a structure toward the surface of the body, while *deep*

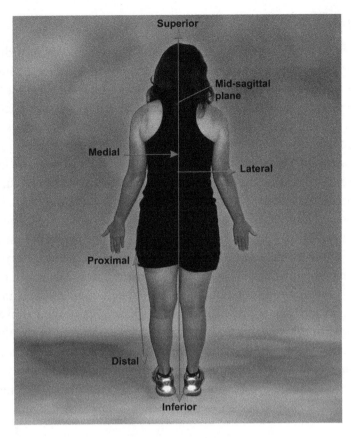

Figure 11.2.   *Posterior view of the body.*

refers to beneath the surface of the body. Skin would be superficial to bone, and bone would be deep to muscle. Superficial and deep are often used to describe the position of muscles, such as the soleus muscle is deep to the gastrocnemius, and the biceps brachii is superficial to the brachialis.

Any of the aforementioned terms can be combined to refer to a structure, generally by the addition of a combining vowel, such as the letter "o." The term *anteromedial* would refer to a structure that is located on the front of the body and toward the midline, such as the nose and sternum. *Superolateral* would refer to a structure near the head and away from the midline, such as the ears (3).

Terms of Laterality

Some structures have left and right members (kidneys), which is referred to as a *bilateral* relationship; however, some structures occur only on one side of the body (spleen), which is referred to as being *unilateral*. These terms are also used by health care professionals during examinations. For instance, if an athletic trainer is examining a patient who has sustained a knee injury, he or she will examine the uninjured knee first to establish normal parameters. With this base information, the trainer then examines the injured knee. This procedure is designated as bilateral examination of the knees. Other terms include *ipsilateral* and *contralateral*. Ipsilateral refers to the same side of the body, and contralateral refers to the opposite side of the body. For example, if an athlete who has previously sprained her right ankle also sprains her right knee, this knee sprain would be on the ipsilateral side. If she were to sprain her left knee instead of her right knee, this injury would be on the contralateral side (7).

Terms of Movement

When analyzing the various joint movements, it is helpful to group them according to specific planes of motion. A plane of motion is defined as an imaginary two-dimensional surface through which a limb or body segment is moved. A sound knowledge of the planes of motion makes it much easier to analyze human movement. There are three specific planes of motion in which joint movements can be classified. The specific planes that divide the body into halves are referred to as cardinal planes. The cardinal planes are the sagittal plane, the frontal plane, and the transverse plane (Figure 11.3). The *sagittal* (Latin for arrow) plane, also known as the *anteroposterior* plane, is a vertical plane that bisects the body from front to back, dividing it into right and left symmetrical halves. Generally, flexion and extension movements such as dumbbell curls (Figure 11.4), bending the knee, and sit-ups occur in this plane. The *frontal* plane, also known as the *coronal* plane, is a vertical plane that bisects the body into two symmetrical front (anterior) and back (posterior) halves. Generally, abduction and adduction movements (Figure 11.5) such as jumping jacks and bending from side to side at the waist occur in this plane. The *transverse* plane, also known as the *horizontal* plane, bisects the body from front to back dividing the body into upper (superior) and lower (inferior) halves. Generally, rotation movements such as forearm *pronation* and *supination* and rotating the spine to the right or left occur in this plane (Figure 11.6).

Most movements occur in a combination of the three planes mentioned above. These movements are said to occur in the *oblique* or *diagonal* plane. If movement only occurred in the three cardinal planes, our movements would be similar to a robot's, which would be inefficient and decrease range of motion. For instance, if you were reaching with your right hand for a coffee cup in a cabinet above your head and to the left, the motion would be a combination of shoulder flexion (sagittal plane) and shoulder internal rotation (transverse plane).

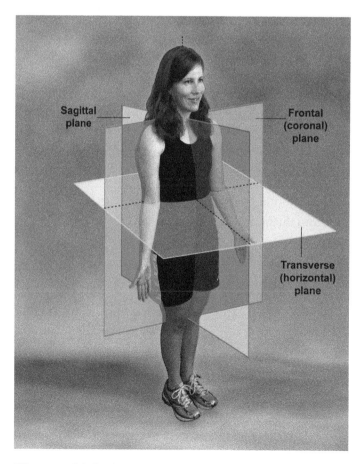

Figure 11.3. *The three cardinal planes of movement.*

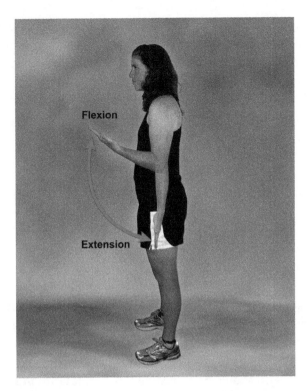

Figure 11.4. *Elbow flexion and extension occur in the sagittal plane about a bilateral axis.*

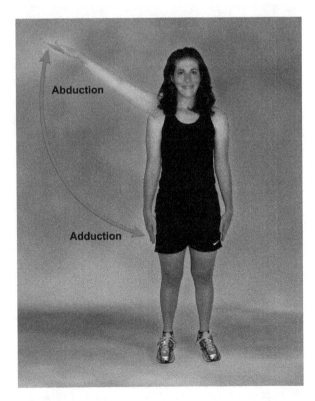

Figure 11.5. *Shoulder abduction and adduction take place in the frontal plane about anteroposterior axis.*

As motion occurs in a given plane, the joint turns around an axis that has a perpendicular relationship to that plane. The axes are named in relationship to their orientation. The four axes include the *bilateral* axis, the *anteroposterior* axis, the *longitudinal* axis, and the *diagonal* axis. Therefore, it can be stated that motion occurs in a plane and about an axis perpendicular to that plane.

The bilateral (also known as the frontal or coronal) axis runs perpendicular to the sagittal plane. Since sagittal plane movements such as flexion and extension occur in an anterior to posterior manner, this axis must run from one side of the body to the other. As the elbow flexes and extends during the motion of a dumbbell curl (Figure 11.4), the forearm rotates about a bilateral axis that runs from the lateral side of the elbow to the medial side of the elbow.

The anterior-posterior axis runs perpendicular to the frontal plane. The primary frontal plane movements are abduction and adduction (Figure 11.5), such as when the shoulder moves away from and then toward the midline. Therefore, the axis for this motion must run from the front of the joint through the back of the joint. The longitudinal, or vertical axis, runs perpendicular to the transverse plane. Most rotational movements, such as internal/external rotation (Figure 11.6) and pronation/supination occur in the transverse plane. As the femur rotates about the pelvis, the axis for this movement runs from the top to the bottom of the femur. The fourth axis, which is the diagonal or oblique axis, runs perpendicular to the diagonal plane. When kicking a ball, the hip moves into a combination of extension and abduction during the backswing and a combination of flexion and adduction during the forward swing. This creates a diagonal motion, and the femur would rotate about the diagonal axis.

When describing joint motion, it should be noted that movement terms indicate the actual change in position of the bones relative to each other with the actual movement occurring in the joint between the articulating surfaces. Depending on the bony arrangement of the joint and the responsibilities of the joint, some joints allow several different movements (shoulder), while others only one movement (elbow). In addition, there is

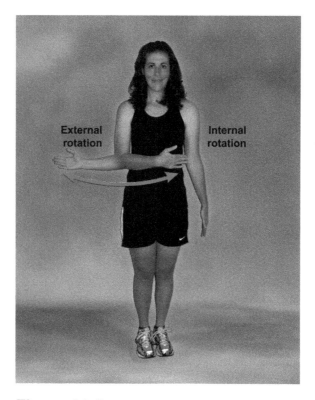

Figure 11.6. *Shoulder internal and external rotation take place in the transverse plane about a longitudinal axis.*

wide variation in the amount of range of motion joints will allow. For instance, the shoulder allows the greatest range of motion, while the joints in the skull allow no motion. Range of motion is dependent on the joint structure, the musculature that surrounds the joint, and associated ligaments (3).

The prefixes *hypo* and *hyper* are movement terms. *Hypo* indicates movement below the normal range of motion, and *hyper* indicates excessive range of motion past normal. Of these terms, *hyperextension* is most commonly used, such as what happens in a whiplash injury during a rear-end automobile collision. When analyzing the movements of a dancer, basketball player, or gymnast, it can seem difficult to identify and classify the various movements. However, if one body segment is taken individually and placed in the correct anatomical position, the task is greatly simplified. When simple movements are combined, they formulate the different patterns for skills such as walking, kicking, throwing a baseball, or performing a handstand. It may seem like activities such chopping firewood, hitting a baseball, sawing logs, or driving a golf ball are completely unrelated. However, their actions are a combination of several simpler motions (7).

General Joint Actions

There are several joint actions that occur at multiple joints. These joint actions are presented in pairs. *Flexion* is a decrease in the angle of the joint, and *extension* is an increase in the angle of the joint. Flexion can also be thought of as a movement that "rolls" the body into the fetal position, while extension is a movement that brings the body out of the fetal position. When a person stands up from a seated position, there is knee extension. The angle between the upper leg and the lower leg increases. When a person sits down in a chair, there is knee flexion. The angle between the upper leg and the lower leg decreases. Likewise, the elbow flexes during the upward phase of a dumbbell curl, and the elbow extends during the downward phase of the movement. Flexion and extension occur in the sagittal plane about a bilateral axis. Other joints where flexion and extension occur are the hip, shoulder, wrist, fingers, toes, neck, and trunk. An example of shoulder flexion and extension can be seen in Figure 11.7.

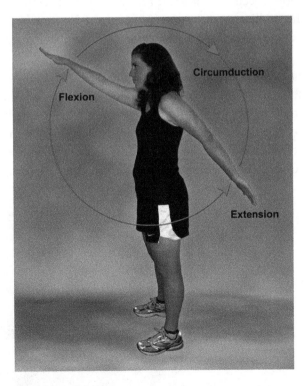

Figure 11.7.   *Flexion and extension of the shoulder.*

Abduction and adduction are motions that take place in the frontal plane about an anteroposterior axis. In abduction, the segment moves away from the midline in the frontal plane, and for adduction, the segment moves toward the midline in the frontal plane. Abduction and adduction take place at the shoulder and the hip during jumping jacks (Figure 11.5). *Circumduction* is a combination of movements that occurs at the hip and shoulder. Circumduction refers to a circular movement at the end of a segment that combines flexion, extension, abduction, and adduction (Figure 11.7).

Horizontal abduction and horizontal adduction are movements that take place in the transverse plane about a longitudinal axis. These motions occur at the hip and shoulder. With the segment flexed, movement toward the midline is horizontal adduction, and movement away from the midline is horizontal abduction. During the upward phase of the bench press, there is horizontal adduction at the shoulder, and during the downward phase, there is horizontal abduction. Internal and external rotation, when occurring from the anatomical starting position, takes place in the transverse plane about a longitudinal axis. Internal rotation is when the anterior surface of the bone, such as the humerus or femur, rotates toward the midline, and external rotation is when the anterior surface rotates away from the midline. These motions primarily occur at the hip and the shoulder as well. When someone throws a ball, the shoulder externally rotates during the cocking phase, and internally rotates during the acceleration phase (2).

Specific Joint Motions

There are several joint actions that only occur at a specific joint. At the ankle, the terms *dorsiflexion* and *plantar flexion* are used instead of flexion and extension. Dorsiflexion occurs when there is a decrease in the angle between the lower leg and the dorsum of the foot. This can occur when a person pulls his toes toward his lower leg (Figure 11.8), or when a person squats down and the lower leg moves toward the top of the foot. Plantar flexion occurs when the angle between the lower leg and the dorsum of the foot increases. This can occur when a person points her toes down (Figure 11.9), or when a person stands up from a squatted or seated position. Two additional motions specific to the ankle are *inversion* and *eversion*. Inversion is when the bottom of the foot moves toward the midline, and eversion is when the bottom of the foot moves away from the midline (Figure 11.9). Many ankle sprains occur when a person "rolls" her ankle and has an excessive amount of inversion.

Pronation and *supination* occur at the proximal radioulnar joint, which is located just below the elbow. During these motions, the radius will pivot about the ulna. Supination is when the radius rotates laterally about the ulna. This causes the palm to face up or anterior. Pronation is when the radius rotates medially about the ulna. This causes the palm to face down or posterior (Figure 11.10). Ulnar and radial deviation (flexion) is specific to the wrist. Ulnar deviation is similar to adduction, it occurs when the hand moves toward the ulna. Radial deviation is similar to abduction, it occurs when the hand moves toward the radius. Lateral flexion

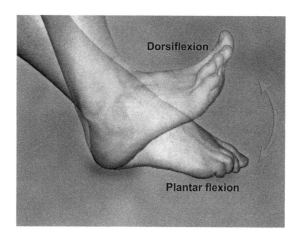

Figure 11.8. *Dorsiflexion and planter flexion of the foot/ankle.*

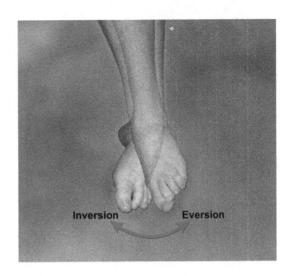

Figure 11.9.   *Inversion and eversion and at the foot/ankle.*

(bending) is a motion that occurs at both the lumbar spine (trunk) and cervical spine (neck). Lateral flexion of the cervical spine occurs when the head moves laterally towards the shoulder, in the frontal plane. Lateral flexion of the lumbar spine occurs when the trunk moves laterally toward the pelvis in the frontal plane. The motion is further defined by adding the direction in which the segment moves. For example, if a person touches her left ear to her left shoulder, the joint motion would be left lateral cervical flexion.

There are six motions that occur specifically at the scapula: *elevation, depression, upward rotation, downward rotation, protraction,* and *retraction*. The scapula must rotate when the humerus moves in order to maintain proper alignment between the humerus and the glenoid fossa. For elevation, the entire scapula moves up, and for depression, the scapula moves down. When performing a shrug, there is scapular elevation during the upward phase and depression during the downward phase. Upward rotation is when the inferior angle, which is at the bottom of the scapula, rotates superiorly and laterally, and downward rotation is when the inferior angle of the scapula rotates medially and inferiorly. Upward rotation occurs when a person abducts his or her shoulder, and downward rotation occurs when a person adducts his or her shoulder. Retraction occurs when the vertebral border of the scapula moves toward the vertebrae, and protraction occurs when the vertebral border moves away from the vertebrae. When performing a bench press, there is retraction of the scapula during the downward phase, and there is protraction during the upward phase (Figure 11.11).

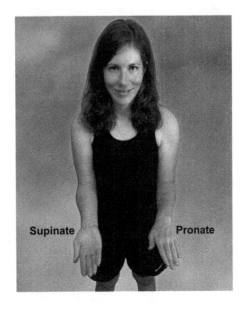

Figure 11.10.   *Pronation and supination of the proximal radioulnar joint.*

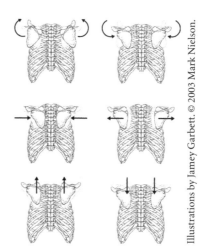

Illustrations by Jamey Garbett. © 2003 Mark Nielson.

Figure 11.11. *There are six motions that occur specifically at the scapula: elevation, depression, upward rotation, downward rotation, protraction, and retraction.*

There are also six motions that occur specifically at the pelvis: *anterior and posterior pelvic girdle rotation, left and right lateral pelvic girdle rotation, left and right transverse pelvic girdle rotation.* When determining the motion of the pelvis, the landmark to focus on is the anterior superior iliac spine. This is typically located at a person's waistline. Anterior and posterior pelvic girdle rotation occurs in the sagittal plane. During anterior rotation, the pelvis rotates forward about a bilateral axis, and during posterior rotation, the pelvis rotates back about a bilateral axis. During the downward phase of a squat, there is anterior rotation at the pelvis, and during the upward phase of the squat, there is posterior rotation at the pelvis. Left and right lateral pelvic girdle rotation occur in the frontal plane around an anteriorposterior axis. During left lateral rotation, the left side of the pelvis moves down, and the right side of the pelvis moves up. During right lateral rotation, the right side of the pelvis moves down and the left side of the pelvis moves up. These motions commonly occur when a person is walking. Left and right transverse pelvic girdle rotation occurs in the transverse plane about a longitudinal axis. For left transverse rotation, the left axis rotates back in the transverse plane, and for right transverse rotation, the right axis rotates back in the transverse plane. When a right handed batter swings a bat, there is left transverse pelvic girdle rotation (4).

OSTEOLOGY

Osteology is the study of bone (*oste* is Greek for bone; *logy* is Greek for the study of). The adult skeleton consists of 206 bones, with 177 actively engaged in voluntary movement. It is divided into two major divisions, the *axial* (Latin for axis) skeleton and the *appendicular* (Latin for to hang on) skeleton. The axial skeleton contains 80 bones, which include the skull, spinal column, sternum, and ribs. The appendicular skeleton contains 126 bones, which include both the upper and lower extremities. The pelvis (Latin for basin) can be classified with either division due to the fact that it is a link between the axial skeleton and the appendicular skeleton.

Bone is continually being formed by specialized bone cells called *osteoblasts*, and old bone is continually removed by *osteoclasts*. In healthy adult bone, the activity of osteoblast cells and osteoclast cells is balanced. However, there is a common condition referred to as *osteoporosis* (Greek: *osteo* is bone and *porosis* is passageway) where excessive amounts of bone are lost, making the bone weak and easy to break. Osteoporosis is most commonly found in postmenopausal women (6).

Skeletal Functions

The skeleton has five major functions. The skeletal system, especially the axial skeleton system, is designed to protect internal organs, such as the heart, brain, lungs, and spinal cord. The skeletal system provides a rigid internal framework that supports upright posture. The skeletal system also facilitates movement by providing attachment sites for muscles and serving as levers. Additionally, the skeletal system produces red blood cells through the process of *hemopoiesis*. This occurs in the red bone marrow found in the vertebral bodies, femur, humerus, ribs, and sternum. Bone also serves as a storage site for minerals such as calcium and phosphorus. These minerals make bone both rigid and flexible (3).

Bone Markings and Formations

Bone markings are a series of cavities, depressions, elevations, projections, and grooves that exist to provide a place of attachment for muscles, tendons, and ligaments. In addition, they serve to stabilize add structural support and provide passageways for nerves and blood vessels. Also, the landmarks are important in helping identify the location and functions of muscles. Common bone markings can be seen in Table 11.1 below (7).

Table 11.1.   Common Bone Markings.

Purpose of Marking	Marking	Description	Examples	
Articulation with other bones to form joint	Condyle	(Latin: knuckle) rounded projection located on the ends of bones that serve as articulation areas	Lateral and medial condyles of the femur and humerus	
	Facet	(French: little face) A small smooth flattened area on the bone	Articular facet of vertebrae	
	Head	Rounded projection on the proximal end of a long bone	Head of the femur and humerus	
Attachment site of muscles, tendons, and ligaments	Epicondyle	(Epi is Greek for above) rounded projection of bone above the condyle	Medial and lateral epicondyles of the humerus and femur	
	Crest	Prominent ridge like projection of bone	Illiac crest of pelvis	

(Continued)

Table 11.1. Common Bone Markings (Continued)

Purpose of Marking	Marking	Description	Examples	
	Angle	Projecting or sharp corner	Inferior angle of the scapula	
	Line	Any long narrow mark less prominent than a crest	Linea aspera of femur	
	Process	Projection or outgrowth of bone	Acromion process of scapula, coranoid process of humerus	
	Spine	Sharp, slender projection of bone	Spine of scapula, spinous process of vertebrae	
	Trochanter	(Greek: to run) A large blunt elevation of bone	Greater trochanter of femur	
	Tubercule	Small rounder projection	Greater and lesser tubercules of humerus	
	Tuberosity	Large rounded elevation of bone	Tibial tuberosity	

Purpose of Marking	Marking	Description	Examples	
Cavities and depressions	Foramen	(Latin: passage or opening) Rounded hole or opening in bone	Vertebral and inter-vertebral foramen	
	Fossa	(Latin: shallow depressed area) Hollow depression or flattened surface	Olecrennon fossa of humerus	
	Groove	Long narrow channel or depression or furrow	Bicipital groove of the humerus	
	Notch	Indentation at the edge of a bone to allow structures to pass through or to stabilize arteries, veins, or tendons	Sciatic notch of the pelvis	

All line drawings in Table 11.1 are by Jamey Garbett. © 2003 Mark Nielsen

Structure of Bone

Bone is composed is a hard, outer covering called *cortical* bone, and a spongier, inner component called *cancellous* bone. Cortical (Latin: bark) bone makes up the outer shaft of long bones and an outer shell for all other types of bones. It is very dense and can withstand high levels of weight bearing. The basic structure of compact bone is referred to as an osteon. An osteon is made up of circular rings known as *lamella* (Latin: thin layer) of which there are 4 to 20 per osteon. When lamella is initially laid in rings, it is known as pre-bone due to the fact that it is a soft pliable gel. Not until calcium and phosphorous are incorporated in the pre-bone does it begin to become rigid and stiff.

Cancellous (Latin: spongy or lattice) bone is located at the ends of long bone and is composed of fine needle-like structures. It is less stiff than compact bone as its purpose is to bend while walking and running to help dissipate force. These needle-like structures have the same osteon structure as compact bone except they are not as dense.

Most people consider bone as a dry, brittle, dead chunk of mineral. However, bone is dynamic living tissue with a rich blood and nervous supply that is constantly being remodeled due to the forces acting on it. Bone responds dynamically to the presence or absence of different forces with changes in its shape, size, and density. This phenomenon was originally described by the German scientist, Julius Wolff in 1892. *Wolff's Law* indicates that bone strength increases and decreases as functional forces on the bone increase and decrease, or that bone will respond to the stresses that are placed upon it. Due to Wolff's Law, bone content is continually being increased, decreased, and reshaped. In addition, bone cells have a lifespan. Generally, a person will replace about 7 to 10% of the skeleton in a year. These additions, subtractions, and reshapings are accomplished by osteoblasts (form bone content) and osteoclasts (decrease bone content). The activity of osteoblasts and osteoclast are usually in balance. However, increased physical activity can cause bones to be denser and larger than normal, while decreased physical activity will have the opposite effect with bone becoming less dense and smaller than normal (bed-ridden patients). Therefore, an individual's activity level and lifestyle will dramatically influence bone density (3).

Types of Bones

There are five primary types of bones. *Long bones* (Figure 11.12) have a long, roughly cylindrical shaft of cortical bone. The ends of long bones consist of cancellous bone. In addition, long bones contain a central cavity known as the *medullary canal*. The canal contains bone marrow, which is responsible for forming red blood cells (important in oxygen transportation). Examples of long bones include the femur and the humerus. Long bones are divided into the *diaphysis* (the shaft) and the *epiphysis* (the end of the bone). At the end of each long bone is a line of cartilage where growth of the bone takes place. This is known as the growth plate, and it is the site of longitudinal growth. Around the entire bone is a layer of tissue known as the *periosteum*, where bone cells are produced to maintain the width of the bone.

Short bones are typically small bones that have a proportional length and width. They function as shock absorbers due to the fact that they are made up of mostly spongy material on the inside with a hard cortical bone shell on the outside. In addition, short bones fit together snugly, which produces stability in a joint. Examples include the carpal bones of the wrist and tarsal bones of the foot (Figure 11.13). *Flat bones* have large, flat surfaces, and are primarily designed for protection. Examples include the bones of the cranium, the sternum, and the scapula (Figure 11.14). Their composition is similar to short bones, which are made mostly of spongy bone on the inside with a hard cortical bone shell on the outside.

Irregular bones have an asymmetric shape in order to fulfill special functions in the human body. For example, the vertebrae carry out several functions: (a) provide a bony, protective tunnel for the spinal cord,

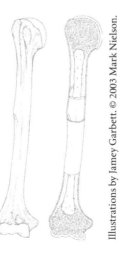

Figure 11.12. *The structure of a long bone. The long, central shaft is the diaphysis, and the ends are the epiphysis.*

Illustrations by Jamey Garbett. © 2003 Mark Nielson.

(b) provide several processes for muscle and ligament attachments, (c) support the weight of the superior body, and (d) enable movement of the trunk in all three cardinal planes. They are similar to short and flat bones in that they are made up of spongy bone on the inside with a hard cortical bone shell on the outside (Figure 11.15).

Seasmoid (Latin for resembling a grain of sesame) *bones*, similar to short bones in shape, are composed of spongy bone on the inside with a hard cortical bone shell on the outside. An example is the patella (Figure 11.16) of the knee, which is imbedded within a tendon. Its primary purpose is to increase the mechanical advantage of a muscle by increasing the angle of pull of a muscle (5).

Articulations (Joints)

Joints are the junctions (articulation) between the bones. The bony configuration of the joint, the ligaments, and the associated musculature that crosses the joint determine the range of motion of the joint. *Diarthroidal* joints are the most common type of joint in the body and are also referred to as synovial joints. Diarthroidal joints have several distinct features. First, the joint is encased in a sleeve-like capsule which has two layers. The outside layer is a strong sheath-like structure that provides stability for the joint. The internal layer contains cells that secrete *synovial* (Latin: egg white) fluid, which reduces friction between the articulating surfaces.

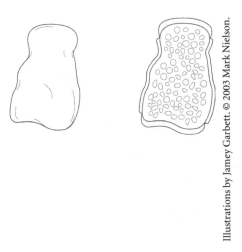

Illustrations by Jamey Garbett. © 2003 Mark Nielson.

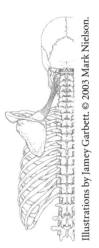

Illustrations by Jamey Garbett. © 2003 Mark Nielson.

Figure 11.14.   *The scapula is an example of a flat bone.*

Figure 11.13.   *Short bone.*

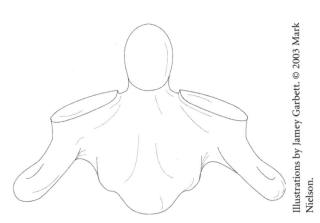

Illustrations by Jamey Garbett. © 2003 Mark Nielson.

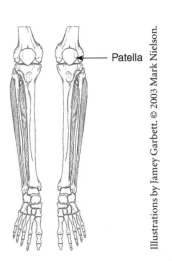

Patella

Illustrations by Jamey Garbett. © 2003 Mark Nielson.

Figure 11.15.   *The vertebrae is an example of an irregular bone.*

Figure 11.16.   *The patella is an example of a seasmoid bone.*

Second, the articular surface of synovial joints is covered in *hyaline cartilage*. Its exterior texture is smooth to decrease friction between articulating structures. In addition, hyaline cartilage is spongy and absorbs synovial fluid. As compression occurs during foot contact with the ground, synovial fluid is squeezed out of the articular cartilage to dissipate force.

Types of Diarthroidal Joints

Diarthroidal joints (Figure 11.17) are classified based on their number of axes. This can range from zero to three. The arthroidal (gliding) joint consists of two flat surfaces that butt up against each other, permitting a limited amount of movement, usually in a straight line. An example would be the carpal bones of the wrist (Figure 11.18). These bones glide past each other as the hand moves. There is no specific axis for this movement. *Uniaxial* joints include the *ginglymus* and *trochoid* joints. A ginglymus (Greek: hinge) joint consists of a concave

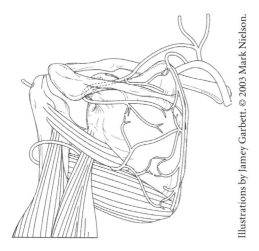

Figure 11.17. *The elbow is an example of a synovial joint. It is also a hinge joint.*

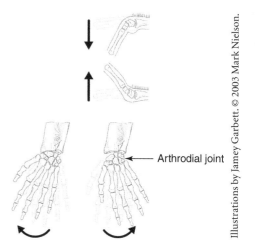

Figure 11.18. *The articulation between the carpal bones is an example of an arthroidal joint.*

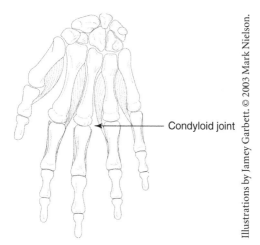

Figure 11.19. *The articulation between the metacarpals and the phalanges is an example of a condyloid joint.*

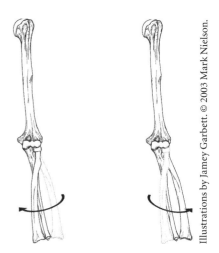

Figure 11.20. *The radioulnar joint is an example of a pivot joint.*

surface articulating with a convex surface. This is similar to the condyloidal joint except hinge joints are usually deeper, therefore only permitting movement in one plane (sagittal). An example would be the humeroulnar joint of the elbow (Figure 11.19). An example of a *biaxial* joint is the condyloidal joint. Condyloidal (biaxial ball and socket) joints consists of an oval *convex* (Latin: arched) surface articulating with an oval *concave* (Latin: hollow) surface. It permits motion in two planes, flexion and extension in the sagittal plane, and abduction and adduction in the frontal plane. An example would be the metacarpophalangeal joints of the hand and the articulation between the radius and the proximal row of carpals at the wrist (Figure 11.19). A *trochoid* (Greek: wheel) or pivot joint permits rotation around a central axis, which allows motion in the transverse plane. An example would be the proximal radioulnar joint, where two long bones fit against each other in such a way that one bone can roll around the other, as the radius rotates around the ulna (Figure 11.20).

Two types of joints are *triaxial*. This includes *enarthroidal* and *sellar* joints. Enarthroidal (multiaxial ball and socket) joints consist of a rounded convex surface articulating with a rounded cup-like structure. It permits motion in all three planes. An example would be the shoulder and hip joints (Figure 11.21). This type of diarthroidal joint provides the greatest range of motion of any joint in the body. A sellar (reciprocal reception) or saddle joint, consists of both ends of the convex surface tipping up like a western saddle fitting in a reciprocal convex–concave articulation. It permits motion in the sagittal plane, frontal plane, and circumduction. An example would be the carpometacarpal joint at the base of the thumb (Figure 11.22) (1).

When referring to movements of joints in planes of motion, the term degrees of freedom is often utilized. For instance, the elbow joint moves in only one plane, the sagittal plane. Therefore, the movement of the elbow would possess one degree of freedom. The femur of the hip joint, on the other hand, can move in three planes. Therefore, the hip joint would possess three degrees of movement (2).

Other Types of Joints

In addition to diarthrotic joints, there are two other primary types of joints. *Synarthroidal* (immovable joint) refers to a joint that has little or no movement, but is important in the stabilization of the skeletal system. The joint has no joint cavity and is connected via fibrous tissue. An example is the sutures between the bones of the skull (Figure 11.23). The other type of joint is *amphiarthroidal* (slightly movable joint), which can be structurally divided into three types.

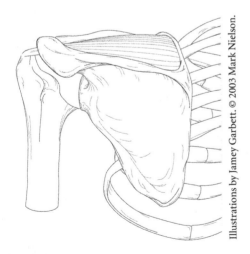

Illustrations by Jamey Garbett. © 2003 Mark Nielson.

Figure 11.21. *The shoulder is an example of an enarthroidal (ball and socket) joint.*

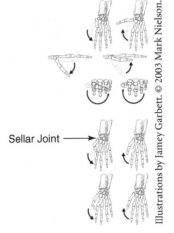

Sellar Joint

Illustrations by Jamey Garbett. © 2003 Mark Nielson.

Figure 11.22. *The first carpal-metacarpal joint at the base of the thumb is an example of a sellar joint.*

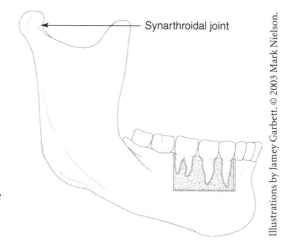

Synarthroidal joint

Illustrations by Jamey Garbett. © 2003 Mark Nielson.

Figure 11.23. *The sutures between the cranial bones are an example of a synarthroidal joint.*

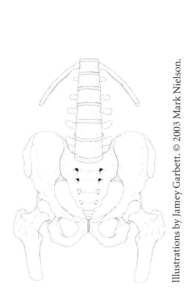

Illustrations by Jamey Garbett. © 2003 Mark Nielson.

Illustrations by Jamey Garbett. © 2003 Mark Nielson.

Figure 11.24. *The tibiofibular joint is an example of a syndesmosis joint.*

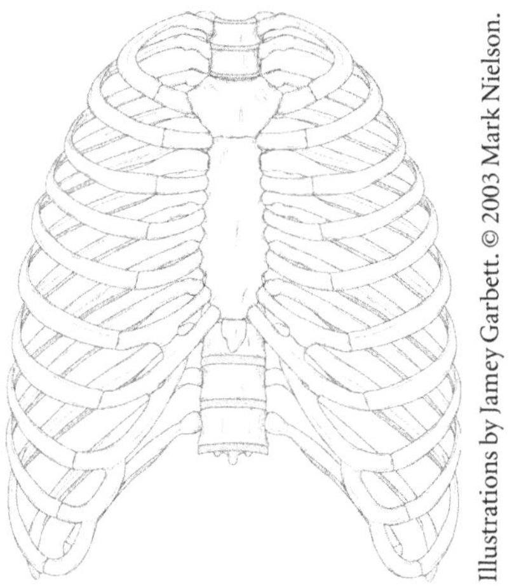

Figure 11.25. *The cartilaginous articulation between the ribs and the sternum is an example of a synchondrosis joint.*

A *syndesmosis* joint is held together by sheets of strong fibrous tissue known as *interosseous* ligaments. The slight movement permitted by this joint is important in dissipating force. An example would be the distal tibiofibular joint (Figure 11.24), which separates slightly to accommodate the talus during weight bearing activities such as walking and running. A synchondrosis joint has hyaline cartilage between the bones that allows some movement. An example would be the cartilage of the ribs (Figure 11.25) as they articulate with the sternum (sternocostal) to allow the thorax to expand to facilitate movement of air. A *symphysis* joint is separated by a fibrocartilage pad that allows slight movement between the bones. An example would be the pubic symphysis (3).

Joint Stability

Joint stability is defined as the ability of the joint to resist displacement. Not all joints have the same stability. This is due to differences in joint structure and the musculature that surrounds a joint. Some joints are fairly stable such as the hip and elbow. However, others such as the shoulder and knees are not as stable and therefore,

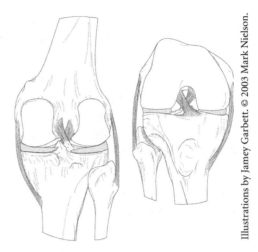

Illustrations by Jamey Garbett. © 2003 Mark Nielson.

Figure 11.26.   *The ligaments of the knee.*

more susceptible to injury. Joint strength and range of motion will follow *Emerson's Law*, which states that "for everything given, something is taken away. " In anatomy, this means that a joint cannot have both a wide range of motion and stability. For example, the shoulder has increased range of motion at the expense of stability. The hip has increased stability at the expense of range of motion." There are five major factors in joint stability: (a) muscular force, (b) ligaments, (c) fascia and skin, (d) atmospheric pressure, and (e) other structures associated with the joint (3).

Muscular force is considered the most important force in joint stability. It is especially important in joints where bony structure contributes little to the stability, such as the knee and shoulder. Ligaments are defined as the structure that connects bone to bone. They can be a strap-like structure, a rounded chord or sometimes not much more than a thickening of a joint capsule, which occurs at the shoulder. They also vary greatly in strength. In the shoulder the ligaments are thin and weak to allow range of motion. However, in the hip they are thick and strong to maintain joint stability. Fascia consists of fibrous connective tissue that forms a sheet like structure around the joint. An example would be the *iliotibial band*, a thickened aspect of the fascia of the thigh that assists in lateral stability of the knee. Atmospheric pressure refers to the gaseous mass surrounding the body that presses on the joints thus increasing joint stability. Other structures associated with the joint that can increase stability include the *joint capsule*, the *labrum* of the hip and shoulder, and the *menisci* of the knee (4).

ROLES OF MUSCLES

Muscles have different responsibilities during the course of a movement. The *agonist* (mover) refers to a muscle or group of muscles directly engaged in movement through concentric development of tension. Agonists are often called prime movers. Due to the fact that several muscles generally contribute to a movement, muscles are also classified as *primary or assistant agonist*. For instance, during elbow flexion, the biceps brachii and brachialis would be the primary agonists and the brachioradialis would be the assistant agonist due to the location of this muscle in relationship to the joint.

The *antagonist* refers to the muscle or muscles that are located on the opposite side of the joint from the agonist and opposing its action. This opposition does not interfere with the agonist's function. Its purpose is to help control agonist movement by slowing the movement down, which helps protect the joint, and to terminate the action of the agonist. An example would be when the hamstring muscles on the posterior aspect of the thigh eccentrically contract to provide braking and controlling actions to the quadriceps muscles located on the anterior aspect of the thigh. The action of the hamstrings would slow down and terminate knee extension.

When a muscle contracts in an antagonist manner, it is more susceptible to injury (tearing). This is due to the fact that the muscle is contracting to slow the limb down, while at the same time being stretched. An example would be the triceps muscle group that helps control and terminate elbow flexion.

Muscles that assist the agonist, but are not the prime movers for the specific joint action are known as *synergists*. For example, while the gastrocnemius and soleus muscles are the agonists for plantar flexion of the foot/ankle, the tibialis posterior, flexor hallicus longus, flexor digitorum longus, peroneus longus, and peroneus brevis muscles also assist with planter flexion. These assisting muscles are not as strong as the gastrocnemius and soleus, and therefore are considered synergists for the joint motion.

Muscles are also utilized as stabilizers in order to fixate a structure so that a specific movement at an adjacent joint can occur. For example, stabilization is very important in the hip joint during gait. When one foot is in contact with the ground in walking or running, the opposite side of the pelvis (of the swing leg) must be stabilized by pelvic girdle muscles, specifically the gluteus medius muscle, to prevent the pelvis from dropping down.

Neutralizer is a term used to describe muscles that counteract or counterbalance. The function of synergist muscle is to contract to eliminate an undesired joint action of another muscle that normally occurs when an agonist develops concentric tension. An example would be if a muscle, such as the tensor fascia latae muscle at the hip causes both flexion and abduction when in it contracts, but only flexion is desired. The adductors of the hip must also contract to eliminate the undesired abduction caused by the tensor fascia latae. When the biceps brachii develops concentric tension, it produces both flexion at the elbow and supination of the forearm. If only elbow flexion is desired, the pronator teres must act as a neutralizer to counteract the supination of the forearm.

Actions of Muscles

When an electrical stimulus is applied to a muscle, it will cause contraction. The classification of muscular actions or contractions into types is based upon whether the muscle shortens, lengthens, or remains the same length, while developing tension. These muscle actions can be used to cause a motion, to control a motion, or to prevent a motion.

A concentric (Latin: toward the middle) muscle action, or contraction, occurs when a muscle generates tension that produces a *torque* (rotary effect of force) larger than the resistive force at the joint. This will cause a

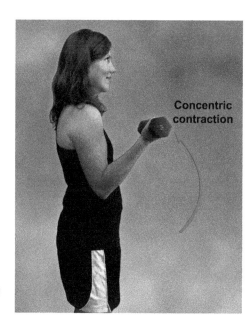

Figure 11.27. *Example of a concentric muscle action (contraction) of the elbow flexors during the upward phase of a dumbbell curl.*

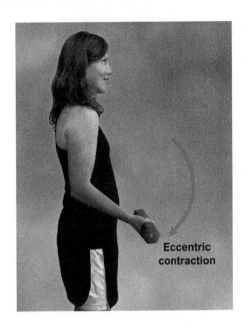

Eccentric
contraction

Figure 11.28.   *An example of an eccentric muscle action (contraction). The elbow flexors develop tension as they lengthen to control the elbow as it extends during the downward phase of a dumbbell curl.*

shortening of the muscle, and the joint angle changes in the direction of the muscular force. An example would be the upward phase of a dumbbell curl. Elbow flexion is caused by a concentric muscle action of the brachialis and biceps brachii muscles. These muscles shorten to overcome the resistance of the dumbbell and cause the elbow to flex. The bone serves as a lever and the joint as a fulcrum (axis).

Eccentric (Latin: away from the middle) muscle actions occur when a muscle lengthens while under tension due to an opposing force greater than the muscle can generate. Eccentric muscle actions usually occur as a force that opposes a concentric muscle to slow the movement down in order to protect the joint and terminate the movement. During the downward phase of the dumbbell curl, the elbow flexors now work eccentrically to control the elbow as it moves into extension. The brachialis and biceps brachii will develop tension as they lengthen to control this movement. Another example would be an eccentric muscle action of the posterior rotator cuff to slow down the shoulder after the release of an object (baseball). When a baseball is released, the shoulder is rotating internally at a very high velocity. The posterior rotator cuff works eccentrically to slow this motion down.

An isometric muscle action occurs when a muscle is active and develops tension, but there is no visible change in joint position. An example would be stabilizing the scapula by the surrounding shoulder girdle muscles. The muscles that attach to the scapula are antagonistic to each other with equal strength, thus counteracting each other in order to stabilize the scapula for shoulder movements to occur. Another example using the dumbbell curl would be holding the elbow in a constant position of 90° of elbow flexion. The elbow flexors would develop tension to maintain this joint position, but their length would not change (2).

SUMMARY

Applied anatomy is defined as that aspect of the discipline of anatomy important for a sound understanding of basic structure and how these structures produce movement. In order to understand, analyze, and prescribe corrections to human movement, one must first understand terminology. This includes the planes and axes of movement, the different types of bones and joints, the different types of joint actions, and the different types of muscle actions. An understanding of this terminology will allow the physical therapist, athletic trainer, coach, or other professionals to use applied anatomy to enhance their analysis of human movement.

REFERENCES

1. Behnke, R. *Kinetic Anatomy*, 2nd ed. Champaign, IL: Human Kinetics, 2006.

2. Floyd, R.T. *Manual of Structural Kinesiology,* 16th ed. Boston: McGraw Hill, 2007.

3. Hall, S. *Basic Biomechanics*, 2nd ed. St. Louis: Mosby, 1995.

4. Hamill, J. *Biomechanical Basis for Human Movement*, 6th ed. Williams and Wilkins, 2006.

5. Kapit, W. *The Anatomy Coloring Book,* 3rd ed. San Francisco: Benjamin Cummings, 2002.

6. Luttgens, K. *Scientific Basis of Human Movement*, 9th ed. Boston: WCB McGraw-Hill, 1977.

7. Moore, K.L. *Clinically Oriented Anatomy*, 6th ed. Philadelphia: Lippincott Williams & Williams, 2010.

8. *Taber's Cyclopedic Medical Dictionary*, 20th ed. Philadelphia: F.A. Davis, 2001.

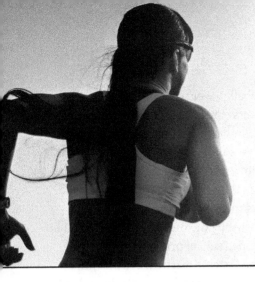

Chapter 12

BIOMECHANICS

 OUTLINE

Objectives
Vocabulary
Units of Measurement/Terminology
Newton's Laws of Motion
Analysis
Applications of Biomechanics
    Sport Biomechanics
    Clinical Biomechanics

Biomechanical Tools
Summary
References

OBJECTIVES

1. Define biomechanics.
2. Understand what type of professionals use biomechanics.
3. Describe the underlying principles of biomechanics.
4. Understand several applications of biomechanics.
5. Define terminology used in biomechanics.
6. Describe how to perform a biomechanical analysis.
7. Describe equipment used to perform a biomechanical analysis.

Have you ever watched a sporting event and questioned how a baseball player was able to hit the ball over 400 feet? Maybe you watched a race and wondered how sprinters can run at such high velocities or questioned how an athlete was able to rehabilitate so quickly following an injury. Human movement is complex and can be difficult to analyze. During movements such as walking and running, there are several joints that are rotating, several muscles that are contracting, and numerous neural signals being sent from the central nervous system to the muscles and from the muscles back to the central nervous system. The science of biomechanics helps us to better understand, describe, analyze, and measure human movement.

Biomechanics is the study of the structure and function of biological systems by the means and methods of mechanics (6). Another good definition of biomechanics is the application of mechanical principles to the study of biological systems (1). Biomechanics limits the study of mechanics to living systems, particularly the human body. To better understand biomechanics, a good starting point is to first understand mechanics, the branch of physics that examines force as the cause of motion, the effects of these forces, and the description of motion produced by the forces (5). Professionals such as engineers, astronomers, and navigation specialists apply the field of mechanics to their work. The laws of motion governing the movement of planets, cars, planes, and other structures also apply to human movement.

In general, the study of biomechanics has been applied to two main areas: clinical settings and sports settings (9). To become proficient in biomechanics, a strong background in anatomy, physics, mathematics, and neural control is needed. The following professionals use biomechanics in their careers: anatomists, athletic trainers, personal trainers, physical therapists, occupational therapists, orthopedists, exercise physiologists, coaches, dancers, physical educators, prosthetists, and ergonomists.

VOCABULARY

An analysis of human movement can be broken down into describing the motion that occurs and the cause of the motion. *Kinematics* is the branch of mechanics that describes motion without regard to the causative forces. Kinematic descriptions of movement include time, displacement, velocity, and acceleration. This includes both straight line or linear kinematics, and rotating or angular kinematics. Displacement, velocity, and acceleration can be considered in terms of individual body parts, individual joints, or the entire body through the center of gravity.

Kinetics is the branch of mechanics examining the forces that cause motion. This includes both internal and external forces. Internal forces include muscle activity, ligaments, joint contact, and friction between the anatomical structures. External forces can include the ground, other persons, external loads, or from passive forces.

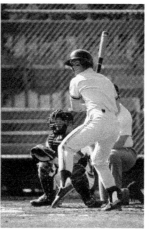

Figure 12.1. *Proper biomechanics is essential for hitting a baseball.*

© Kendall Hunt Publishing Company.

The major source of force within the human body is the muscular system. When muscles contract, they transfer force through their tendons to the skeletal system. Tendons then pull on bones, which allow joints to rotate. Describing these muscular forces is an example of a kinetic analysis, analyzing the joint's angular displacement, velocity, and acceleration is an example of a kinematic analysis (1).

Mechanics can further be broken down into *statics* and *dynamics*. Statics is the study of a system that has zero acceleration. This means that the system is either in a state of rest (no motion) or is moving at a constant velocity. In a static situation, all the forces acting on a system are balanced. Dynamics is the study of a system that is accelerating. In a dynamic situation, the forces acting on a system are unbalanced, and therefore an object will be changing motion or moving from a static position. Work, power, and energy are included in the study of dynamics (5).

Many of the concepts in mechanics are either *scalars* or *vectors*. A scalar quantity only contains a magnitude. Mass, speed, temperature, and time are examples of scalar quantities. Vector quantities contain both a magnitude and a direction. Examples of vector quantities include displacement, velocity, acceleration, and force. In order to describe a force, one must describe the quantity of force applied and the direction in which the force is applied. Vectors can be represented graphically by an arrow. The length of the arrow should represent the magnitude of the vector, the orientation of the vector represents the line of action, and the tip of the arrow represents the direction of the vector. If more than one vector is drawn, the tail of the vector should correspond proportionally to the magnitude of the vector (4).

UNITS OF MEASUREMENT/TERMINOLOGY

Biomechanics uses the metric system as its unit of measurement. Distances are measured in meters (m), mass is measured in kilograms (kg), force is measured in Newton's (N), and time is measured in seconds (s). Weight, which will be discussed later, is a force and is measured in Newton's as well. In the United States pounds (lbs) is the more common unit of measurement for both force and weight (5). It is common to standardized force by a person's body weight in order to make comparisons between individuals that do not weigh the same amount.

Understanding terminology is vital when performing biomechanical analyses. Distance is a scalar quantity that describes the amount of space covered. For example, if a person walks 8 m to the east, and then 6 m to the north, the distance covered would be 14 m. Displacement is a vector quantity that describes a change in distance with respect to a reference or starting position. If a person walks 8 m to the east, and then 6 m to the north, the displacement is 10 m with respect to his or her starting position. Displacement does not represent how far a person or object travels (that is distance), only the final change in position. As seen in Figure 12.2 below, one line is drawn to represent walking 8 m to the east, and another line is drawn to represent walking 6 m north. The displacement would be the change in position from where the person started to where the person finished. This is represented by a line from the starting point to the ending point, which is the hypotenuse of a right triangle. Using the Pythagorean theorem, if both 6 m and 8 m are squared and then summed, and the square root is taken of that value, the displacement if 10 m.

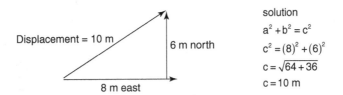

Figure 12.2. *If a person walks 8 m to the east and 6 m north, then his or her displacement is 10 m.*

If we want to describe how displacement is changing over a period of time, we would measure velocity (v). If an individual's displacement is 50 m and it takes him or her 10 s to achieve this displacement then the velocity would be 5 m/s. This indicates that displacement has changed, on average, by 5 m every second. The person's initial displacement is subtracted from the final displacement and divided by the amount of time to calculate velocity.

If we want to describe how velocity changes, we would examine acceleration (a). If a person's velocity is 3 m/s and 4 seconds later their velocity is 7 m/s, their acceleration over this time period would be 1 m/s^2. This indicates that velocity is increasing by 1 m every second. The initial velocity is subtracted from the final velocity and divided by the amount of time in order to calculate acceleration. When velocity is not changing acceleration would be 0 m/s^2. This would occur when an object is at rest and when it has a constant velocity (1, 4, 5).

These terms can also be applied to situations that involve angular or rotational motion. If we were to examine the change in the orientation of a line segment, this would be the angular displacement (θ), which is measured in radians. For example, if we were to measure the amount of change in the angle of the knee during a squat, we would examine the joint's angular displacement. If we wanted to look at how angular displacement changed over a period of time, we would examine the joint's angular velocity (ω). If a joint's angular displacement changed by 3 radians over a period of 2 seconds, the joint's angular velocity would be equal to 1.5 rad/s. If we wanted to examine how a joint's angular velocity was changing, we could measure the angular acceleration (α) of the joint. If the joint's angular velocity changed from 2 rad/s to 8 rad/s over a period of 2 seconds, then the angular acceleration would be equal to 3 rad/s^2. Angular displacement, angular velocity, and angular acceleration can readily be observed in Figure 12.3 as a pitcher delivers a pitch.

Kinetics is the study of the cause of motion, including both *force* and *moment of force*. Force (F) is the effect of one object on another or the effect of one body on another. If the forces are unbalanced, the object or body will accelerate. When 1 N of force is applied to an object with a mass of 1 kg, the object will accelerate at 1 m/s^2 in the direction in which the force is applied. A moment of force (M), also referred to as *torque*, can be considered a rotational force—the rotational effect a force has about a fixed point. A moment of force is equal to the product of the force and its perpendicular distance from its line of action to the axis of rotation. In Figure 12.4 the biceps brachii exerts a turning force on the forearm that causes the forearm to rotate and results in the joint action of elbow flexion. The moment of force here would be equal to the magnitude of force applied by the biceps brachii on the forearm multiplied by the perpendicular distance from the line of action of the biceps brachii to the elbow's axis of rotation (9).

The human body is a series of rigid links (bones) that are connected at joints. Thus, the body can be labeled as a system of levers. A lever is a simple machine that can perform one of four functions: (a) balance two or more forces, (b) change the direction of the applied force, (c) favor force production, and (d) favor speed

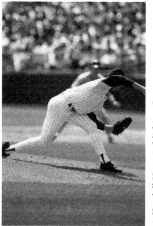

Figure 12.3. *The glenohumeral joint experiences very high angular velocities during the overhead throwing motion.*

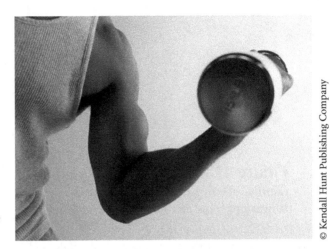

Figure 12.4. *The moment of force will be equal to the magnitude of the muscular force applied by the elbow flexors multiplied by the perpendicular distance from the insertion of their tendons on the forearm the to the axis of rotation of the elbow (moment arm).*

and range of motion. A lever consists of five components: an axis of rotation, the applied force, the resistive force, the force moment arm, and the resistance moment arm. In the human body the force is supplied by the muscles with the point of force application being the attachment of the muscle's tendon. Resistance is often the weight of the body, body segment, or an external resistance. The axis is the joint center of rotation. The force moment arm is the perpendicular distance from the point of force application to the axis of rotation. The resistance moment arm is the perpendicular distance from the point of resistance application to the axis of rotation (4, 5). The components of a lever can be seen below in Figure 12.5.

There are three types of levers. In a *first-class lever* the axis is between the force and the resistance. A first-class lever can potentially perform all four functions of a simple machine, depending on the placement of the axis (which affects the length of the moment arms) and the magnitude of the applied force and resistance. In Figure 12.5 if both forces are equal, this lever will balance the two forces because their moment arms are equal. If the downward directed force is greater than the upward directed force, then the lever will move down on one end and up on the other end. An example of a first-class lever in the body is elbow extension. The axis is the elbow, the applied muscular force is supplied by the triceps to the posterior elbow at the olecrennon process, and the resistance is the weight of the hand and forearm (Figure 12.6). In this configuration, the resistance moment arm is much longer than the force moment arm. This arrangement of a first-class lever will favor speed and range of motion. The proximal end of the forearm will only move a small distance, but the distal end of the forearm and the hand will move a much greater distance. Neck extension is another example of a first-class lever, where the force is applied to the posterior aspect of the head by the neck extensor muscles. The axis of rotation is the cervical vertebrae and the resistance is supplied by the weight of the head.

In a *second-class lever* the resistance is always between the force and the axis of rotation. Since the force moment arm will always be longer than the resistance moment arm, this type of lever will favor force production. There are very few examples of second-class levers in the human body. One example is a toe raise.

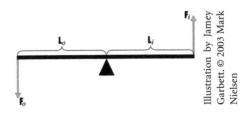

Figure 12.5. *An example of a lever.*

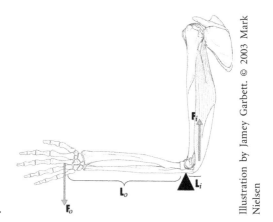

Figure 12.6. *Elbow extension is an example of a first-class lever. The axis is between the muscular force and the resistance.*

The axis is at the ball of the foot (metatarsal-phalangal joint), the resistance is the body weight through the center of gravity, and the force is supplied by the gastrocnemius and soleus muscles through the Achilles tendon (Figure 12.7).

In a *third-class lever* the applied force is between the axis of rotation and the resistance. The resistance moment arm will always be longer than the force moment arm. A third-class lever will always favor speed and range of motion. The human body is primarily composed of third-class levers, because we are designed to be able to run, throw, and kick things. Some examples of third-class levers include elbow flexion, knee flexion and extension, and wrist flexion and extension. In Figure 12.8 the resistance is supplied by the weight of the hand and forearm, the force is supplied by the elbow flexors, and the axis is the elbow.

NEWTON'S LAWS OF MOTION

Newton's three laws of motion apply to any type of movement, including all aspects of human movement. The effects of these laws on human movement is readily observed, whether it is in the flight of a batted ball, the way people are able to run and jump, or the amount of force needed to move a heavy object (4).

Newton's *first law of motion* states that objects in motion tend to stay in motion and objects at rest tend to stay at rest unless acted upon by an outside force. Simply put, it takes an unbalanced force to start, stop, or change an object's motion. Resistance to change in motion is known as *inertia*. An object's inertia is measured by its mass. The more massive an object, the greater amount of force it will take to begin moving it, to stop its motion, or to change the direction of the motion. Mass is measured in grams (g) or kilograms (kg) and is a scalar quantity. An offensive lineman in football is typically more massive than a running back. If a running back and offensive lineman were running at the same velocity, it would take a greater amount of force to stop the motion of the offensive lineman (1).

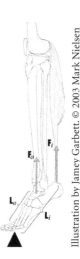

Figure 12.7. *A toe raise is an example of a second-class lever.*

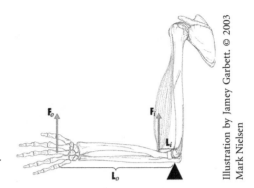

Illustration by Jamey Garbett. © 2003
Mark Nielsen

Figure 12.8.   *Elbow flexion is an example of a third-class lever.*

Examples of Newton's first law are readily observable in everyday life and in sports. If a running back wants to change the direction of his run, he has to apply an unbalanced force to the ground to change his motion. A bowling ball will continue rolling down a lane until an outside force stops its motion. When we are riding in a car and it suddenly brakes, we continue moving forward until an outside force stops our motion. Hopefully this force is provided by the seatbelt and not the dashboard.

Newton's *second law of motion* is known as the Law of Acceleration and can be represented by the equation: $F = ma$. The law of acceleration states that the acceleration of an object is proportional to the force causing it, in the same direction as the force, and is inversely proportional to the object's mass. In order to change the velocity of an object (acceleration), a force must be applied to the object. This change in velocity will occur in the same direction in which the force is applied. In order to roll a bowling ball down a lane and toward the pins, a force must be applied to the ball and the ball will move in the direction in which the force is applied at the time of release.

Newton's second law of motion also describes the principles of *momentum* and *impulse*. Since acceleration is a measure of the change in an object's velocity over change in time, it can be expressed as $a = v/t$. When v/t is used in the equation instead of acceleration, and when both sides of the equation are divided by t (time), the resulting equation is $Ft = mv$, or force multiplied over the time in which the force is applied is equal to the object's mass multiplied by its velocity.

Momentum is the product of an object's mass and velocity. It describes the motion of the object. Any object or person in motion has momentum and any object or person at rest does not possess momentum. Momentum is equal to the amount of force applied and the time over which this force is applied. This concept is known as Impulse. In order to change the momentum of an object an impulse must be applied. This includes the application of force to increase or decrease an object's momentum, such as when running, or the application of force to stop an object, such as when landing from a jump. Oftentimes to increase the chances of being successful in sports, a person needs to apply as much force as possible over a very short period of time. This is true of sprinters in track in field. The foot is only in contact with the ground for a few milliseconds, but in order to run at a high velocity, the sprinter needs to apply a large amount of force over that time period. When landing from a jump, it is beneficial to apply the force over as long of a time period as possible, which will help reduce the stress placed on the joints of the lower extremity. This is why people are encouraged to flex their knees and hips when they land (1).

Newton's *third law of motion* is the law of reaction—for every action there is an equal and opposite reaction. Whenever a person or object exerts a force onto another person or object, the second person or object will exert an equal and opposite force on the first person or object. A plate resting on a dinner table exerts a downward force onto the table, and the table exerts an equal force in the upward direction onto the plate. Since these two forces are balanced, no motion will occur. Whenever a person walks or runs, the feet push down and back into the ground, and the ground pushes back with equal force, but in an upward and forward direction. If a person wants to decrease their walking or running velocity, they push down and forward into the ground, and the ground applies an equal force in an upward and backward direction. The force from the foot is

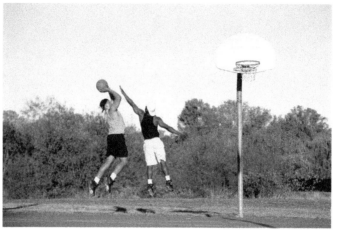

Figure 12.9. *In order to jump, basketball players apply a force down into the ground, and the ground will apply an equal force back in the upward direction. This is the ground reaction force.*

© Kendall Hunt Publishing Company

considered the action force, and the force from the ground is considered the reaction force. In locomotion, the force from the surface is known as the *ground reaction force*. The vector of the ground reaction force is equal in magnitude and opposite in direction to the force vector that is applied to the ground. An example of ground reaction force can be seen in Figure 12.9 when a person jumps.

Examples of Newton's third law of motion are all around us. When we push a door open with our hands, the door pushes back on our hands with an equal amount of force. When we hit or strike an object with a bat, club, or racquet, the ball applies an equal amount of force to the bat, club, or racquet that the bat, club, or racquet applies to the ball. When a linebacker tackles a running back, he applies a certain amount of force to the running back in a specific direction, and the running back applies an equal amount of force back in the opposite direction.

ANALYSIS

There are several purposes of a biomechanical analysis. One purpose is to identify any movement errors. Another purpose is to identify any movements that might increase the chances of the person sustaining an injury. An additional purpose is to increase the efficiency of the movement in order to improve performance.

In order to perform a biomechanical analysis, there are several steps that must be taken. The first step is to identify the overall goal of the skill. This is a relatively simple, but necessary step that will help the analysis. Is the goal of the skill to run or swim as fast as possible over a certain distance? Is the goal of the skill simply to walk efficiently after a hip replacement? Is the goal to place a tennis shot in a location that is difficult for the opponent to return? The goal of the skill could be to place a ball or puck inside a net. Identifying the goal of the skill will help determine the requirements of the skill. In some skills, production of large amounts of force may be the most important component. In other skills, accuracy is the most important component. In many skills, both speed and accuracy are critical.

The second step when analyzing a skill is to break it down into its component parts. Typically, it is beneficial to break skills down into at least three component parts, although more complex skills, such as the overhand throwing motion, walking gait, and running gait may require more components. Many skills can be broken down into a *preparatory phase*, an *action/force phase*, and a *follow through phase*. Walking can be broken down into two main phases—a single support phase when only one foot is on the ground and double support when both feet are on the ground. Within these two main phases, several secondary phases can also be identified.

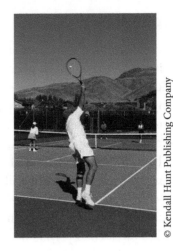

Figure 12.10.   *In order to properly analyze the tennis serve, it must first be broken down into different components.*

© Kendall Hunt Publishing Company

In Figure 12.10, the tennis serve can be broken down into a stance phase, the ball toss phase, the backswing, the forward swing (and contact), and the follow through.

The third step is to determine the optimal placement to observe the skill and perform the analysis. For skills that are primarily performed in the sagittal plane, such as walking, running and jumping, standing to the side of the performer will provide the optimal viewing angle. For skills that are primarily performed in the frontal plane, standing in front or behind the performer will offer the best viewing angle. For skills that are primarily performed in the transverse plane, a superior view will offer the best angle. Many skills take place in multiple planes, so it may be necessary to view the skill from several different positions.

The fourth step is to identify the joints where movement occurs during performance of the skill and to determine what actions take place at those joints. It is necessary to have a thorough understanding of anatomical terminology in order to perform a biomechanical analysis. One must know all the different joint actions and be able to identify them. After identifying joint actions, the next step is to identify muscle actions and the muscles that are used during the performance of the skill. This includes concentric, eccentric, and isometric muscle actions.

The fifth step in the biomechanical analysis would be to identify flaws or errors associated with the movement. These errors could lead to a decrease in performance, injury, or both. If the errors are large, or the performer is a novice, they can often be detected strictly with a visual observation. A runner may have a great deal of frontal plane motion that is easily observable. If it is an elite level athlete, oftentimes the errors will be small, and it may be difficult to detect them without the use of a video camera. Regardless, it will likely take several observations of the skill to detect all of the possible errors.

The sixth and final step in the biomechanical analysis is to prescribe corrections. These corrections may be simple and easily implemented. However, the corrections may require the assistance of a coach or physical therapist who specializes in the specific sport skill or in rehabilitation techniques. Many times, the biomechanist can identify errors and provide suggestions for solutions, but the coach or therapist will decide what type of drills and training plans to assign to the specific athlete or patient based on the errors he or she is making. As a follow up to the initial analysis, the biomechanicst should evaluate the athlete or patient's movement again after he or she has had time to practice and implement the recommended changes.

APPLICATIONS OF BIOMECHANICS

Biomechanical principles apply to the sport and clinical setting. Sport biomechanics is more concerned with analyzing biomechanical issues contributing to sport performance, while clinical biomechanics is more involved with rehabilitation, surgical repair, and orthopedic issues. Regardless of the application, the overall goal is to prevent injuries or improve performance by either changing techniques or equipment (2).

Sport Biomechanics

Biomechanics has long been used to analyze and improve sport performance and technique, but only recently have advanced tools been introduced to greatly assist in analysis. A biomechanical analysis of sport performance can be conducted without any equipment. Whenever a coach, athletic trainer, or biomechanist observes a person performing an athletic skill and provides feedback, they are likely using a touch of biomechanics to conduct the analysis. This can be as simple as a youth basketball coach instructing a player to bend her knees more when she shoots a basketball. Another example would be a baseball coach instructing a pitcher to keep his hand on top of the ball when taking it out of the glove. Advances in equipment, such as high-speed video cameras, force platforms, and electromyography allow for a much more in depth analysis of sport performance. A pitcher can have his throwing motion analyzed and a biomechanist can determine the angular velocity of his shoulder. A biomechanist could also determine the amount of stress placed on the medial side of his elbow. Biomechanical studies of baseball players have found that pitchers throwing with high velocity, when compared with pitchers throwing lower velocity balls have a greater amount of external rotation at the shoulder, greater anterior tilt of the trunk when the ball is released, and a higher amount of angular velocity of the pelvis and torso.

Sport biomechanics also investigate the equipment used by athletes. This can include enhancing equipment to improve performance, such the design of speed skates and hockey sticks. Equipment may also be modified for safety reasons after undergoing a biomechanical analysis. A recent development by biomechanists at the University of Delaware led to the design of a new figure skate that allowed the skater to land toe-first and then bring the rest of the foot down to the ice. This allows the ground reaction force from the ice to be spread over a much greater time and reduces the peak forces transmitted up the lower extremity. Prior to this new design, the old figure skate limited the motion at the ankle and caused the skater to land in a flat footed position, which would decrease the amount of time the impact force from the ice is applied to the foot and increase the peak impact forces. In addition to helping reduce stress in the lower extremity, this new skate also may help performance (4).

Other sports and activities that have been improved recently by advances in sport biomechanics include golf and running. Golf biomechanics can identify flaws in a person's swing and help correct them to improve club head speed and ball contact, which will result in greater distance and accuracy. Footwear has greatly changed over the past few years. Shoes are now specifically designed for different types of feet in order to help prevent an overuse injury and increase the running velocity of the athlete. A biomechanical analysis can also identify small errors with an athlete's running gait that could potentially be the difference between winning or losing the race. Current athletic wear has been designed to increase athletic performance by providing less resistance to movement.

Clinical Biomechanics

Clinical biomechanics is more concerned with *mechanopathology*, the mechanics that cause an injury, and *pathomechanics*, the mechanics that are the result of an injury (2). A person may step down off a curve onto an uneven surface and "roll" his ankle, resulting in a lateral ankle sprain. The mechanopathology of this injury would be the ground reaction force causing excessive inversion at the ankle joint, resulting in the sprain. After sustaining the injury, the person may lose some range of motion at his ankle and change his walking gait. This change in walking gait would be an example of pathomechanics. Specialists that use clinical biomechanics are concerned with understanding and possibly eliminating the mechanopathology that may cause an injury (Figure 12.11). They also are able to predict and identify the pathomechanics that will occur as a result of an injury and develop interventions to correct these faulty mechanics.

There are several different types of specialists that use clinical biomechanics. An orthopedic surgeon needs an understanding of biomechanics to make surgical repairs of ligaments and tendons. Athletic trainers and physical therapists need an understanding of biomechanics to understand the injury mechanopathology

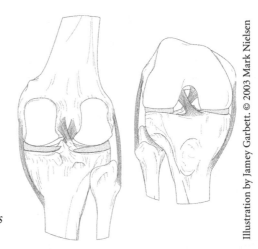

Figure 12.11. *Understanding the mechanopathology of knee ligament injuries is crucial for clinical biomechanics.*

Illustration by Jamey Garbett. © 2003 Mark Nielsen

and the resulting pathomechanics that may occur after an injury. An example would be understanding how the different ligaments of the knee protect it against specific forces and the typical mechanopathology that would cause a specific knee injury. A prosthetics and orthotics specialist will need an understanding of biomechanics when he is designing and fitting a prosthetic limb. To treat and rehabilitate patients after injury or disease, these specialists must first understand the normal biomechanics of human movement, such as walking, running, and prehension. With a basic understanding of what is normal, the specialists will be much more efficient when presented with a patient with a specific disease or disorder that affects movement. Ergonomists are also clinical specialists that utilize biomechanics in the occupational setting. This includes evaluating a wide range of movement and loading patterns, from workers on a factor assembly line to people that primarily work at a desk. Many orthopedic issues, such as low back pain and carpal tunnel syndrome, may be the result of unnecessary stress placed on the musculoskeletal system due to improper workstation design. An ergonomist can evaluate the interaction between the person and their workstation and make recommendations to reduce the risk of injury.

An area that is critical for both sport biomechanics and clinical biomechanics is balance and stability. These are crucial for optimal sport performance, and often times after an injury, disease or disorder there is a loss of balance and stability. Balance can be defined as the ability to control the body (center of gravity) over the base of support (2). Our base of support is normally our feet, but can also include the hands, particularly in sport like gymnastics or if a person puts his or her hand on the ground to prevent a fall.

Balance can be further broken down into static balance and dynamic balance. In static balance, all the forces acting on the body are in equilibrium. When a person is standing, there are two external forces acting on them: the person's weight and the ground reaction force. As long as the vector from the vertical component of the ground reaction force, which is the center of pressure, stays directly under the person's center of gravity, the person will remain in static equilibrium. An example of static balance would be when a person is standing still, either on one leg or both legs.

During a dynamic situation, the center of pressure is not always going to be directly under the center of gravity, because the person is moving. The ability of the person to return the center of pressure under the center of gravity is crucial for athletic performance. Examples of dynamic balance include walking, running, cutting, and landing from a jump. Dynamic balance is more challenging and will suffer more following an injury, disease, or with aging.

The size of a person's base of support has a large influence on balance. The larger the base of support, the more stable the person is. With the increase in stability, however, comes a decrease in mobility. A person cannot walk or run very fast if they have a wide base of support. Toddlers and the elderly will oftentimes walk with a wide base of support because they need the extra stability. With a narrow base of support, a person can walk or run at a much faster speed, however, stability will suffer. Therefore, the more stable a person is, the less mobile he or she is, and the more mobile a person is, the less stable he or she is. Whenever a person's center of gravity moves outside of his or her base of support, they will become unstable, and a corrective move (oftentimes a step) must take place to restore equilibrium. If this corrective measure does not occur fast enough to move the center of gravity back within the base of support, the person will fall.

In sports, it is necessary for an athlete to learn how to maintain balance in a way that also maximizes mobility. A running back must know how to change directions quickly while maintaining balance in order to be successful. A hockey goalie must maintain balance while moving around on the ice to stop a slapshot. A basketball player must maintain balance after landing from a jump so he or she can move in another direction as quickly as possible. These movements must be analyzed to ensure that the athletes are maximizing their mobility while also gaining optimum stability. In the clinical setting, most lower extremity injuries, such as ankle sprains, knee sprains, and muscle strains will have a negative effect on balance. The clinician must understand how to evaluate balance after an injury and what exercises to prescribe in order to restore balance. Many neurological disorders, such as Parkinson's disease, multiple sclerosis, and cerebellar disorders will have a negative impact on balance. There are a number of tools that can be used to evaluate balance, including force platforms, the BalanceMaster, and Biodex balance system. Balance can also be easily evaluated by having a person stand on both or one legs with the eyes open or closed, and observing the amount of sway that is present. There are also simple tests that can be performed to evaluate dynamic balance.

BIOMECHANICAL TOOLS

There are many different tools and equipment that can be used to perform a biomechanical analysis. The most commonly used tool is the video camera. Because human movement is so inherently complex, a video imaging system is the only piece of equipment that captures all of the data (9). Eadweard Muybridge was the first person to use cinematography to analyze human movement. Today there are several different types of video cameras used to capture human movement, ranging from the standard home video camcorder to high-speed cameras that can record at several thousand frames per second. Most video cameras used to shoot home movies have an adequate frame rate to capture everyday movements, but the rate is not high enough to adequately capture many athletic movements, such as hitting or throwing a baseball.

The goniometer is another tool used in a biomechanical analysis. A goniometer is an electrical potentiometer that is attached to the limbs and is used to measure joint angles. The goniometer has two arms: One is attached to the proximal limb segment, and the other arm is attached to the distal limb segment. For example, if one wanted to measure knee flexion and extension, one arm of the goniometer would be attached to the lateral portion of the thigh and the other arm would be attached to the lateral portion of the lower leg. The axis of the goniometer would be positioned over the axis of the knee joint. Goniometers are relatively inexpensive and the data is available for interpretation immediately after it is collected. However, there are some disadvantages. Goniometers can require a large amount of time to be placed properly over a joint, they can affect movement, especially if multiple goniometers are used, and they measure relative angles, not absolute angles. Goniometers are effective at hinge joints such as the elbow and knee, but not as effective at more complex joints like the hip and shoulder (9).

To analyze human movement in all three dimensions, a multi-camera motion capture system is a necessity. There are several different types of motion capture systems. A television imaging camera system is used with retroreflective markers placed over various bony landmarks. Issues can arise when using this type of system to measure fast movements because of the tendency for the picture to be blurry. In order to help eliminate the problem of blurriness, infrared cameras may be used. Infrared cameras do not use visible light and are not affected by reflections from other light sources. Infrared cameras can also capture data at much higher frequencies than television video cameras. A typical infrared motion capture system will consist of six to 12 cameras mounted around a biomechanics laboratory. The light reflected from the infrared camera is the only light picked up by the camera, thus freezing each image and eliminating blurriness (9).

There are several pieces of equipment that can be used to measure force. This includes dynamometers, force transducers, and force platforms. A force transducer outputs an electrical signal that is proportional to the force applied to it. Some examples of force transducers include piezoelectric, piezoresistive, strain gauge, and capacitive. When force is applied to the transducer, it causes a certain amount of strain. A force platform is a very useful tool for measuring the most common type of force acting on the body, which is the ground. Any time we walk, run, jump, or stand, we apply a force to the ground through our foot, and the ground applies a force back on our feet. This force is three dimensional, and includes a vertical component, an anterior-posterior component, and a medial-lateral component. A force plate measures the ground reaction force, and it measures the center of pressure. This is very useful for analyzing a variety of skills, including walking, running, jumping, landing, balance, and a variety of sports skills. A typical force platform is approximately 2 feet by 2 feet and can be mounted within the floor of a biomechanics laboratory. It consists of four triaxial force transducers located at the four corners of the plate. This allows for the measurement of the ground reaction force in all three dimensions, the center of pressure, and the moments about the x, y, and z axis (9).

A force plate is a very useful tool for evaluating a person's walking gait. There are two peaks to the vertical component of the ground reaction force. Each of these peaks is greater in magnitude than the person's body weight. The vertical force rises at heel contact and peaks once full weight bearing occurs. It then decreases during the middle portion of the stance phase as the knee flexes, and peaks again during pushoff as the ankle plantar flexors become active to propel the body forward. The force will decrease as the foot moves off of the force plate. The anterior-posterior force, depending on the orientation of the force plate, will peak in either the positive or negative direction at heel strike, and then it will shift direction and peak in the opposite direction at toe off. At heel strike, the anterior-posterior force is considered to be a braking force, and at toe off, it is a propulsive force. The medial-lateral component of the ground reaction force is useful in analyzing the amount of pronation and supination present at the foot during walking. A person with a flat foot will have excessive pronation and will display a great deal of medial force. The path of the center of pressure will also be more medially directed in a person with flat feet.

In addition to analyzing walking and running gait, a force plate can also be useful for analyzing a person's balance. By measuring the person's center of pressure, characteristics of balance such as sway area, sway velocity, and radial displacement can be calculated. Force plates are also useful tools for analyzing jumping and landing. The propulsive force during the upward phase of a jump can provide useful data that when combined with kinematic data from a motion capture system can help an athlete to jump higher. Landing forces can also be measured in order to analyze impact to ensure proper technique is being used and equal stress is being placed on both of the limbs.

If a biomechanist or clinician wants to examine patterns of muscle activity, electromyography (EMG) is the tool of choice. A motor unit consists of an alpha motor neuron and all the muscle fibers it innervates. It takes an action potential to activate a motor unit. This action potential is the result of an electrochemical process and this electrical component of the signal can be amplified and recorded.

There are two types of EMG: surface and intramuscular. Surface EMG uses adhesive electrodes that are placed parallel to the muscle fibers. Surface EMG is noninvasive and relatively easy to use. However, it can only measure the average activity of several motor units, it can only record the activity of muscles close to the surface, and it is prone to movement artifact because the skin oftentimes is subject to movement when a person is moving. Intramuscular EMG involves inserting a needle directly into the muscle. It can measure the electrical activity of a single motor unit. It is also very useful for examining deeper muscles, such as the muscles of the rotator cuff. Intramuscular EMG is invasive and requires specialized training to use. Surface EMG is oftentimes beneficial for laboratory studies that involve a great deal of movement, such as walking, running, jumping, and other sports activities. Intramuscular EMG is more beneficial for clinical studies to determine if a nerve is functioning properly.

Electromyography may be used to measure reaction time, muscle latencies, and muscle activation patterns. Reaction time is a measure of the amount of time it takes a person to prepare and initiate a response to a specific stimuli. It is a critical component of many athletic skills. By using EMG, a biomechanist can determine how long it takes a muscle to activate after a person is presented with a specific stimulus. Measuring the activity of the hip extensors during the start of a track race would be one example.

Muscle latencies, especially during reflexive movements, can also be measured using EMG. When the ankle is forced into inversion, which is the common mechanism of a lateral ankle sprain, the muscle spindles in the peroneus longus and peroneus brevis are activated due to these muscles lengthening. This rapid lengthening causes a reflexive shortening of these muscles to counteract the inversion at the ankle. The amount of time it takes these muscles to become active after the onset of the inversion moment can be measured using EMG, and EMG can be used to determine how different injuries affects this latency (7).

Electromyography can also be used to determine muscle activation patterns during more complex movements, such as walking, running, and throwing. A biomechanist may be interested in determining the relationship between the hip flexors and hip extensors during running or examining the activation patterns of the elbow flexors and elbow extensors during the overhead throwing motion.

SUMMARY

Biomechanics is the study of the structure and function of biological systems by the means and methods of mechanics. Biomechanics has strong roots in anatomy, physiology, physics, and motor learning. Several different specialists use biomechanics to analyze human movement, including exercise scientists, orthopedic surgeons, coaches, athletic trainers, physical therapists, and occupational therapists. The goals of a biomechanical analysis are safety, effectiveness, and efficiency. Several different pieces of equipment are useful for performing a biomechanical analysis, including video cameras, force plates, and electromyography. However, a biomechanical analysis can be conducted simply be watching a person move. There are different branches of biomechanics, including clinical biomechanics and sport biomechanics. Clinical biomechanics is used to analyze issues related to injuries, rehabilitation, surgical reconstruction, and biomechanical issues related to the workplace. Sport biomechanics is used to improve sport performance.

REFERENCES

1. Enoka, R.M., *Neuromechanics of Human Movement*. Champaign, IL: Human Kinetics, 2002.

2. Flanagan, S.P., *Biomechanics: A Case Based Approach*. Burlington, MA: Jones & Bartlett Learning, 2014.

3. Floyd, R.T., *Manual of Structural Kinesiology*. New York: McGraw-Hill, 2007.

4. Hall, S.J., *Basic Biomechanics*. New York: McGraw-Hill, 2007.

5. Hamilton, N., W. Weimar, and K. Luttgens, *Kinesiology: Scientific Basis of Human Movement*. New York: McGraw-Hill, 2008.

6. Hatze, H., "The meaning of the term biomechanics." *Journal of Biomechanics* 7(1974): 189–190.

7. Knight, A.C., and W. H. Weimar, "Effects of inversion perturbation after step down task on the latency of the peroneus longus and peroneus brevis." *Journal of Applied Biomechanics* 27(2011): 283–290.

8. Nordin, M., and V. H. Frankel, *Basic Biomechanics of the Musculoskeletal System*. Philadelphia, PA: Lippincott Williams & Wilkins, 2001.

9. Winter, D.A., *Biomechanics and Motor Control of Human Movement*. Hoboken, NJ: John Wiley & Sons, 2005.

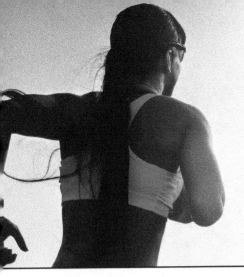

BEHAVIORAL KNOWLEDGE BASE

O ur understanding of human movement would be incomplete without delving into the mental and emotional processes that are part of our basic natures as humans. Thus, two important disciplines of kinesiology, Exercise and Sport Psychology (Chapter 13) and Motor Behavior (Chapter 14), seek to understand human movement in behavioral terms.

Science can ascertain many factors that lead to world record sport performances, including nutritional, physiological, and biomechanical factors. However, unless we understand what motivates athletes to pursue and achieve top performances or why certain individuals continue to exercise while others do not, our understanding of human movement would be lacking. The psychological makeup of individuals, then, is an important realm of study. Likewise, kinesiology is concerned with understanding the processes that lead to movement, both skilled and unskilled. These processes involve the central and peripheral nervous systems and the neural circuits that innervate muscle groups. This, coupled with how developmental factors across the lifespan changes human movement, is the topic of this section.

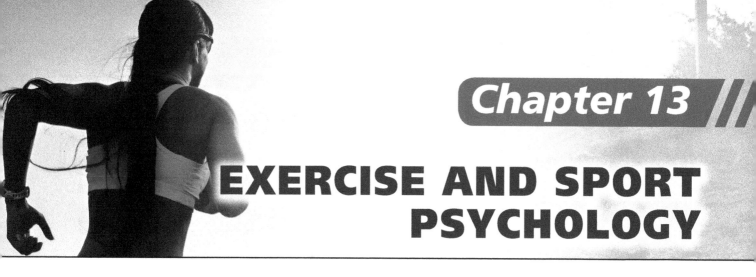

Chapter 13

EXERCISE AND SPORT PSYCHOLOGY

OUTLINE

OBJECTIVES

1. Distinguish between exercise and sport psychology.
2. Describe how exercise might influence thoughts and emotions.
3. Describe some underlying principles common to exercise and sport psychology.

"Just Do It"— "Impossible is Nothing"—"Be Your Own Champion"—"It's What's Inside"

What do these slogans mean to you? Do they inspire? Do they make you want to get up off the couch and go work out? Do they make you want to compete harder against the competition? Why does a simple three- or four-word slogan influence some to start exercising and others to practice harder? And for those who aren't motivated by a simple phrase (or even concern for their own health), how do we get them to become physically active or help them compete at a higher level? The answers to these questions are found within the discipline of exercise and sport psychology.

Simply stated, exercise and sport psychology involves taking the theories and research of psychology and putting these ideas into practice in the paradigm of sport, exercise, and physical activity. The goals of exercise and sport psychology are twofold:

1. To help participants optimize their involvement, performance, and enjoyment of sport and exercise
2. To help individuals change their behavior during recovery and rehabilitation from injury or illness and improve their quality of life

Regarding the quality of life, exercise has long been recognized as having the potential to influence moods and emotions, thus there is thought to be a link between mental health and physical health. The sidebar on anxiety and depression examines the case for exercise and mental health.

Concepts from exercise and sport psychology are often utilized in advertising and marketing across a wide variety of business and industry. Although there are many specific areas of concern within exercise and sport psychology (goal setting, concentration, motivation, relaxation, imagery, team building, and teamwork), the general goal is to teach the mental skills necessary to perform consistently in training and competition, increase adherence to exercise programs, and/or to help individuals realize their potential.

Anxiety and Depression

Research has clearly shown that acute and chronic exercise is associated with reductions in anxiety and depression. These effects hold for those suffering from mild-to-moderate levels of anxiety and depression and for those who have normal levels of anxiety and depression. Endurance and resistance forms of exercise reduce depression, while only endurance (aerobic) exercise has been shown to be effective in alleviating anxiety. Few research studies have examined the dose-response nature of exercise effects. To do this, the study would have to vary exercise dose by manipulating *intensity, duration,* and *frequency,* then study the impact on psychological status.

Unfortunately, the research is still fairly equivocal, because some suggests that durations of as little as 5 minutes may result in favorable psychological changes. The main problem with making any conclusive statements about minimal durations and intensities is the overall failure of the research to systematically examine these variables. However, it does seem that as the length of chronic exercise training increases, greater reductions in anxiety and depression occur. This suggests that making exercise a regular lifestyle habit improves mental health, but carrying this healthy habit to an extreme could prove to be problematic (see Overtraining and Mental Health).

CASE STUDY Overtraining and Mental Health

Although a regular regimen of exercise is healthy, taking it to the extreme can lead to problems. Athletes involved in heavy training can sometimes experience significant mental health disturbances; sports like swimming and distance running are an example. Overtraining in these sports involves high mileage so that when the athlete tapers (reduces the training load) before competitions, the body responds with faster times.

Intensive training changes the psychological state so that the individual experiences increased tension and depression and decreased feelings of vigor and energy. This is not unexpected given such intensive training, but some athletes may become clinically depressed. In such a response, the athlete should reduce training and seek assistance.

Such negative psychological changes are tightly linked with the training load in swimming. The athlete's mental health is negatively affected when the training load increases, but it is positively affected with the training load decreases. It has been proposed that psychological monitoring of the athletes during the course of their season could help prevent some cases of more severe psychological disturbances.

WORKING WITH CLIENTS

It should be remembered that there is no "one size fits all" program for clients (whether athletes or individuals who exercise) or patients. Any type of intervention, rehabilitation program, or performance enhancement strategy must be customized for the individual. Much of what exercise and sport psychology entails is getting to know the individual, their circumstances, goals, and desired outcomes.

In working with individuals, groups, or teams, the performance enhancement consultant or exercise psychology consultant will often perform an initial interview. An initial interview may also entail meeting with other individuals who may be involved or have a significant interest. These stakeholders can include parents, spouses, coaches, physicians, team owners, employers, or others who may have a vested interest in the client's health or performance. Oftentimes, it is critical for the PEC or exercise psychology consultant to ensure client confidentiality and to be sure that stakeholders understand what will and can be discussed with them. This will build trusting relationships with clients, which can then be used to provide a customized program.

There are some individuals who are beyond the area of expertise and scope of practice for the sport and exercise psychologist. Clients, patients, and athletes who display evidence of poor coping, depression, or anxiety that interferes with their ability to function, who seem to be abusing recreational or prescription medication or drugs, or who have chronic complaints of being overwhelmed may need referral for further, more specialized assistance. Additionally, people dealing with a life crisis of some type (marital issues, unemployment, financial issues, familial health problems) need to be referred to a mental health professional.

UNDERLYING PRINCIPLES

Many of the concepts and ideas used in exercise and sport psychology originate from research and theories within the parent discipline of psychology. Underlying theories from psychology provide the foundation for effective practice and use of counseling techniques and motivational skills.

The use of various assessments, including discussion of an individual's goals, motivations, and likes/dislikes assists with an initial plan of action. In addition to information gained from the meeting, questionnaires, or other psychometric instruments can be utilized to focus on specific needs (improving self-confidence, decreasing anxiety, evaluating possible depression). Once the client—practitioner relationship has been established, the PEC can begin to apply theoretical underpinnings in the development of a suitable program.

A Brief History of Exercise and Sport Psychology

The discipline of exercise and sport psychology is not all that new. The first recognized research study is attributed to Norman Triplett (1861–1931) in which he observed that cyclists riding in a group tended to have faster times than those riding by themselves. Further, G. Stanley Hall (1844–1924) reported on the benefits of physical education in childhood development in 1908. Both Triplett and Hall are noted for their contributions to the founding of social psychology and educational psychology, respectively. G. Stanley Hall is also noted for founding the American Psychological Association (APA) in 1892.

Coleman Griffith (1893–1966) is largely recognized as the "father" of sport psychology. In 1925 he founded the Research in Athletics Laboratory at the University of Illinois. His research involved studies of personality, motor learning, and motivation in reference to performance in sport. In 1938 P. K. Wrigley, owner of the Chicago Cubs, hired Griffith to help improve the team's performance, which involved filming and measuring the players' skills in an attempt to build a "scientific" training program. The information derived from these studies resulted in more than 600 pages of published reports.

Unlike sport psychology, exercise psychology was not formally recognized as an area of study until the late 1960s and early 1970s. William P. Morgan expanded the psychological study of physical performance beyond that of sport performance. His research originated in work psychology and expanded further to include highly influential studies on the role of exercise on anxiety and depression. His research also provided the foundation for understanding and studying exercise adherence and exercise addiction.

As may be derived from the history of sport and exercise psychology, both interest areas can be traced from their origins in the parent disciplines of psychology and physical education, with further later contributions from exercise science, social psychology, educational psychology, and ergonomics. As the fields of sport and exercise psychology continued to evolve, other specialty areas developed (health psychology, rehabilitation psychology, performance psychology). These fields continue to aid advances in exercise and sport psychology today (Figure 13.1).

It should be noted that study in either exercise or sport psychology will not result in an individual becoming a licensed clinical psychologist. In many states individuals are not allowed to call themselves an exercise or sport psychologist unless they are licensed clinical psychologists.

The preferred term for individuals who practice exercise or sport psychology, but are not clinically licensed, is performance enhancement consultants (PEC). PECs are professionals trained in sport and exercise, but they are not licensed psychologists or counselors. They also may be known as exercise or sport psychology consultants or mental coaches.

There is an assortment of theories from which performance enhancement, injury rehabilitation, or behavior change programs can be constructed. Each of these theories and models is briefly described as applied to exercise and sport psychology.

Learning Theories

Learning theories are based on the idea that more complex behaviors, such as shooting a free-throw accurately or successful weight loss, are the result of many smaller and simpler behaviors. By targeting the smaller components with reinforcement (such as saying good job or providing rewards for achieving a predetermined goal), the individual will associate the new behavior with the reinforcement. Reinforcement can be both positive and negative in nature and may result in an individual performing or not performing the desired behavior. Positive reinforcement is typically the most effective way to motivate individuals toward desired behaviors (5).

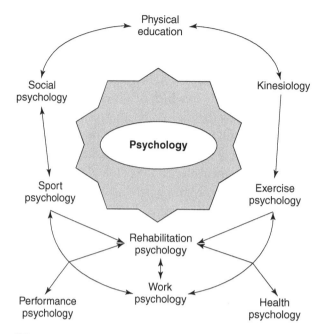

Figure 13.1. *The disciplines of exercise psychology and sport psychology are each influenced by a number of disciplines/professions, including psychology, physical education, and kinesiology. In turn, exercise psychology and sport psychology have influenced other disciplines and led to the development of additional fields of study.*

Health Belief Model

Theoretically, an individual will engage in a behavior, such as exercise, in response to a perceived threat to one's health. While the health belief model is typically employed more in exercise psychology, it may also apply to sports. Underlying the health belief model is the belief that the benefits of an action must outweigh its costs. Hence, individuals must feel they can change their behavior and will be successful in accomplishing their goals. This concept is known as self-efficacy, which may be defined as an individual's self-confidence in his or her ability to perform a task or complete a goal (9).

Transtheoretical Model

The transtheoretical model, also known as the stages of change, is a theory that is used almost exclusively in exercise psychology. The model consists of three key components: (a) people progress through five stages of change at varying rates, (b) throughout the process of change, people will move back and forth through the stages at various rates, and (c) people will use various cognitive and behavioral processes and strategies to facilitate change. Within the transtheoretical model there are five cognitive and five behavior processes (see Table 13.1). It is typically suggested that the cognitive processes are best utilized during the early stages of change and that the behavioral processes are more effective during the latter stages (8).

Relapse Prevention Model

The relapse prevention model involves the development of plans and interventions for coping with situations that may result in lapses or relapses in behavior changes or rehabilitation, or self-destructive type behaviors. In simple terms, this model suggests that we help individuals plan for things that may upset their plans or goals.

Table 13.1. The Transtheoretical Model.

Cognitive Processes	Behavioral Processes
Consciousness Raising—increasing knowledge	*Counterconditioning*—substituting alternatives
Dramatic Relief—warning of risks	*Helping Relationships*—enlisting social support
Environmental Reevaluation—caring about the consequences to oneself and others	*Reinforcement Management*—rewarding yourself
Self-Reevaluation—comprehending benefits	*Self-Liberation*—committing yourself
Social Liberation—increasing healthy opportunities	*Stimulus Control*—reminding yourself

These things may be holidays, vacations, illness, or injury. Or in the case of sport, the relapse prevention model can be utilized in helping an athlete cope with losing a game, becoming injured, or other unexpected events like a suspension or not making a team.

In either situation, it is incumbent upon the practitioner to help the client realize that missing a workout session, or losing a game or whatever the case may be, is not the end of the world. Rather, the client is assisted in creating plans and strategies to move forward. If the client is unable to move past certain issues, it may be necessary to find further assistance for him or her, such as a licensed counselor or psychologist (6, 7).

Reasoned Action

The theory of reasoned action suggests that an individual's intentions are the most important factors in determining behaviors. Thus, the individual's attitude toward the behavior or action will influence his or her success. For example, if a team believes they will win or lose, this will influence their attitudes toward their performance. If an injured athlete believes he or she will never return to full abilities this will impact his or her attitudes toward rehabilitation.

These attitudes can be influenced by the individual's own confidence and the attitudes of others around them, which is known as subjective norms. Subjective norms can include the attitudes, feelings, and support (or lack thereof) of family members, coaches, friends, fans, therapists, and others who the client may interact with in some manner—including social media (10).

Planned Behavior

The theory of planned behavior extends the theory of reasoned action by incorporating behavioral control. Behavioral control includes perceived power and control, which is the suggestion that the individual has a perceived amount of control over the behavior or action in question. As with reasoned action theory, the intentions of the individual can greatly influence the outcome. However, with the inclusion of behavioral control, the individual takes a greater role in determining and thus influencing the outcome.

This theory can manifest as, for example, a client providing input in his or her exercise prescription or athletes taking it upon themselves to organize extra practice sessions. These strategies are intertwined with motivation and self-efficacy (confidence) building, which can assist the individual in taking control of his or her situations (1).

Social Cognitive Theory

Social cognitive theory is one of the most widely known and used theories to assist in behavior change, and includes behavioral, personal, and environmental factors (see Figure 13.2). Within these three factors are a range of influences that can be used by clients/patients/athletes to assist them in achieving their goals.

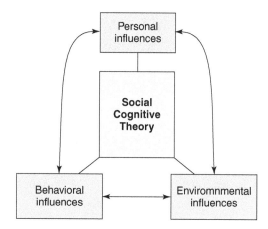

Figure 13.2. *The social cognitive theory includes considerations for how the relationship between personal, behavioral, and environmental influences can impact an individual's motivations and actions.*

These influences range across an array of interventional strategies from observational (vicarious) learning to goal-setting to management of emotional arousal. Each of these influences can assist the individual in achieving the desired outcome (11).

DIFFERENCES BETWEEN SPORT AND EXERCISE PSYCHOLOGY

Exercise and sport psychology are two separate fields of study with unique characteristics, although they also share some commonalities. First examined are the differences before discussing what these disciplines have in common.

Sport Psychology

Sport psychology involves the study of how psychological factors can affect performance and how participation in sport and exercise affect psychological and physical factors. In addition to performance improvement, sport psychology may be used to assist athletes, coaches, and parents when dealing with injuries, rehabilitation, communication, team building, and career transitions (4).

Sport psychology can be divided into academic and applied focus areas. Academic sport psychologists typically focus on performing research, teaching basic concepts of sport psychology to practitioners (coaches, athletic trainers, strength and conditioning coaches), and training future academics and certified sport psychology consultants. Those who work in the academic area of sport psychology will most typically hold a doctorate (Ph.D. or Ed.D.) degree in sport psychology.

Practitioners of applied sport psychology assist individual athletes or teams perform at an optimal level. Typical scenarios involve the use of a sport psychologist to help athletes overcome a "slump," recover from an injury, or work with a team through performance-related issues preventing their best effort. Sport psychologists are expected to have an understanding of psychological issues as well as the demands and challenges of the sport in which the athlete performs.

The Association for Applied Sport Psychology (AASP) serves as a unifying body to promote the development of science and ethical practice in the field of sport psychology. AASP offers a certified consultant designation in sport psychology to members with a master's or doctoral degree who meet specific course requirements in the sport and exercise sciences at both the graduate and undergraduate level. They also complete an extensive (a minimum of 400 hours) supervised work experience in the area.

Those involved in the applied sport psychology may work in a variety of settings. Some colleges and universities have certified consultants on staff in athletic departments to assist their athletes, while other consultants may have private practices. Those individuals with private practices may consult with both amateur and professional athletes for either a set hourly fee or on retainer. Additionally, the majority of private sporting academies (International Management Group [IMG] Academy) and national athletic development groups

(U.S. Olympic Committee [USOC], Australian Institute of Sport [AIS]) will have sport psychology consultants on staff to help train their athletes in performance enhancement techniques.

Exercise Psychology

Formally, exercise psychology includes the study of behavioral, physiological, cognitive, and social factors that serve as the antecedents to and consequences of acute and chronic exercise. What this basically means is that exercise psychologists attempt to answer various questions such as determining how exercise affects behavior and learning, why people do or do not engage in exercise and physical activity, and how to motivate individuals to be more active or change unhealthful behaviors. These questions are just a small sampling of what exercise psychologists research to find new ways to assist clients and patients.

Like sport psychology, exercise psychology can be divided into both academic and applied areas; however, the career prospects do not follow the same model. Within the academic side of exercise psychology, the focus is typically on performing research, teaching classes, and mentoring students. This avenue serves as the most common area of employment for those interested in exercise psychology, because there is not currently a market for hiring exercise psychologists in private industry. Rather, the information taught to students in introductory level exercise psychology courses is intended to assist them in their future profession. A course in exercise psychology provides students basic knowledge they can use to assist clients or patients in becoming more active, changing behaviors, or achieving goals.

CONCEPTS COMMON TO EXERCISE PSYCHOLOGY AND SPORT PSYCHOLOGY

It is easy to recognize how sport psychology and exercise psychology are different—one deals primarily with exercise motivation and adherence, while the other primarily works with athletic performance enhancement. However, they both share similar roots and thus have much more in common than one might realize. The largest difference between these two areas is the clientele involved and how the information is applied (2).

The similarities between the exercise and sport psychology are quite extensive. Many of these skill sets and ideas used in one area are easy to transfer into the other, when modified appropriately. Concepts such as goal-setting and motivation are used in sport, exercise, injury and health rehabilitation, as well as in advertising and business. These two concepts—goal-setting and motivational strategies—are key components in any interventional or performance enhancement—type program. They are also essential components in many marketing campaigns. The motivational slogans at the start of this chapter are also slogans for various sporting goods companies.

The concepts underlying exercise and sport psychology are regularly employed in many industries and everyday life. The following are basic examples of how ideas originating from exercise and sport psychology can be utilized to assist patients or clients in improving their health or performance and serve to assist an individual in changing their behavior.

Goal Setting

The establishment of a goal-setting program includes setting specific, measurable goals that are realistic and challenging, but still achievable. These goals should be tangible (important) to the person setting the goal and should include a deadline for achievement. People commonly set goals that omit portions of these guidelines, making the goal vague or difficult to evaluate or determine when it has been reached. Further, individuals often need assistance and support in trying to achieve their goals, so practitioners in fields related to kinesiology are often called upon to assist clients or patients in setting, evaluating progress on, revising, and ultimately achieving their goals. Understanding the concepts of goal-setting and having the knowledge and experience in helping someone to achieve those goals is a focus area in exercise and sport psychology programs.

Motivational Strategies

Assisting clients, patients, and athletes to work toward their goals, make positive behavioral changes, and continue to put forth the effort needed to improve performance or health is an essential element of both exercise and sport psychology. A practitioner should be able to find ways to encourage and motivate clients and patients. However, these methods need to be specific to each individual. What might work for one person may not work for another.

Talking with clients, athletes, and patients to determine their reasons for coming to you, discussing factors that may interfere or inhibit progress, and developing the best means and methods for helping them achieve their specific goals is critical in determining an exercise, rehabilitation, or performance enhancement program.

Time Management and Organization

The ability to plan and maintain one's regular schedule in a way that allows for the inclusion of exercise or practice while reducing or avoiding confusion, conflict, and undue stress is quite common between exercise psychology and sport psychology. Exercise and sport psychologists teach clients or patients time management techniques, including managing life demands and assisting them to determine possible exercise interventions that can be done throughout the day.

Anxiety or Energy Management

Individuals who have knowledge of techniques in exercise or sport psychology are often called upon to assist clients, patients, or athletes manage anxiety, stress, and anger. Anxiety management skills are most commonly used to help individuals who experience anxiety, stress, or activation at levels that are not effective (too high or too low) for optimal performance. Techniques may include: (a) breathing exercises (diaphragmatic breathing, rhythmic breathing), (b) progressive relaxation, (c) meditation, (d) imagery or visualization, and (e) cognitive techniques (thought stopping and cognitive restructuring). These techniques can be used to increase performance, reduce awareness of evaluative factors, and assist individuals in reducing pain or fear of a situation.

Imagery, Visualization, Mental Practice

Imagery, visualization, and mental practice are used to help enhance individuals' performance, assist in rehabilitation, and learn new skills. While these skills are more commonly used in sport performance enhancement, they can be useful in many areas outside of sport:

- Imagery and visualization of structures, routes, or procedures to assist in learning and processing of information
- Mental practice to help students remember facts, concepts, or skills

Regardless of the context in which these skills are used, they can be a very effective means of helping an athlete perform better, an injured patient regain confidence in his or her abilities, or a client learn a new lift or imagine him or herself completing a desired goal.

Self-Talk

Self-efficacy is an important concept in exercise and sport psychology. Self-efficacy is the ability to complete tasks and reach goals. In exercise and sports, it is the belief that you can run and complete a 5K race or make the critical hit to win the game. Within the idea of self-efficacy is *self-talk*. Self-talk is what you say or think before, during, and after a task. Self-talk patterns are often related to how people feel and act. Self-talk is commonly used for (a) prompting specific behaviors, (b) improving self-confidence, (c) attention control, (d) motivation, and (e) arousal control.

In using self-talk to enhance performance, common components include the identification of negative or irrelevant thoughts, challenging these thoughts, and then creating positive thoughts, substituting them for the negative thoughts.

Team Building

One idea that started primarily in the sport setting, but has now become popular in industry is team building. Team building has crossed over into exercise settings, as many charities are now using teams to help in fundraising. For example, Ride-for-the-Cure and Run-for-the-Cure teams recruit individuals to participate in marathons, triathlons, and other similar events. These events provide training opportunities, social support (being a member of the team), and entry into the event in return for raising a certain amount of money for the organization in question. The American Heart Association and the American Diabetes Association are two organizations using team building.

Team building helps members of a group enhance their ability to work cohesively through the improvement of communication, group objectives, trust, and respect. It can also be used to build social support and provide individuals with someone they are accountable to during their efforts.

Team-building strategies in sport are often used at the beginning of a season to help group members become more familiar and trusting of each other. However, team-building activities are now becoming more common in business and industry. It takes skill to enhance teamwork and team building. Common techniques include group introductions of each other, challenge courses, and individual and team goal setting.

PROFESSIONAL ASSOCIATIONS

As mentioned previously, the Association of Applied Sport Psychology is an international, multidisciplinary, professional organization that offers certification to qualified professionals in the field of sport, exercise, and health psychology. While AASP tries to encompass both exercise and sport psychology, the focus of the organization is directed more toward sport, rather than exercise psychology (3).

Division 47 of the American Psychological Association (APA) was established in 1986 to further the clinical, educational, and scientific foundations of exercise and sport psychology. Division 47 tends to emphasize areas of scientific inquiry including motivation to persist and achieve; psychological considerations in sport injury and rehabilitation; counseling techniques with athletes, clients, and patients; talent assessment; exercise adherence and well-being; self-perceptions related to achieving; expertise in sport; youth sport; and performance enhancement and self-regulation techniques (2).

While these are the two most notable groups to specifically support sport and exercise psychology, other groups such as the American College of Sports Medicine (ACSM), the National Athletic Trainers' Association (NATA), and the American Public Health Association (APHA) also serve as outlets for the distribution of information regarding exercise and sport psychology.

SUMMARY

This chapter outlined the role and activities typically involved with exercise psychology and sport psychology. Exercise and sport psychology has a history that extends back to the 19th century with theoretical underpinnings taken from the parent discipline of psychology and specific applications made to exercise and sport. There are commonalities between exercise and sport psychology and also differences.

REFERENCES

1. Ajzen, I. From Intentions to Actions: A Theory of Planned Behavior. Springer Berlin Heidelberg, 1985.

2. APA Division 47: Society for Sport, Exercise & Performance Psychology. 750 First St. NE, Washington, DC 20002-4242.

3. Association for Applied Sport Psychology. 8365 Keystone Crossing, Suite 107 Indianapolis, IN 46240.

4. Bandura, A. Social Foundations of Thought and Action: A Social Cognitive Theory. Prentice-Hall, Inc., 1986.

5. Hall, C. S., Gardner, L. Theories of Personality. Hoboken, NJ: John Wiley & Sons, Inc., 1957.

6. Marlatt, G.A., Donovan, D. M. (Eds.). Relapse Prevention: Maintenance Strategies in the Treatment of Addictive Behaviors. Guilford Press, 2005.

7. Marlatt, G. A., George, W. H. Relapse prevention: Introduction and overview of the model. British journal of addiction, 1984: 261–273.

8. Prochaska, J.O., Velicer, W.F. The transtheoretical model of health behavior change. American Journal of Health Promotion, 1997: 38–48.

9. Rosenstock I.M. The health belief model and preventive health behavior. Health Education Monograph. 1974: 354–386.

10. Sheppard, B.H., Hartwick, J., Warshaw, P.R. The theory of reasoned action: A meta-analysis of past research with recommendations for modifications and future research. Journal of Consumer Research, 1988: 325–343.

11. Weinberg, R.S., Gould, D. Foundations of Sport and Exercise Psychology. Champaign, IL: Human Kinetics, 2010.

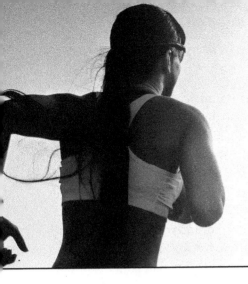

Chapter 14

MOTOR BEHAVIOR

OUTLINE

OBJECTIVES

1. Understand the historical background of motor behavior.
2. Understand the disciplines (motor development, learning, and control) of motor behavior.
3. Understand the academic and professional opportunities that are available within motor behavior.

ndrew is a former high school athlete and currently an undergraduate student employed by his city's Parks and Recreation Department as a coach for the children's basketball program. The participants are 5–6 years of age. The goal of his first practice is to obtain an assessment of the children's initial skill level. The coach has set up a series of stations that consist of basic basketball drills and skills. For example, some of the stations consist of stationary dribbling, dribbling around cones, passing the basketball to one another, and taking a shot a few feet from the basketball goal. However, this first practice is not beneficial because he failed to consider the motor and developmental level of the children along with basic principles and concepts related to the teaching, learning, and assessment of motor skills. There are principles and concepts that Andrew would have learned in any motor behavior course. Motor behavior is a discipline that has practical application to all individuals from researchers to clinicians to parents, because one must remember that all parts of our daily lives encompass some aspect of movement.

What if you were asked to identify a young child who has the potential to be an Olympic athlete or select applicants to serve in the Navy Seal Training Program? What deductive reasoning will you use to make this selection? Principles for the discipline of motor behavior have often been used to make these decisions. For example, during World War II, the U.S. military used a battery of personality, intelligence, and perceptual-motor tests to identify top applicants for the Aviation Cadet Program and these assessments are still used today (1). Principles and assessments as they relate to motor behavior and the science of how human and in some cases animals learn and control movement skills are extremely valuable to a wide range of professionals (physical education teachers, coaches, researchers, sport psychologists, physical and occupational therapists) and individuals whose ultimate outcome is motor (sport) performance. Motor performance refers to observable behaviors indicative of one's capability to complete motor tasks or skills. So, if you want to identify the next Serena Williams, Cameron Newton, Lindsay Vonn, or Albert Pujols, it would be imperative for you to have a thorough understanding of motor behavior.

BRANCHES OF MOTOR BEHAVIOR

The three branches of motor behavior are *motor development, motor control,* and *motor learning.* The following is a breakdown of the specific goals of each branch:

- Motor Development: Studies the progression and regression of one's movement ability and motor performance across the lifespan.
- Motor Control: Studies the neurological mechanisms and the mechanical functions that influence motor performance.
- Motor Learning: Studies how individuals learn and improve their motor skills and performance.

The ultimate goal of each area is to enhance and optimize skill performance and acquisition. There is a wide range of research questions that are commonly explored within motor behavior. Some questions investigate the type of practice that is most effective as it relates to skill learning, factors that influence the learning and retention of motor skills in young learners, the role of motor performance in physical activity across the lifespan, the neurological benefits of movement-related activities along with the movement demands (costs) for individuals with physical limitations or handicapping conditions (amputees, those with Parkinson's disease).

Although motor development, learning, and control are often considered three separate academic fields, researchers must possess a specialization in one of the fields, along with a basic competence in the other two. Research often overlaps. For example, a researcher may explore the relationship of motor skills competence or the learning and retention of motor skills on changes within the brain. Or she may investigate the neurological damage following stroke on an individual's activities of daily living or movement patterns. As you can see, motor behavior has a wide reach and researchers often take a similar approach to answering questions related to this academic discipline of exercise science.

CONSTRAINTS APPROACH TO MOVEMENT

There are three key questions that motor behaviorists often use to shape research investigations. It is important to understand:

1. What is the behavior you what to change or assess?
2. What are the factors that influence the behavior?
3. How can you control or measures factors to see how the behavior changes?

To answer these questions, motor behaviorists have created an approach to understanding motor performance through examining the constraints surrounding the movement task. Kugler and colleagues proposed the development of constraints that are caused by the interaction of a learner with their environment (the constraints model) (13).

> Karl M. Newell is the Marie Underhill Noll Chair and Professor of Kinesiology and Biobehavioral Health at Penn State University. His research area focuses on the coordination, control and skill of normal and abnormal human movement across the life-span along with the development of coordination. Dr. Newell's 1986 paper that focuses on constraints on the development of coordination is one of the most cited papers in motor behavior.

Dr. Newell further proposed a theory suggesting that how movement is accomplished is the result of three different constraints acting on that movement (18, 19). In this model, do not think of a constraint as negative, but rather as a guiding factor that can either elicit or repress movement. According to Newell, the three constraints acting on movements are *environment, task,* and *individual.*

Environmental constraints are factors external to the individual that shape our movement. These constraints are either physical or sociocultural factors. *Physical environmental factors* are external conditions like the temperature, lighting, and weather. For example, think about how rain, wind, and snow alters how a quarterback throws a football or how a softball player fields a ball. Various factors within our society also shape our motor patterns and behaviors. *Sociocultural factors* entail various social or cultural norms that greatly influence our movement. You might ask, How do norms and society influence movement? In the United States the passage of Title IX supported girls' and women's participation in movement, sport, and physical activity. However, in cultures where there are no laws supporting women's athletics, women may not be able to participate in sports due to a sociocultural constraint.

Task constraints are specific aspects of the task that may affect the outcome of the movement. Task constraints include the goals of the movement, rules, and equipment (19). All movement is constrained by the goal of the task. For example, take the sport of swimming: The stroke you are competing in will determine what movement pattern you must undertake. You would not perform the backstroke to compete in the free-style event. Hence, the task itself helps constrain the movement you choose to complete. Another example is football, where the goal is to outscore your opponent by accumulating more points through touchdowns and field goals. Imagine how athletes will have to alter their motor patterns and coaches change their strategy if the dimensions of the field or the size of the ball were to change.

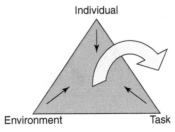

Figure 14.1. *Newell's constraints on movement.*

The last constraint in Newell's model is *individual constraints.* Individual constants consist of various structural and functional constraints. Specifically, structural constraints include physical characteristics like height, weight, body composition/size, and sex. Think how the structural constraint of height influenced the motor performance of two of the NBA tallest and shortest basketball players: Yao Ming (7 ft 6 in) and Earl Boykins (5 ft and 5 in). Functional constraints are a range of psychological and cognitive factors like motivation, drive, anxiety, and arousal that influence our mobility. Think of how an athlete's performance would be influenced if a person has either too much or too little anxiety. Hence, if motor behaviorists can understand the constraints surrounding a movement, they can better understand the movement itself.

MOTOR DEVELOPMENT: HOW WE DEVELOP MOTORICALLY

As stated previously in this chapter, motor development (Figure 14.2) is the study of movement changes across the lifespan and the underlying factors that affect these changes. Imagine your best friend has just had a baby. Everyday your friend bombards you with information about the amazing things her child has accomplished: rolling over, sitting up, pulling on a table to stand, crawling, and finally the first steps. Although you may not share your friend's endless joy, it is quite remarkable when you take a moment to think about how a newborn infant progresses from having little to no control over his motor coordination and movement skills to accomplishing bipedal walking and intentional grasping—two skills used on a daily basis across the lifespan.

Humans develop in four major domains: *physical, cognitive, affective,* and *motor* (21). As you can see, there is an overlap of developmental domains, indicating that all four domains are critical. Thus, it is important from a motor development standpoint to have a thorough understanding of all of three domains. Quite often research that evolves from motor development encompasses aspects of one if not all of the other domains. For example, young children demonstrate a positive relationship between self-perceptions of their physical ability (how they feel about how well they can perform a movement task) and their actual fundamental motor skills (how well they perform a movement task) (22). Additionally, self-perceptions of obese children are significantly lower than those with healthy weights (28). Data from the Framingham Heart study clearly demonstrates how aspects of physical growth (obesity) adversely affect one's cognitive performance in males. Thus, it is critically important to understand that we do not development within one silo or domain; humans simultaneously develop and grow within all four domains. So, take a moment and think back to the newborn baby developing from no control of movement to basic movement skills. The infant will continue to develop motor skills until she is proficient. Hence, researchers in the field of motor development seek to understand why and how we learn to move and how our learning to move impacts all facets of our development.

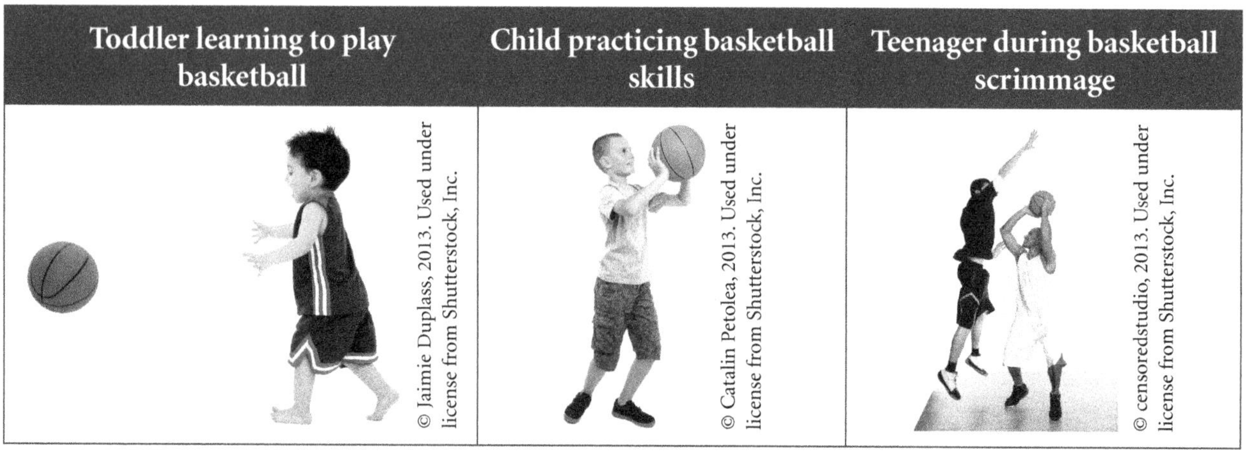

Toddler learning to play basketball	Child practicing basketball skills	Teenager during basketball scrimmage
© Jaimie Duplass, 2013. Used under license from Shutterstock, Inc.	© Catalin Petolea, 2013. Used under license from Shutterstock, Inc.	© censoredstudio, 2013. Used under license from Shutterstock, Inc.

Figure 14.2. *Motor development.*

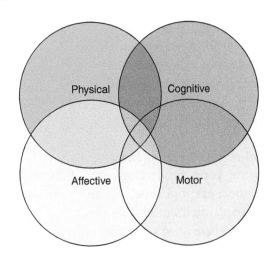

FIGURE 14.3.   *Domains of human development: how we learn intellectually (cognitive domain), how we perceive our self-worth (affective domain), how we grow (physical domain), and how we move (motor domain).*

Although we commonly think of humans gaining motor skills within the first years of life, motor skills continue to develop and decline across the lifespan. This chapter embraces the definition of motor development as "the changes in motor behavior over the lifespan and the process which underlie these changes" (6). This definition incorporates both the progression and regression of our motor behavior and all of the factors that promote and/or deter these behaviors throughout our life. With age, our motor abilities decline. Think about how your parents and grandparents move in relation to when they were younger. They might still be able to complete the task, but not with the same ease. The field of motor development stretches across the lifespan.

With time, the discipline began to see that the nature approach did not take into consideration the environmental and social factors that influence motor development (nurture approach). An excellent explanation of the combination of both nature and nurture affects on development can be seen in Gallahue's Triangulated Hourglass (10).

Gallahue's Triangulated Hourglass depicts two pitchers—*Heredity* (nature) and *Environment* (nurture)—that contain "sand" or what makes us who we are in terms of our motor behavior (reflexive, rudimentary, fundamental, and specialized motor skills). As you can see, there is a lid on the heredity pitcher. At conception, our genetic contribution to our motor development is determined, but the "sand" from the environment pitcher is endless. Youth sports, physical education programs, and the number of siblings are an example of environmental factors that influence our motor behavior. Thus, the model provides a great representation of the interaction between both the environment (nurture) and heredity (nature) on development.

Although the hourglass model is specific to motor development, applications can be made across various aspects of human development. During the mid-1940s, there was a shift from the centralized nature-nurture debate to the understanding on when and how certain movement skills develop. Researchers (Anna Espenschade, Ruth Glassow, Lolas E. Halverson) began to establish normative data to gain an understanding of the emergence of motor skills along with the order of progression. Specifically, researchers strived to describe the process of when motor skills emerge, how new skills are developed, and how these skills are maintained. Historically, Halverson's research began by examining the effect of environmental and learning factors on patterns of movement and many researchers continued to take this interactionist approach (integration of the environment with motor performance) to research (11).

Lolas Halverson graduated from the University of Northern Iowa in 1944 with a Bachelor of Arts degree in physical education, thereafter serving the teaching profession in Michigan, Iowa and Minnesota before joining the Department of Physical Education for Women, University of Wisconsin-Madison in 1948. She earned a Master of Science degree in 1949 and a Doctor of Philosophy degree in 1959 from the University of Wisconsin-Madison. She chaired the undergraduate major program during her tenure and served as chair of the Department of Physical Education for Women from 1963 to 1971 and as coordinator of the motor development laboratory from 1971 until her retirement in 1988. She authored or co-authored numerous articles, chapters, books and films. She was nationally known and respected for her research in motor development and her efforts to improve movement and physical education programs for young children. She was a firm believer that the carefully designed and developmentally appropriate environment will bring about positive changes in their movement responses.

The environment surrounding our learning to move is complicated web of people, places, and policies all simultaneously acting upon our development. Think about the infant from the beginning of the section. It will learn to move under environmental influences surrounding it, such as the floor surface in its home, the amount of toys or other play items nearby, the amount of time mothers hold them, and the muscular strength the baby has developed. There are a myriad of environment influences that shape our motor development.

Historical Periods of Motor Development

Precursor Period (1787–1928)
Maturational Period (1928–1946)
Normative/Descriptive Period (1946–1970)
Process Oriented Period (1970–present)

The history of motor development has deep roots in both psychology and biology and was historically grounded in the nature-nurture debate regarding what influenced development. The first motor developmentalist held firm to the belief that human movement was the result of preprogrammed changes in the nervous system (i.e., nature). A scientist from the maturational period would claim that if a person did not develop a movement pattern at the anticipated time, it was a failure of the central nervous system due to some sort of genetic defect. Scientists such as Arnold Gesell and Myrtle McGraw, who held this strict view that nature controlled movement, are called *maturationalists*. McGraw was a child psychologist who investigated the biology of development with one of the most famous twin studies ever published (Jimmy and Johnny Twin Study (16). In the study, one twin (Johnny) received daily movement experiences that consisted of both universal (sitting and walking) and culturally specific (swimming and skating) activities for the first 22 months of life while the other twin (Jimmy) stayed in the crib for most of the day and just matured without any planned movement experiences. Between the 22nd and 25th month Jimmy was exposed to the same movement experience as Johnny. Findings concluded the early training did have a positive effect on Johnny's motor performance initially and long term.

Nature vs. Nurture Debate

On the nature side, whatever measure of individual differences has been discovered, two children with the same characteristics can have quite different outcomes and two children with different characteristics can have the same outcome.

On the nurture side, whatever measure of the social environmental has been discovered, two children with the same experiences can have different outcomes and two children with quite different experiences can have the same outcome.

To learn more about the Jimmy and Johnny study visit the following URL: http://archive.org/details/growth_study

Researchers in motor development have started to examine how environment factors shape our motor abilities. For instance, researchers have examined the role of sibling relationships and how siblings affect motor performance (31).

The increase in obesity personal factors, such as weight status and its effect on mobility, have been investigated (20). Another line of research is the effect of footwear on motor performance (24). These are just a small sample of the studies being done to better understand the role the environment plays on a child's motor development.

Process and Product Approach

From the conception of motor development, two distinct approaches have been taken as it relates to how we observe motor patterns: process and product. The *process* of movement focuses on the execution or mechanics of one's motor performance (processes or patterns of movement). The *product* approach focuses on the outcome of movement. Take, for instance, a child learning to throw a ball. A product approach would be how fast the child throws the ball (velocity) or if she is able to hit a target. A process approach would focus on the child's movement during the throw: stepping forward with opposition, hip and trunk rotation, and follow-through upon release of the ball. Thus, it is possible for a person to have great mechanics as it relates to throwing a ball (process), but demonstrate very low speed and the inability to hit the intended target (product). In the same light, a person may have poor throwing mechanics (process), but have a high throwing speed and hit the intended target (product). Both the process and product of movement are of critical importance. Researchers today continue to debate which approach is more appropriate, but many are incorporating assessments that focus on either the process (24, 30), product (7, 31), or both approaches to movements (14).

The *Motor Performance Study* began at Michigan State University in 1967 (4). This longitudinal study collected normative data on both product and process measures in children and youths between the ages of 2.5 and 13.0 years. Specifically, the study examined the relationship among seven motor skill tasks and 13 physical growth and biological maturity assessments. This study concluded before the turn of the century with growth and motor performance variables being conducted on over 1,200 participants and included over 20,000 data sets of growth and more than 17,000 data sets on motor performance. The *Motor Performance Study* project provided valuable data as it relates to understanding growth and developmental changes in children.

Categories of Motor Skills

Despite the approach that individuals take to assess movement, motor skills tend to fall into basic categories: fine motor, gross motor, object control, and locomotor. The two broadest categories are *fine motor skills* and *gross motor skills* (Figure 14.4).

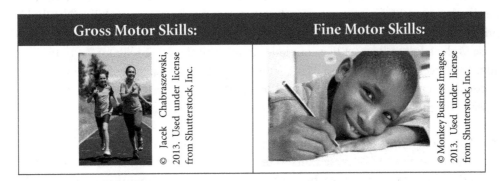

Figure 14.4.   *Motor skills.*

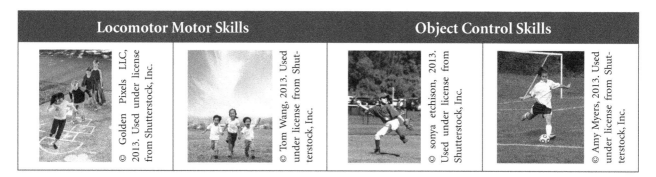

Figure 14.5. *Categories of gross motor skills.*

Fine motor skills are smaller movements that require the recruitment of small motor units. Fine motor skills include writing, brushing your teeth, and moving your eyes. Gross motor skills are larger movements requiring recruitment of larger motor units. These are movements used to propel ourselves or objects through space. Examples of gross motor skills include running, jumping, leaping, throwing, and kicking. Gross motor skills can be further broken down to either *locomotor* or *object control skills* (Figure 14.5).

Locomotor skills are those skills used to propel our bodies through space moving from one location to another. Locomotor skills include running, jumping, leaping, skipping, galloping, and sliding. Object control skills are skills used to propel an object through space. Examples of object control skills include throwing, catching, kicking, striking, and rolling. Both locomotor and object control skills are important to become a proficient mover. Various assessments are used to assess motor skills. The most widely used assessment is the Test of Gross Motor Development—2nd Edition (TGMD-2) (29).

The TGMD-2 is a validated, criterion-based, process-oriented assessment that is designed to qualitatively assess gross motor skills in children. Specifically, motor performance is based on the performer's ability to complete three to five performance criteria for each motor task. Another popular assessment, the Movement Assessment Battery for Children-2 (MABC-2), is a validated, product-oriented assessment that quantitatively evaluates motor competence in children (12). Motor performance is based on a quantitative scoring system of the number of successful trials or the amount of time to task completion.

A Mountain of a Metaphor to Describe Motor Development

Now that you have a basic understanding of the terminology and foundational aspect of motor development, there is one last thing to cover—a metaphor to describe motor development (5).

> Dr. Jane E. Clark received her Ph.D. from the University of Wisconsin—Madison and is the current Dean of the University of Maryland School of Public Health. Her work focuses on understanding the development of movement control and coordination in motor skills. Dr. Clark's work is grounded in the dynamic systems approach and demonstrates that the newly walking infant's limbs, like those of the adult walker, act like coupled nonlinear limit cycle oscillators at both the intralimb and interlimb levels of coordination. Her current projects examine the role of sensory information in the development of upright posture and locomotion in infants along with perception-action relationship for children with developmental coordination disorder (DCD).

The mountain metaphor is both eloquent and practical and provides an excellent explanation of motor development and the application of these skills in the grand scheme of human development. First, the model recognizes the critical importance of both biology (nature) and environment (nurture) in skillful movement. Additionally, a person's motor skill repertoire resembles a mountain range with various peaks and valleys. In

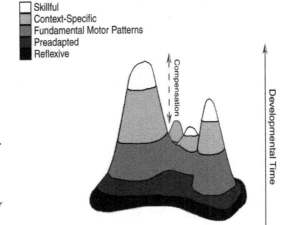

Figure 14.6. *The mountain of motor development: A metaphor.*
Reprinted with permission, from V. Seefeldt, 1980, Development of motor patterns: Implications for elementary school physical education. In *Psychology of Motor Behavior and Sport-1979*, edited by C.H. Nadeau, W.R. Halliwell, K.M. Newell (Champaign, IL: Human Kinetics), 317.

this mountain range an individual mountain peak represents each motor skill, and the layers of the mountain represent different levels (states) of movement competence or ability. Just as some mountain peaks are higher than others, a person will have some motor skills or tasks that are more highly developed than others. Despite the fact that some peaks are higher (skills are more developed), all the peaks share a foundation. Without a solid foundation, the mountain range could not exist. For the case of humans, a solid foundation is needed for us to reach our full potential as it relates to motor skill development.

The base of the motor skills mountain has three divisions or layers: *reflexive, preadaptive* and *fundamental motor skills*. The first level of the base is the reflexive motor skills period. Reflexes are involuntary responses that found at birth and are universal. Reflexes are needed for our survival. These motor behaviors are biologically driven (nature), but the gravitational forces within the environment (nurture) continue to shape the behaviors or "primitive reflexes" (e.g., stepping).

Around 2 weeks of life until the first year or the onset of walking, infants enter the preadaptive period. This period begins when an infant's movement behaviors are no longer reflexive and ends when infants begin to apply these skills as independent movers. These skills include rolling, crawling, creeping, and walking. These skills are necessary for even the most rudimentary form of independence and often seem to develop (mature) on their own. We all know that children are not taught to walk. A child's first tottering steps might not be taught (instructed), but a great deal of practice goes into making them. Babies first pull themselves up to a stand or hold onto a table or caregiver as they cruise around. Doing these moments, the child is actually practicing and improving her balance skills while improving her strength.

Around 1 until 7 years, a child begins to make his way up to the next level of the mountain: fundamental motor pattern. Here he masters the basic fundamental motor skills that will be applied to various forms of movement, physical, and recreational activities across the lifespan. Thus, these skills are considered to be building blocks (throwing, catching, and running) for future movements. If a person does not firmly master these skills, he cannot advance to a more context (sport)-specific adaptation of these skills. Ironically, some people still think that the development of basic fundamental motor skills is a naturally occurring phenomenon, but research clearly indicates that these must be taught, practiced, and reinforced (15, 23).

After the fundamental movement pattern, peaks start to advance at different rates due to changes both environmental (instruction and access) and biological (growth and maturation). Two more layers that can be achieved are *context specific* and *skillful*. In the context-specific phase, an individual begins to refine and combine basic motor skills (running, jumping, galloping, sliding, hopping, leaping, throwing, catching, striking, dribbling, rolling, and catching) to more specific movement patterns. This refinement allows a person to perform a sport-specific task with proficiency for applications in real-life settings, recreational or sports-related. For instance, before one can kick a penalty shot in soccer, she must master the basic skills of kicking and leaping from the fundamental motor period. It is critically important to understand that children who do not acquire basic fundamental motor skills might experience difficulty transitioning their movement repertoire into specific contexts. Thus, they might never reach the next level of the mountain.

Most people will end in the context-specific strata of movement. With countless hours of practice, some individuals will reach the mountain's summit, called *skillfulness*. Some researchers suggest that it takes 10,000 hours of practice to become an expert in any skill (9). The expert layer is only found in those who have completely mastered their sport. For instance, Tiger Woods is in the skillfulness layer for golf, and Mia Hamm is in the skillfulness layer for soccer. However, Tiger Woods is not in the skillfulness layer for soccer just as Mia Hamm is not in the skillfulness layer for golf. People are likely to be skillful in only some movement skills. Think about the athletes in the previous example: Could you imagine each playing the other's sport?

You should characterize the *Mountain of Motor Development* more accurately as a mountain range. A person may be near the peak in some skills (high competence) and lower on the mountain in other skills (low competence). For example, Gabrielle Douglas is the 2012 Olympic All-Around Champion in Women's (Artistic) Gymnastic (the Mountain Summit), but might be at a significantly lower level of skill proficiency in Rhythmic Gymnastics.

One final aspect of in the Mountain for Motor Development metaphor is *compensation*. Compensation refers to adjustments in motor performance that might occur during aging, injury, loss of strength, or for other reasons, including disease. Thus, performers have to compensate or relearn a movement. Following an injury and during rehabilitation, a performer might find himself traveling down the mountain, but with improved strength and practice, the performer might be able to return back to the mountain's summit.

MOTOR CONTROL: HOW WE CONTROL MOVEMENT

Throughout our daily lives, humans complete a variety of seemingly simple tasks like pouring their coffee in the morning, walking out to their car, or typing a paper. Although these tasks are done almost automatically, they are far from simple. The neuromuscular system works to coordinate the muscles required for movement.

If a child is learning to dribble a basketball, the science of motor control seeks to understand how the brain is communicating with the muscles to control that movement. Motor control also examines the cognitive processes that are devoted to the action and how can we alter or repair these neural pathways to become more proficient performers or in recovery from stroke or injury. To date, researchers are still unable to fully explain how movement occurs. However, scientists are gaining new and exciting knowledge in this field as technology is advancing.

Key Concepts in Motor Control

All movement starts at the central nervous system. We are able to move our arms and legs because our brain tells us to do so. We take information from our environment and use it to calculate our movements. Hence, a brief overview of our nervous system is needed for a firm understanding of motor control.

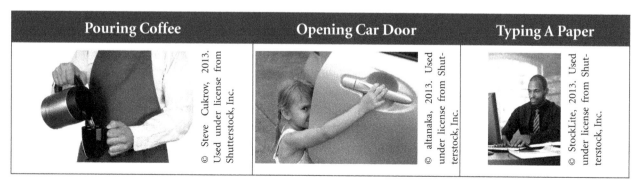

Figure 14.7. *Depictions of motor control in action.*

Historical Background

Like motor development, the study of motor control is fathered by two distinct fields: biology and psychology. Biologists have long wondered at how the body is able to create movements and psychologists have questioned how the brain interacts and functions. Hence, a merging of interests from the two fields contributed to the discipline of motor control. Sir Charles Sherrington is a famous researcher in the field of motor control. In the early 1900s, Sherrington discovered one of the most influential foundations to motor control, the *motor unit*. His important discovery not only gave great insight into the working of the nervous system, but also to the physiology behind the production of human movement. From the initial discovery of the motor unit, science has made great progress in the science of motor control. Today, scientists are using motor control in a variety of practical ways to help retrain the brain after a stroke or help patients control robotic limbs with the mind.

Sir Charles Scott Sherrington (27 November 1857–4 March 1952) was a neurophysiologist, histologist, bacteriologist, and a pathologist. He was a Nobel laureate and president of the Royal Society in the early 1920s. Sherrington received the Nobel Prize in Physiology and Medicine with Edgar Adrian in 1932 for their work on the functions of neurons. Prior to his work, it was widely accepted that reflexes occurred as isolated activity within a reflex arc. Sherrington received the prize for showing that reflexes require integrated activation and demonstrated reciprocal innervation of muscles (Sherrington's Law).

Brief overview of Sherrington's work:

1. The Liddell-Sherrington reflex is the tonic contraction of muscle in response to its being stretched. When a muscle lengthens beyond a certain point, the myotatic reflex causes it to tighten and attempt to shorten. This is the tension you feel during stretching exercises.
2. The Schiff-Sherrington reflex describes the rigid extension of the forelimbs after damage to the spine. It may be accompanied by paradoxical respiration—the intercostal muscles are paralyzed and the chest is drawn passively in and out by the diaphragm.
3. Sherrington's First Law states that every posterior spinal nerve root supplies a particular area of the skin, with a certain overlap of adjacent dermatomes.
4. Sherrington's Second Law—Reciprocal Innervation. When contraction of a muscle is stimulated, there is a simultaneous inhibition of its antagonist. It is essential for coordinated movement.
5. The Vulpian-Heidenhain-Sherrington Phenomenon describes the slow contraction of denervated skeletal muscle by stimulating autonomic cholinergic fibers innervating its blood vessels.

Our nervous system can be divided into two parts: *central nervous system* and *peripheral nervous system*. The central nervous system (CNS) includes the brain and spinal cord.

The peripheral nervous system (PNS) includes the rest of the nervous system outside of the central nervous system (Figure 14.9). In the case of movement, information from the peripheral nervous system is transmitted to the central nervous system. The central nervous system will interpret the information and send back the instruction for the appropriate movement. For example, if you place your hand on a hot stove, thermal (heat) receptors from the PNS will fire and will send the information to the CNS. In return, the CNS will respond with instructions to remove your hand from the stove. Although it sounds like this process may take a while, it actually occurs in a matter of milliseconds and without conscious thought—you do it automatically. Think about it: Your body has to send and interpret information that quickly or your hand would be damaged.

As with many systems in the body, the nervous system has a unique set of specially designed cells called *neurons* (Figure 14.10). Neurons have four main components: dendrite, cell body, axon, and synapse. Information enters the neuron via the dendrites, is interpreted in the cell body, and is transferred to the synapse via the

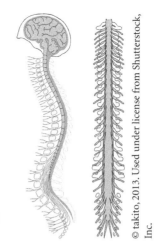

Figure 14.8. *The central nervous system.*

© takito, 2013. Used under license from Shutterstock, Inc.

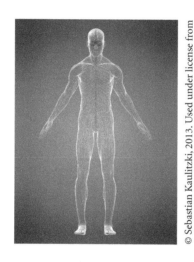

Figure 14.9. *Peripheral nervous system.*

© Sebastian Kaulitzki, 2013. Used under license from Shutterstock, Inc.

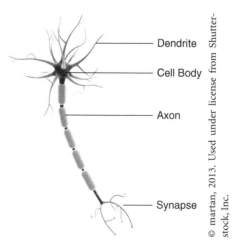

Dendrite

Cell Body

Axon

Synapse

© martan, 2013. Used under license from Shutterstock, Inc.

Figure 14.10. *The neuron.*

axon. The synapse is a small gap between each neuron. In order for the signal to continue across the gap, a neurotransmitter is released from the ends of the axon, travels across the synapse, and will stimulate the dendrites of the next neuron. In this manner information is transmitted through the nervous system.

Crucial to the study of movement is how are we able to perceive the world around us. Our vision, hearing, touch, smell, taste, even knowledge of where our body is in space (proprioception) are all mechanisms our PNS uses to interpret our surrounding environment. The body has special receptors designed to gather information about the environment surrounding us. Sensory receptors come in all shapes and sizes. Some are found within the layers of our skin, within the muscle body, in tendons, in our eyes, and even our ears. Information gathered within the receptors is transmitted to the CNS where interpretation and selection of movement occurs.

One of the most applicable sensory receptors to motor control is proprioceptors. Proprioceptors help us better understand where our body is in space. Muscle spindles are found locked in among muscle fibers. Muscle spindles are able to detect length of the muscle while the Golgi tendon organs, found within the tendon of the muscle, detect the change in muscle tension. Working together, these two proprioceptors allow us to understand where our body is in space even without the aid of vision or hearing. Try it, close your eyes and flex your elbow. Did you have an understanding of where your body was in space or where you nose is without the aid of vision? However, you should note that these proprioceptors lose their efficiency (ability to signal) with age.

After information is gathered from the sensory portion of the PNS, it travels to the CNS. Here the body interprets the information and decides what action to take. Two different reactions are possible. The body may choose a reflexive or voluntary movement. Reflexive movements occur without any conscious effect (cognitive processing). They just happen and are the infant reflexive skills that were discussed early in the Mountain for Motor Development metaphor. Think of when you see a newborn and touch her palm with your finger. Her hand then grasps your finger (i.e., palmar grasp reflex). Another example is when you go to the doctor and he taps your knee and your knee extends (i.e., patellar reflex) (Figure 14.11). These are examples of reflexes and the sensory information travels to the CNS, which responds with an automated response.

On the other hand, most movement is voluntary. These tasks include things such as performing various motor skills, completing a sudoku puzzle, or playing the piano. Although it may seem to occur automatically, it is not a preprogrammed response. Sensory information travels to the CNS and through stimulation of different brain centers, and your body cognitively chooses which response should occur. It is important to note that due to ethical concerns (and rightly so), the direct stimulation of different brain centers to see what movement patterns they elicit is not done frequently. Hence, truly understanding what part of the brain is activated is predominately studied through "reading" the brain with functional magnetic resonance imagining (fMRI) or electroencephalography (EEG) (Figure 14.12) as movement occurs.

After the CNS has decided what movement should occur, it will send a signal back down the PNS. Motor neurons travel from the CNS and will innervate or enter the muscle and stimulate multiple muscle fibers. A motor neuron and all the muscle fibers it innervates is called a motor unit (Figure 14.13).

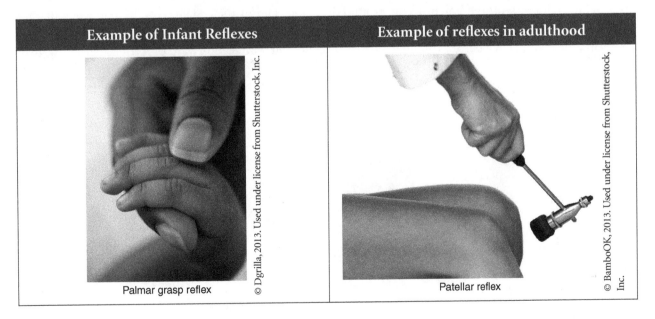

Example of Infant Reflexes	**Example of reflexes in adulthood**
Palmar grasp reflex	Patellar reflex

© Dgrilla, 2013. Used under license from Shutterstock, Inc.

© BamboOK, 2013. Used under license from Shutterstock, Inc.

Figure 14.11. *Reflexes.*

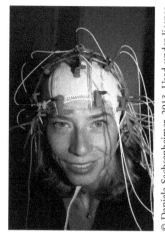

Figure 14.12. *Person set up for a EEG "reading."*

© Daniela Sachsenheimer, 2013. Used under license from Shutterstock, Inc.

When a motor neuron is stimulated, all the muscle fibers it innervates will fully contract. Therefore, if you are lifting a light bag of groceries, you will recruit fewer motor neurons than when lifting a heavy box of books. It is also important to note that not all motor neurons innervate the same number of muscle fibers. Muscles used in fine motor tasks, such as eye and hand movements, will have smaller motor units, typically between 10 or 20 muscle fibers. In a similar fashion, muscles used in gross motor tasks such as walking or throwing will have larger motor units involving the innervation of hundreds of muscle fibers. Hence, sensory information plays a huge role in the number of motor units recruited for a task. Have you ever bent down to pick up a box and unbeknownst to you the box was empty? Due to the sensory input, your body recruited enough motor units to pick up a heavy load only to find out you did not need them all. It must quickly correct its mistake or the box could fly out of your reach.

Using the example above, after you lift the box, you will be provided with feedback. Proper interpretation of feedback is important to correct movement. Did you recruit too many motor units or too few motor units? How fast were you able to move the box through space? Through properly evaluating the movement task you just completed, you can start to prepare to be more efficient at that movement in the future. These examples are just one means of describing feedback.

Feedforward is another type of feedback that uses sensory information to plan a particular movement. Before lifting the box, you used your sensory input to judge multiple characteristics about the box such as its weight, whether to lift the box from the ground or a table, and/or the distance you have to carry the box. Hence, movement is refined through both the process of feedback and feedforward. If for some reason, injury or stroke, for example, if a person can no longer provide himself with feedforward or feedback, his movement efficiency will suffer.

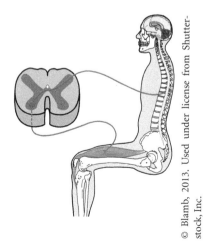

© Blamb, 2013. Used under license from Shutterstock, Inc.

Figure 14.13. *The motor unit.*

MOTOR LEARNING: HOW WE LEARN MOTOR SKILLS

The final area of motor behavior is motor learning. Just as motor control and motor development focuses on the neurological aspect of movement and the changes of motor patterns across our lifespan, respectively, motor learning is the study of how to make permanent changes to specified movement patterns. Motor learning is a set of processes associated with practice experience leading to relatively permanent changes in the capability for movement (25).

Take again the child learning to dribble a basketball. The science of motor learning seeks to explain the different stages and processes that child will progress through to becoming a proficient dribbler. What types of practice will create permanent improvement? What kind of feedback should a coach or therapist employ? These are just a few of the questions researchers in the field of motor learning are seeking to understand.

Stages of Learning

Have you ever watched a young child try to dibble a ball for the first time? Their movements are choppy, uncoordinated, and appear to take every ounce of concentration and visual feedback. However, eventually the child will progress and be able to dibble fluidly without requiring nearly as much concentration. The changes a performer undergoes can be categorized into three phases: *cognitive, associative,* and *autonomous* (Figure 14.14).

It is important to understand that the progression through phases is not age dependent, but is dependent on movement experience and opportunities. Most of you have to take prerequisite courses before taking a more advanced level class. The same is true for a performer who must have accomplished certain prerequisites before progressing into the next stage of learning.

The initial stage of learning is referred to as the *cognitive phase.* In this phase, an individual is first learning a skill; hence, performance of the skills requires maximal cognitive processes. In this stage the performer will exhibit a choppy, deliberate movement with unpredictable outcomes. Much as computer technicians write code to instruct a computer what function to perform, at this stage of learning a performer is starting to write a code for a particular skill, in our case, dribbling. The code she is writing is referred to as a motor program. The cognitive phase ends after a performer is able to complete the skill as demonstrating. For a child learning to dribble, the cognitive phase will end when he is able to continuously dribble the ball without having to catch the ball in between each dribble.

If that same child continues to be exposed to learning opportunities and experiences related to dribbling, he will enter the *associative phase* of learning. This phase is all about refining the movement. Through continued practice, the skill will become more automatic and require fewer cognitive processes. With less concentration required to complete the task, the performer can begin to divert his attention to performing the task in the environment around him (the defensive player in front of him or the movement of his teammates). In this stage, movement tasks are categorized along a continuum between two extremes: closed skills and open skills (Figure 14.15).

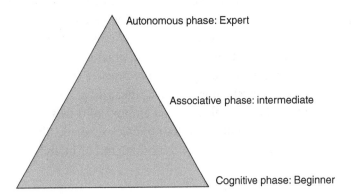

Figure 14.14. *Phases of learning.*

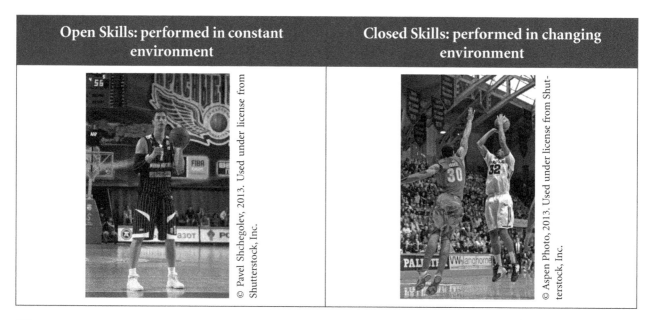

Figure 14.15. *Open and closed skills.*

Closed skills are performed in a relatively stable environment: basketball free throw, golf putt, or target shooting. The refinement of closed skills requires consistent execution of a particular task, fixation. On the other hand, an open skill is performed in an environment that is constantly changing or adapting. Examples of open skills include shooting a goal in soccer or driving to the net in basketball. A skilled performer of open skills should be able to successfully perform the task in whatever particular environment is provided to her. Hence the goal of the refinement of a task is diversification. A performer may or may not ever progress past the associative phase. The only individuals who progress past the associative phase are those who have fully mastered the skill.

The final learning stage is the *autonomous phase*. As stated above, only individuals who have mastered a skill will ever enter this phase. This is reserved for the high-level players. In this stage a performer will focus little attention on the learned task and be able to adjust to any environmental situation. The motor code is complete and fully refined. In this stage, little is left to improve. However, a performer requires motivation to continue at his or her current level of ability.

Types of Practice

One question that remains consistent within the field of motor learning is, What type of practice will elicit the best changes in performance? Additionally, researchers have to ask, Will the changes be only specific to practice or can they be generalized to alternate situations? As such, there are three main situations researcher considers: *blocked vs random practice*, *variable vs constant practice*, and *whole vs part practice*. These are questions that students with a desire to be the coach or physical education teacher would like to know.

The first consideration, blocked vs random practice, seeks to answer if performers should practice one skill per practice (blocked) or a variety of skills per practice (random) (Figure 14.16).

In a blocked practice schedule the performer will practice her serve in one practice, backhand in another, forehand in another. This can also be a set amount of time within one practice session (30-minute blocks for each task/skill). However, with a random practice schedule, the tennis player will devote a little time in each practice to his serve, his backhand, and his forehand or interchange the strokes of a backhand, forehand, and volley.

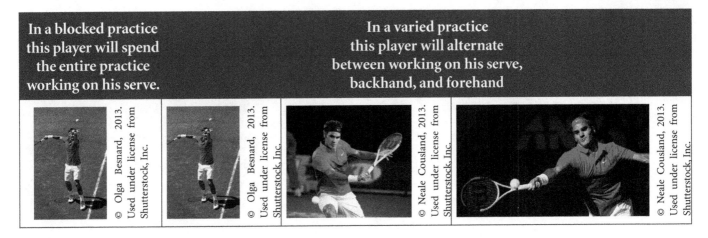

In a blocked practice this player will spend the entire practice working on his serve.

In a varied practice this player will alternate between working on his serve, backhand, and forehand

Figure 14.16. *Blocked versus random practice.*

Completing a block practice schedule will result in better initial performance, but a random practice schedule will result in better long-term learning during retention tests and transfer of skills trials (32). One method of scheduling random practice may be conducted using *contextual interference*, which refers to the interference that results from practicing a task within the context of the typical practice situation. This is extremely important as it relates to game play (2, 3). Take a moment and think about the variation of strokes in one rally of play in a tennis game. It might be more beneficial for Serena Williams to incorporate more random practice to her training schedule while an individual coaching in a children's youth tennis camp will use more blocked practice.

The second consideration is deciding between a constant or variable practice. In a constant practice a skill is practiced through a specific delivery pattern. In a variable practice the skill is practiced with a variable delivery pattern. For example, if a tennis player was practicing his backhand in a constant practice, the ball coming toward the performer would be placed at the same speed and location on the court for each repetition. In a variable practice, the ball would be placed in a variety of locations and speeds on the court. It is logical to conclude that a variable practice will produce better long-term results and application to sport settings than the constant practice (8, 26). The variable practice not only helps the player with acquisition of the skill, but also forces her to apply the skill to various situations. Hence, better long-term performance in game-like situations is seen. Again, based on the skill and developmental level of the learner, think back to motor development, a coach or physical education teacher will design a practice that meets the performer's ability while manipulating constraints to make her more proficient.

The third and final practice consideration is whole vs part practice. Should you learn a new skill in its entirety or break it down into distinct components? Unlike the former considerations, research suggests that the type of practice you choose should be based on the nature of the skill being taught. In general, a whole practice approach should be used under the following conditions:

1. If the skill is not too complicated
2. If the skill is safe and can be practiced with moderate success
3. If the skill is being completed by a competent athlete
4. If the athlete has the attention span required
5. If the skill is naturally comprised of interdependent components

Take, for instance, a gymnastic floor routine and a basketball layup. Due to the nature of a gymnastic floor routine, using a part approach is more appropriate. The skill can be broken down into its components (the whole routine has far too much information to process at one time). On the other hand, a basketball layup is

Table 14.1. Examples of Feedback.

	Motivation	Reinforcement	Punishment	Error Correction
Augmented Feedback	"Good shot!"	"Excellent shot on goal"	"Stop tossing the ball so far in front of your body before you serve"	"Make sure you pull your elbow in on your shot"
Intrinsic Feedback	Accomplishing a personal best time at 100 m dash	Scoring the winning free-throw shot	Pain from strained shoulder during baseball pitch	Consciously reminding yourself to pull your elbow in

a very fluid skill that has highly interdependent components, can be practiced with moderate success, and is not too complicated; therefore, it lends itself to a whole practice technique.

The last topic of motor learning to discuss is the concept of feedback. In motor control the sensory system was used to provide feedback for a particular skill (in the case relayed early, picking up the box). In this example, the feedback being employed is an example of intrinsic feedback. The body was receiving feedback of the movement completed through its own sensory input. Intrinsic feedback is extremely important for the learning of movement. An athlete must be aware of the "feelings of motion" and must use his intrinsic feedback to perfect a skill. However, in addition to intrinsic feedback, motor learning also examines augmented feedback on motor skill performance. Augmented feedback is feedback not naturally provided by our sensory input, but rather is given from an outside source such as a coach or therapist. Proper use of augmented feedback from a coach or any other outside source is crucial for the learning of a skill and development of movement (17, 27).

Feedback has three important functions: motivation, reinforcement/punishment, and error correction. Coaches and therapists need to make sure to be properly motivating their players or clients. Feedback as motivation is strongly tied to goal setting and achieving. Performers in the autonomous stage of learning are especially in need of motivating feedback. Through the use of feedback as reinforcement/ punishment, a skill can be fine-tuned and refined. Reinforcement is used to continue a desired behavior and punishment to stop a negative behavior. Through utilizing feedback as reinforcement and punishment, a player can continue with good practices and discard movements that are harmful. The final use of feedback is error correction. Through both augmented and intrinsic feedback, motor skills and tasks can be performed correctly. It is important to remember that only expert performers know how a movement is supposed to be performed and therefore are the only ones who should be providing augmented error correction feedback. Table 14.1 gives some examples of feedback.

SUMMARY

Motor behavior is a diverse branch of kinesiology incorporating the study of motor development (how movements emerge and diminish throughout the lifespan), motor control (how the nervous system controls movements and postures), and motor learning (how skills can be taught or adapted). All three branches are distinct and important. In motor behavior, movement is seen as a result of constraints surrounding the movement specifically environmental, task, and individual constraints. Hence, through better understanding of each constraint, we can understand movement. Motor behavior is applicable both inside and outside the classroom. Physical educators, physical therapists, coaches, and even parents can benefit from a basic knowledge of this science.

REFERENCES

1. Ashcroft, B., "We wanted wings: A history of the Aviation Cadet Program." (2005). Retrieved February 20, 2013, from www.scribd.com/doc/1446022/US-Air-Fprce-AFD061109026.

2. Brady, F., "Contextual interference: A meta-analytic study." *Perceptual and Motor Skills* 99(2004): 116–126.

3. Brady, F., "The contextual interference effect and sport skills." *Perceptual and Motor Skills, 106*(2008): 461–472.

4. Branta, C., J Haubenstricker, and V. Seefeldt, "Age changes in motor skills during childhood and adolescence." *Exercise and Sport Science Review* 12(1984): 467–520.

5. Clark, J. E., and J. M. Metcalfe, "The mountain of motor development: A metaphor." In J. E. Clark & J. H. Humphrey (Eds.), *Motor Development: Research and reviews.* Reston, VA: NASPE Publications, 2002, pp. 163–190.

6. Clark, J. E., and J. Whitall, "What is motor development: The lesson of history." *Quest* 41(1989): 183–202.

7. D'Hondt, E., B. Deforche, L. De Bourdeaudhuij, and M. Lenoir, "Relationship between motor skill and body mass index in 5–10 year old children." *Adapted Physical Activity Quarterly* 26(2009): 21–37.

8. Douvis, S. J., "Variable practice in learning the forehand drive in tennis." *Perceptual and Motor Skills* 101(2005): 531–545. Elias, M. F., P. K. Elias, L. M. Sullivan, P. A. Wolf, and R. B. D'Agostino, "Lower cognitive function in the presence of obesity and hypertension: The Framingham heart study." *International Journal of Obesity* 27(2003): 260–268. doi:10.1038/sj.ijo.802225

9. Ericson, K. A., R. T. Krampe, and C. Tesch-Römer, "The role of deliberate practice in acquisition of expert performance." *Psychological Review* 100(1993): 363–406.

10. Gallahue, D., "Motor development: A theoretical model." In D. Gallahue, J. Ozmun, & J. Goodway, eds., *Understanding Motor Development: Infants, Children, Adolescents, Adults.* New York: McGraw Hill, 2012, pp. 46–63.

11. Halverson, L. E., M. A. Roberton, and C. J. Harper, "Current research in motor development." *Journal of Research and Development in Education* 6(1973): 56–70.

12. Henderson, S. E., D. A. Sugden, and A. L. Barnett, *Movement Assessment Battery for Children –2.* London: Harcourt Assessment, 2007.

13. Kugler, P. N., J. A. S. Kelso, and M. T. Turvey, "On the control and coordination of naturally developing systems." In J. A. S. Kelso & J. E. Clark, eds., *The development of movement control and coordination.* New York: Wiley, 1982, pp. 5–78.

14. Logan, S. W., L. E. Robinson, M. E. Rudisill, D. D. Wadsworth, and M. Morera, "The comparison of school-aged children's performance on two motor assessments: The Test of Gross Motor Development and the Movement Assessment Battery for Children." *Physical Education and Sport Pedagogy* (2012): 1–12.

15. Logan, S. W., L. E. Robinson, A. E. Wilson, and W. A. Lucas, "Getting the fundamentals of movement: A metaanalysis of the effectiveness of motor skill interventions in young children as assessed by the Test of Gross Motor Development." *Child: Care, Health and Development* (2011). doi: 10.1111/j.1365-2214.2011.01307.x.

16. McGraw, M. B., *Growth: A study of Johnny and Jimmy.* New York: Appleton Century-Crofts, 1935.

17. Molier, B. I., E. H. F. Van Asseldonk, H. J. Hermens, and M. J. A. Jannink, "Nature, timing, frequency and type of augmented feedback; does it influence motor relearning of the hemiparetic arm after stroke? A systematic review." *Disability and Rehabilitation* 32(2010): 1799–1809.

18. Newell, K. M., "Physical constraints to development of motor skills." In J. R. Thomas, ed., *Motor development during childhood and adolescence.* Minneapolis: Burgess, 1984, pp. 105–120.

19. Newell, K. M., "Constraints on the development of coordination." In M. D. Wade & H. T. A. Whiting, eds., *Motor development in children: Aspects of coordination and control*. Dordrecht, The Netherlands: Martinus Nijhoff, 1986, pp. 341–360.

20. Okely, A. D., M. B. Booth, and T. Chey, "Relationships between body composition and fundamental movement skills among children and adolescents." *Research Quarterly for Exercise and Sport* 75(2004): 238–247.

21. Payne, G. V., and L. Isaacs, *Human motor development: A lifespan* approach. New York: McGraw-Hill, 2011.

22. Robinson, L. E.,. "The relationship between perceived physical competence and fundamental motor skills in preschool children." *Child: Care, Health and Development* 37(2010): 589–596. doi:10.1111/j.1365-2214.2010.01187.x

23. Robinson, L. E., and J. D. Goodway, "Instructional climates in preschool children who are at-risk. Part I: Object control skill development." *Research Quarterly for Exercise and Sport* 80(2009): 533–542.

24. Robinson, L. E., M. E. Rudisill, W. H. Weimar, C. H. Breslin, J. F. Shroyer, and M. Morera, "Footwear and locomotor skill performance in preschoolers." *Perceptual and Motor Skills* 113(2011): 534–538.

25. Schmidt, R. A., and T. D. Lee, *Motor Control and Learning: A Behavioral Emphasis*, 4th ed. Champaign, IL: Human Kinetics, 2005.

26. Shoenfelt, E. L., L. S. Snyder, A. E. Maue, C. P. Mcdowell, and C. D. Woolard, "Comparison of constant and variable practice conditions on free-throw shooting." *Perceptual and Motor Skills* 94(2002): 1113–1123.

27. Sigrist, R., J. Schellenberg, G. Rauter, S. Broggi, R. Riener, and P. Wolf, "Visual and auditory augmented concurrent feedback in a complex motor task." *Presence* 20(2011): 15–32.

28. Spessato, B. C., C. Gabbard, L. E. Robinson, and N. C. Valentini, "Body mass index, perceived and actual physical competence: The relationship among young children." *Child: Care, Health and Development* (2012). Doi:10.1111/cch/1204.

29. Ulrich, D. A., *Test of Gross Motor Development*, 2nd ed. Austin, TX: PRO-ED, 2000.

30. Williams, H. G., K. A. Pfeiffer, J. R. O'Neill, M. Dowda, K. L. McIver, W. H. Brown, and R. R. Pate, "Motor skills performance and physical activity in preschool children." *Obesity* 16(2008): 1421–1426.

31. Wrontinak, B. H., S. J. Salvy, L. Lazarus, and L. H. Epstein, "Motor proficiency relationships among siblings." *Perceptual and Motor Skills* 108 (2009): 112–120.

32. Wu, W. F. W., D. E. Young, S. L. Schandler, G. Meir, R. L. M. Judy, J. Perez, and M. J. Cohen, "Contextual interference and augmented feedback: Is there and additive effect for motor learning." *Human Movement Science* 30(2011): 1092–1101.

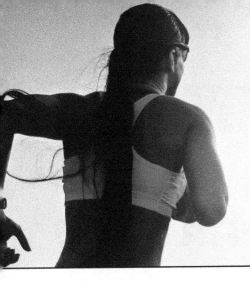

THE PROFESSIONS OF KINESIOLOGY

Part Three of *Fundamentals of Kinesiology* overviews those academic fields that have gained professional status. Practitioners of these professions apply their knowledge of movement, exercise, physical activity, and/or sport to better the human condition and make life more enjoyable.

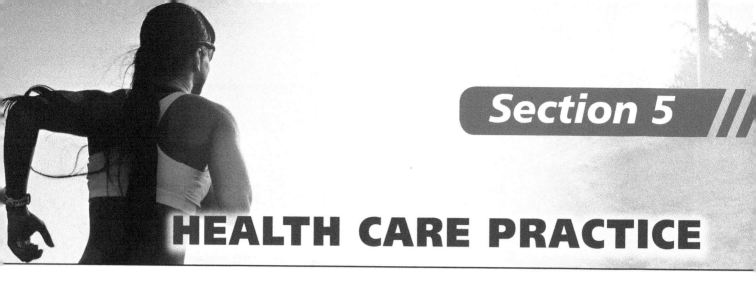

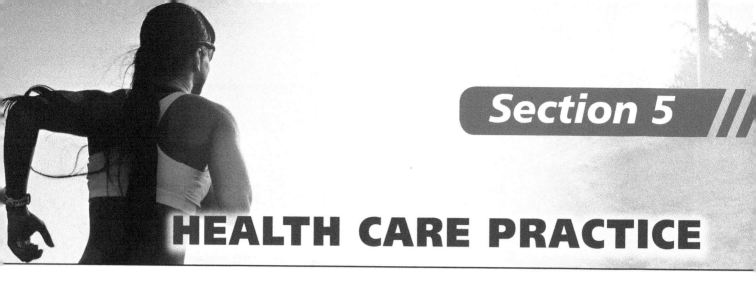

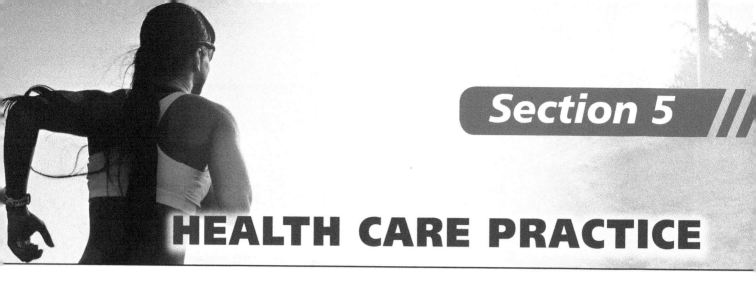

Section 5

HEALTH CARE PRACTICE

Five of these professions (Chapters 15–18) have gained the status of a health care practice field. What each has in common is the use of some form of movement or exercise in the treatment of individuals with acute or chronic movement dysfunction. Each professional practice builds on and is grounded in one or more of the disciplines of kinesiology presented in Part Two of the text. To be sure, these professions, more or less, rely on other parent disciplines from which they derive clinical practice standards. Yet, at their core, each profession presented in Section 5 is inexorably tied to the study of movement.

Chapter 15

PHYSICAL AND OCCUPATIONAL THERAPY

OUTLINE

OBJECTIVES

1. Recognize the importance of the principles of kinesiology to the practice of occupational and physical therapy.
2. Describe the fields of both occupational and physical therapy and identify basic interventions utilized by therapists.
3. Gain a basic understanding of the history of occupational and physical therapy.
4. Describe the educational requirements currently in place to obtain a degree in occupational and physical therapy.
5. Recognize opportunities for further education after obtaining an entry-level degree in occupational and physical therapy.

KINESIOLOGY IN THE PRACTICE OF OCCUPATIONAL AND PHYSICAL THERAPY

Knowledge of movement is essential for the practicing occupational and physical therapists. The goal of these health professionals is to assist individuals to achieve the highest level of function despite a variety of health and injury challenges. To do this, an extensive knowledge of the basis of human movement is required. Physical and occupational therapists possess knowledge of pathology at the tissue level, of impairments that occur as a result of improper static and dynamic postures, and of disability that affects an individual's ability to participate in important life activities.

For example, individuals who have sustained a spinal cord injury resulting in loss of mobility in the lower body must learn a new array of movement strategies to perform basic functional activities including moving from a wheelchair to a bed, propelling a wheelchair over a variety of environmentally challenging surfaces (inclines, curbs, and gravel), and dressing (Figure 15.1). Physical therapists must teach these individuals the skills necessary to master those tasks.

Imagine an elite baseball pitcher or concert violinist who has developed shoulder or arm pain (Figures 15.2 and 15.3). Intervention directed at managing inflammation of the rotator cuff or subacromial bursa in the athlete's or musician's shoulder or elbow will certainly help his or her symptoms. Failure to address abnormal mechanics such as faulty scapulohumeral rhythm during shoulder abduction leading to tissue breakdown will undoubtedly result in recurrent pain, further tissue damage, and ultimately loss of the ability to perform at the same elite level. The ability to analyze and athlete's pitching motion or a musician's performing position will enable a health care practitioner to direct treatment toward the faulty biomechanics that resulted in tissue breakdown, pain, and loss of performance. The following case study is an example of a physical therapy case to correct shoulder pain.

INTRODUCTION TO THE FIELDS OF OCCUPATIONAL AND PHYSICAL THERAPY

Occupational Therapy

Occupational therapy is an allied health profession that focuses on maximizing an individual's ability to participate in life independently. Occupational therapists center on enabling persons of any age to participate in activities of daily life—or occupations—that are vital to maintaining overall health and wellness.

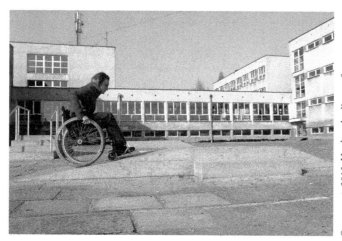

© pryzmat, 2013. Used under license from Shutterstock, Inc.

Figure 15.1. *Wheelchair navigation up a ramp.*

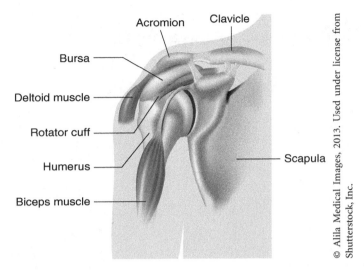

Figure 15.2.   *Subacromial structures of the shoulder at risk of impingement.*

An individual's occupation is an activity that occupies his or her time and is meaningful (2). Occupations may include self-care activities, home-management tasks, socialization, work, leisure, or tasks related to a specific life role such as parenting. Impairments resulting from developmental delay, trauma, illness, and/or progressive disease can interfere with one's ability to complete daily life tasks or occupational performance. Occupational therapists are experts at analyzing occupations. The following case study is an example of the type of maladies occupational therapists see.

Occupational therapy services are provided to individuals, groups, populations, and organizations to increase participation in roles within various settings including home, school, work site, and community. Screenings and evaluations focus on determining current and potential level of occupational performance. Based on the information gathered, an intervention plan is developed in collaboration with the client to achieve goals. Interventions may address the specific physical, sensory, cognitive, and psychosocial factors interfering with the independent performance of an occupation. Examples include improving upper extremity weakness, restoring fine motor coordination, or remediating a cognitive deficit such as attention. Interventions may also compensate for deficits through environmental changes, task modifications, or through use of adaptive devices to maximize function in an occupation. To increase independence in basic activities of daily living (ADL) such as feeding or bathing, an individual may be instructed in the use of a built-up utensil to

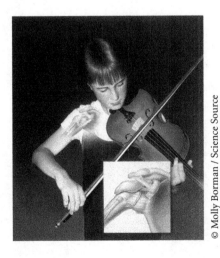

Figure 15.3.   *Shoulder positioning of a violinist.*

CASE STUDY: Right Shoulder Pain

Patient profile: Age: 37

Occupation: Architect
Recreational activities: Volleyball, running

History:

- Gradual onset of right shoulder pain while playing volleyball six months ago
- Symptoms have progressively worsened; unable to play more than games during practice over the past two weeks
- Started a vigorous weight training program three weeks prior to symptom onset
- Previous similar problem seven years ago; played through it and it resolved in ~ six months.
- Past Medical History: Unremarkable

Subjective Examination:

- **Nature of symptoms:** Constant mild ache in right shoulder that increases with certain activities. Also reports some stiffness with UE elevation.
- **Aggravating factors:** Extremes of right shoulder movements, Hitting/setting/serving in volleyball. Pain lasts 30–40 minutes after ceasing play.
- **Easing factors:** Morning shower helps to loosen the shoulder, ice
- **24 Hour Behavior:** Stiff in AM; pain increases with vigorous activity; occasional sleep disturbance 2° pain
- **Pain Rating:** Current: 2/10; increases to 5/10 with activity
- **Medication:** None

Objective/Physical Examination

- **Observation:**

  (R) shoulder slightly anterior with a mild anterior tilt and downward rotation of the scapula, otherwise generally good postural alignment and symmetry noted. In supine, the (R) shoulder more anterior than the (L).

- **Active Range of Motion:**

Shoulder	(R)	(L)
Flex	160°*	175°
Abd	160°*	175°
ER	75°	80°
IR	70°	70°
Flex/abd/ER	T3*	T5
Ext/add/IR	T8	T7

  * = pain reported at end range.

- **Passive Range of Motion:**

Shoulder	(R)	(L)
Flex	170°	180°
Abd	170°	175°
ER	75°	75°
IR	75°	75°

- **Resisted Isometric Tests:**

  All negative except (R) shoulder resisted abduction is strong and painful

- **Manual Muscle Testing:**
  5/5 (L) Upper extremity
  All 5/5 in (R) Upper Extremity except:

  Abduction: 4/5, Scapular Protraction: 4/5, Scapular Adduction: 4/5
  Scapular Depression: 4-/5

- **Special Tests (R) shoulder:**

  (+) Empty can
  (+) Hawkins-Kennedy

- **Palpation:**

  (+) tenderness over (R) greater tubercle and (R) supraspinous fossa

Assessment:

- **PT Diagnosis:** Patient presents with impaired posture, impaired motor control, and impaired muscle performance of the right scapulohumeral muscles, all contributing to positive signs and symptoms of right shoulder impingement involving the supraspinatus muscle.

- **PT Prognosis:** Patient's prognosis for achieving painfree mobility of the right shoulder is good; however, his current recreational pursuits are adversely affecting his shoulder symptoms. While the patient appears motivated to participate in a conservative program to address the right shoulder symptoms, his outcome may depend on his willingness and ability to modify his current activity. Anticipate patient's return to full activity in ~ 1 month or 6–8 PT sessions.

- **Treatment:** Treatment should focus on addressing postural imbalances, improving scapular muscle strength/motor control to improve scapulohumeral rhythm, and local treatment of the supraspinatus (transverse friction massage, iontophoresis, gradual progressive resistive exercise). Patient should limit overhead activity until he demonstrates pain-free ROM.

reduce pressure over painful arthritic joints or an elevated toilet seat to prevent excessive hip flexion following a joint replacement. Retraining in instrumental activities of daily living (IADL) such as meal preparation and homemaking may incorporate work simplification and/or energy conservation techniques into a task such as sitting down to dry off after a shower. Occupational therapists may also incorporate health promotion and prevention activities into a plan of care including training in relaxation techniques to reduce anxiety during stressful situations.

CASE STUDY: Occupational Therapy

Lynn, a 22-year-old graduate student, is admitted to the inpatient rehabilitation unit this afternoon to maximize her recovery from a diving accident. After reviewing the medical record, the occupational therapist (OT) learns that Lynn acquired a C5 (cervical) vertebral burst fracture with an incomplete spinal cord injury after diving and hitting the bottom of an above ground swimming pool. Her past medical history is unremarkable.

(Continued)

Evaluation

From an interview with Lynn, the OT develops a profile of her occupational roles, performance level, and current and future goals. Lynn lives with her partner in a multilevel townhouse. She was a collegiate volleyball player in undergraduate school and is pursuing a graduate degree in social work. Lynn enjoys outdoor activities with her friends and family and would like to return to her home life and continue graduate school. She hopes to play recreational volleyball again. She and her family are concerned about the wheelchair accessibility of her home environment.

The OT completes an initial evaluation and finds that Lynn presents with tetraplegia. She has the ability to move her scapulae and activate her deltoids. Her biceps are extremely weak and she has no forearm, wrist, and hand movement at this time. She has paralysis of her trunk and lower extremities. At this time, she requires total assistance for self-care and mobility activities. Lynn is able to sit in a reclining wheelchair for 15 minutes at a time.

Intervention Plan

In collaboration with Lynn, her family, and the interprofessional rehabilitation team, the OT develops goals to increase Lynn's ability to participate in the management of her self-care activities. Intervention methods include: client and family education on the effects of spinal cord injury; modifications using assistive technology and adaptive equipment; splinting and positioning to prevent additional impairments to musculoskeletal and skin systems; and self-care retraining to restore abilities. Expected outcome from occupational therapy interventions include improved participation and performance in daily occupations at home, school, and the community for health and quality of life.

Intervention Activity

In this session, the OT works on self-feeding. Since her deltoids and biceps are weak, Lynn's upper extremity needs to be supported so she can work toward feeding herself. The OT uses a mobile arm support to accommodate for the weight of the arm so Lynn can use her existing upper extremity muscle strength to move her hand toward her mouth. Because Lynn lacks grip, the OT applies a universal cuff with a utensil to her hand. The universal cuff is a type of orthosis that sits on the palm of the hand and has a place for attaching tools like utensils, writing implements, or devices used in daily activities. Lynn practices the feeding movement pattern while in the mobile arm support; overtime her muscles will strengthen.

Physical Therapy

Physical therapy is described by *The Guide to Physical Therapist Practice* as a "dynamic profession with an established theoretical and scientific base and widespread clinical applications in the restoration, maintenance, and promotion of optimal physical function (6)." Physical therapists are an integral part of the health care team, and they serve an important role in the diagnosis and management of movement dysfunction. Physical therapy treatment aims to improve mobility, decrease pain, improve or restore function, and minimize disability in individuals with a variety of medical and health conditions. Treatment is also directed at preventing mobility problems *before* they occur in many individuals. Optimization of physical performance and functional capabilities is a primary concern for physical therapists.

Similar to occupational therapists, physical therapists address movement dysfunctions through a patient/client management process that includes five elements: examination, evaluation, physical therapy diagnosis, prognosis, and intervention. Examination includes both general screening and comprehensive testing designed to identify the appropriate physical therapy diagnostic classification and to determine if the patient/client needs to be referred to another health care practitioner. Evaluation refers to the informed clinical judgments the therapist makes based on the findings of the examination. Physical therapists do not make medical diagnoses. Rather, the therapist evaluates the information from the examination and makes a physical therapy diagnosis that is reflective of a movement system disorder.

Examples of movement disorders include gait abnormalities that occur as a result of weakness, abnormal, and/or inefficient extremity movement that may result from spasticity or joint contractures, and peripheralization of leg pain with specific movements that cause compression of the nerve root. The therapist does not diagnose the cause of the spasticity (for example, a stroke or spinal cord compression) or the nerve root compression (intervertebral disc herniation or foraminal facet compromise), but is concerned with the movement dysfunction occurring as a result of those pathologies. Prognosis attempts to identify the predicted level of improvement a patient/client is expected to achieve within a specific timeframe. The last component of the patient/client management process is intervention. The therapist determines the most appropriate, individualized plan of care to administer in order to achieve the predicted outcome levels.

There are many types of interventions used by physical therapist. One example of a common physical therapy intervention is therapeutic exercise. Knowledge of normal and abnormal human movement is imperative in determining the correct exercise prescription for an individual. Goals for this intervention include increasing strength, flexibility, endurance, and range of motion. The therapist must take into account the current capabilities of the muscle system to generate an adequate contraction that results in sufficient force to produce the desired movement; however, the therapist must also consider the effects that the patient's medical condition may have on the musculoskeletal system when prescribing appropriate exercises. Manual therapy techniques such as joint mobilization are frequently used by physical therapists to address joint mobility limitations.

Knowledge of arthrokinematics allows the therapist to apply accessory motions to the joint in order to assess and treat a range of motion limitation. For example, a patient/client may have a limited amount of knee extension that interferes with his ability to walk with a normal gait pattern. Loss of knee extension could be the result of decreased quadriceps muscle strength, hamstring muscle tightness, or knee capsule tightness. Muscle weakness and tightness may be addressed with therapeutic exercise, but capsular tightness may need to be addressed through the use of passive accessory joint mobilization techniques. In this case, recognition that knee extension involves the arthrokinematic movement of an anterior glide of the tibia relative to the femur allows the therapist to apply that glide to improve capsular extensibility (Figure 15.4).

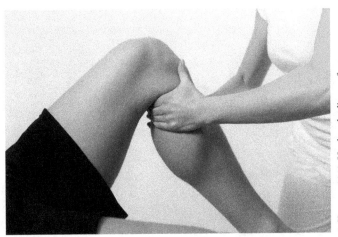

© Kzenon, 2013. Used under license from Shutterstock, Inc.

Figure 15.4. *Manual therapy technique: Anterior tibial glide to improve knee extension.*

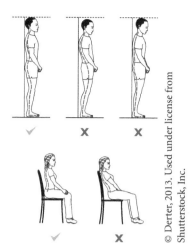

Figure 15.5. *Sitting/standing posture.*

© Derter, 2013. Used under license from Shutterstock, Inc.

Other examples of typical physical therapy interventions include:

1. Therapeutic activities for improving functional activities utilizing optimal posture/body mechanics to improve efficiency and minimize risk of injury. Examples of this include lifting, pushing, pulling, and transferring between a variety of surfaces: wheelchair to bed, floor to chair, car transfers (Figure 15.5).
2. Neuromuscular reeducation to promote balance, optimal movement patterns, and facilitation and/or inhibition of muscle activity.
3. Physical agents such as mechanical spinal traction and heat/cold application.
4. Electrotherapeutic modalities to modulate pain or facilitate muscle contraction (Figure 15.6).
5. Gait training over a variety of surfaces and with a variety of assistive devices (Figure 15.7).
6. Airway clearance techniques.
7. Wound care.

Physical therapists practice in a wide array of settings. Acute care physical therapists provide service to patients admitted in a hospital setting for short-term care. Patients discharged from an acute care hospital may go to a rehabilitation hospital or sub-acute rehabilitation facility. Both physical therapists and occupational therapists working in rehabilitation hospitals provide intensive therapy with the overarching goal of maximizing functional independence. Therapy services provided in a sub-acute rehabilitation facility are typically

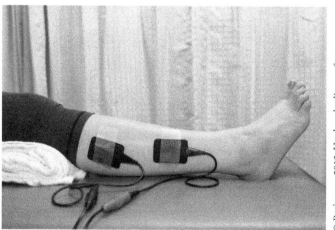

© Praisaeng, 2013. Used under license from Shutterstock, Inc.

Figure 15.6. *Lower Extremity Muscle Stimulation.*

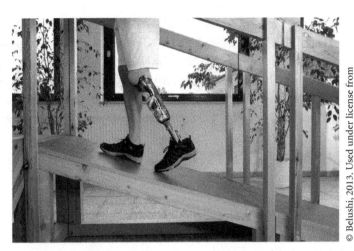

Figure 15.7.   *Patient with lower extremity amputation walking up a ramp.*

less intensive. Additional settings for physical therapy practice include nursing homes, outpatient/private practice clinics, home-health, wellness/fitness centers, industrial/workplace clinics, and schools. Physical therapist education and knowledge in movement dysfunction as well as disease, injuries, and various medical conditions enables the practitioner to prevent or minimize the deleterious effects of these conditions in order to improve quality of life.

HISTORICAL PERSPECTIVE

Occupational Therapy

Formalized in 1917 as The National Society for the Promotion of Occupational Therapy (NSPOT), the profession of occupational therapy developed from the belief that individuals were healthier if they were involved in meaningful occupations that stimulated them both physically and cognitively (11–13, 15). The primary modalities used by early occupational therapists, initially nurses in psychiatric hospitals, were arts and crafts and simple work (12, 15). Physicians and nurses noticed that even simple projects resulted in improved mental health. This was only a small part of the repertoire of those currently used in the profession (9).

The profession changed through the years, responding to societal influences including the war, deinstitutionalization, and advancements in science and technology. Occupational therapists assisted returning soldiers with disabilities in developing vocational and independent living skills. They provided those managing mental illness with strategies to reintegrate into community living. Occupational therapists adapted toys and computers with switches to enable children to better participate in school activities. Today, occupational therapists can be found providing similar interventions within hospitals, outpatient clinics, nursing homes, school systems, companies, and community practice settings.

Physical Therapy

The evolution of the practice of physical therapy in the United States is related to major events that challenged the health and well-being of its citizens. Some of the earliest references to the practice of physical therapy describe the use of physical modalities and procedures in the treatment of infantile paralysis in the late 1800s and early 1900s (14). Like the occupational therapy profession, World War I and the move to a more industrialized society brought about additional societal needs that were addressed by the earliest practitioners of physical therapy.

Most early practitioners did not receive formal education or training. Mary McMillan was educated and trained in England prior to returning to the United States to practice and is recognized as the first physical therapist in this country. The polio epidemic and World War II further increased the need for additional practitioners of physical therapy during the 1940s and 1950s. As advances in medicine occurred throughout the last century and life expectancy increased, individuals survived longer with injuries or illnesses that would not have previously been the case. As a result, the need for physical therapists continued to grow.

PROFESSIONAL ORGANIZATIONS

Occupational Therapy

In 1921, NSPOT changed its name to the American Occupational Therapy Association (AOTA) and began working toward safeguarding the profession by establishing a national registry of occupational therapists and minimum educational essentials. AOTA is now the professional organization responsible for the promotion and advancement of the occupational therapy profession in the United States. Individual state associations promote occupational therapy at the local level by participating in advocacy and educational efforts. State organizations also represent local constituents to the national organization.

Physical Therapy

The first professional organization for physical therapists was the American Women's Physical Therapeutic Association formed in 1921 and led by Mary McMillan (4). This organization evolved into the American Physical Therapy Association (APTA) by the late 1940s and continues to serve as the professional organization representing more than 85,000 members throughout the United States today. The stated goal of this organization is to "promote advancements in physical therapy practice, research and education (4)." The organization has played an important role in representing its members and the profession in the legislative arena to protect both providers and consumers of physical therapy services.

Each state and the District of Columbia are represented at the local level by a Chapter. Additionally, the organization currently has 18 Sections representing various special interest areas within the profession. Section membership provides opportunities for therapists to stay current in their specific area of practice and to

Occupational Therapist Entry-Level Education

Occupational Therapist

A post-baccalaureate degree in occupational therapy from an accredited program is required to enter the profession and to be eligible to sit for the national certification examination. Typically, state licensure is required prior to practicing. Entry-level occupational therapist degrees are either at the master's or doctoral level. Admission requirements include a competitive GPA and prerequisite coursework in the natural and social sciences. The education program consists of didactic and clinical components followed by a six-month fieldwork experience.

Occupational Therapy Assistant

An associate degree in occupational therapy from an accredited program is required to enter the profession and be eligible to sit for the national certification examination. State licensure is typically required prior to practicing. Admission requirements include a high school diploma and natural science coursework. The education program consists of didactic as well as clinical components and a four-month fieldwork experience.

Physical Therapist Education

Entry-level (or first professional degree) programs in physical therapy are offered at the master and doctoral levels, but there is a move toward doctoral-level programs only. Eligibility to practice physical therapy in the United States requires graduation from an accredited physical therapy program and a passing score on a licensure exam. Most physical therapy programs are approximately three years in length and consist of a combination of classroom and clinical learning experiences.

Physical therapist assistant programs are typically two years long and are offered at the associate degree level. Physical therapist assistants work under the direction and supervision of the physical therapist. In order to practice as a physical therapist assistant in the United States, most states require that the individual is licensed; graduation from an accredited physical therapy assistant program is a prerequisite for the licensure exam.

connect/network with other practitioners in that specialty area of practice. Examples of sections in the APTA include Acute Care, Geriatrics, Neurology, Orthopaedics, Sports Physical Therapy, and Women's Health. A full list and brief description of each section can be found at the APTA website (5).

EDUCATION REQUIREMENTS

Occupational Therapy

An occupational therapy practitioner may be an occupational therapist or an occupational therapy assistant. An occupational therapy assistant practices under the direction of an occupational therapist. An entry-level degree from an occupational therapy program accredited by the Accreditation Council for Occupational Therapy Education is required to enter the occupational therapy profession and be eligible to sit for the required national examination administered by the National Board for Certification in Occupational Therapy (3).

For the occupational therapist, the entry-level degree is post-baccalaureate and can either be a master's or doctoral degree. Admission to entry-level professional education programs is competitive and applicants must complete prerequisite courses in the biological, physical, behavioral, and social sciences. The occupational therapy assistant entry-level degree is at the associate's level. There are two components to the professional preparation of occupational therapy practitioners: academic and fieldwork or clinical (1). The academic portion consists of occupational therapy specific courses covering foundational knowledge, theory, assessments, and interventions. The fieldwork component is the supervised application of classroom knowledge within areas of practice; students are mentored by practicing occupational therapists. Most states require licensure or certification to practice.

Physical Therapy

Physical therapy services are provided by licensed physical therapists or physical therapist assistants. Entry-level physical therapist education is offered at two degree levels: Doctor of Physical Therapy (DPT) and Master/Master of Science in Physical Therapy (MPT/MSPT). All physical therapy programs must award the DPT degree by 2015 in order to be accredited. To practice physical therapy in the United States requires (a) possession of a PT degree from a program that has been accredited by The Commission on Accreditation in Physical Therapy Education (CAPTE) and (b) passing a licensure exam.

Traditional entry-level PT programs are approximately three years in length and require a bachelor's degree and required prerequisites prior to admission into the program. Some nontraditional programs offer admission after three years in a pre-professional program. Admission requirements vary among the PT educational programs, so interested applicants should access program information on the APTA website. Current information regarding accredited programs and a centralized application service are available on that website. Admission into programs is very competitive. Students interested in pursuing a degree in physical therapy are encouraged to gain exposure to the profession via observation/volunteer hours in PT practices and to seek counseling regarding appropriate undergraduate coursework required for admission. During the three-year professional program, approximately 80% of the time is spent in lecture/lab activities while the remaining 20% of the time is devoted to clinical education rotations in a variety of physical therapy practice settings (8).

Physical therapist assistant degrees are awarded at the associate level. As is the case with OTs and COTAs, PTAs are required to work under the direction and supervision of a licensed PT. Entry-level PTA programs are approximately two years long and consist of both classroom (lecture/lab) experiences in addition to clinical education in a variety of clinical settings. Most states require that a PTA practice with a license; only PTA students who have graduated from an accredited program (CAPTE) are eligible to sit for the licensure exam (5).

While earning a degree in either occupational or physical therapy requires significant time and financial commitments, the job outlook is reliably good. Both professions consistently rank high in surveys that consider employment opportunities, salary, and job satisfaction (7). The Bureau of Labor Statistics predicts a much faster than average growth in physical therapist employment compared to other occupations (10). The same is true for the employment outlook for physical therapist assistants, occupational therapists, and occupational therapist assistants.

POST-PROFESSIONAL EDUCATION/TRAINING OPPORTUNITIES

Occupational Therapy

Many occupational therapy practitioners continue their formal education beyond the entry-level degree. Practitioners may choose to advance their practice skills by obtaining a clinical doctorate in occupational therapy. Those choosing to become researchers or enter academia may obtain a doctorate in occupational science or another field.

The American Occupational Therapy Association (AOTA) acknowledges advanced practice knowledge and skills through Board Certification in four major areas: gerontology, mental health, pediatrics, and physical rehabilitation. Specialty certification is available to occupational therapists with unique therapy intervention skills in five areas: driving and community mobility; environmental modifications; feeding, eating, and swallowing; low vision; and school systems. Specialty certification is available from organizations other than AOTA as well. For example, therapists who work in pediatrics may seek advanced evaluation and intervention training in sensory integration while those working in upper extremity rehabilitation may choose to become certified hand therapists.

Physical Therapy

Following attainment of an entry-level degree in physical therapy, many practitioners opt to pursue additional training to further advance their knowledge and skill set. Clinical residency, clinical fellowship, and specialty certification are some of the current opportunities available to licensed physical therapists. Similar to the medical/physician model, a residency is an initial postprofessional program that provides both clinical and didactic education opportunities in a specific area of practice while a fellowship is designed to further advance the knowledge/skills of individuals who already possess a certain level of expertise in an area of clinical practice. The American Board of Physical Therapy Specialties administers the process by which a therapist can become board-certified clinical specialists in a particular area of physical therapy practice. Specialist certification is not required to practice as a physical therapist.

There are many additional opportunities for physical therapists to continue their education following attainment of an entry-level degree. Continuing education opportunities are often required to maintain competency and licensure. Certification programs in manual therapy and seating/mobility are just two examples of advanced training opportunities available to therapists. Therapists with a strong desire to teach or engage in clinical research may opt to pursue a doctoral degree such as a PhD, DSc, or DPH.

SUMMARY

Movement provides the basis for functional mobility. Humans face a variety of movement challenges that may be the result of injury, disease, aging, poor posture/body mechanics, and environmental obstacles, to name a few. Skilled activities such as high-level sports or performing arts can also present unique movement demands. Occupational and physical therapists possess key knowledge and training to help individuals achieve optimal function, efficient movement, and improved quality of life. The ability to integrate knowledge of pathology, injury, kinesiology, movement assessment, and functional training makes physical and occupational therapists important components of health care and wellness efforts for a variety of populations. Despite competitive application into occupational and physical therapy programs, the need for therapists remains high resulting in a positive job outlook for individuals seeking a challenging and rewarding career.

REFERENCES

1. Accreditation Council for Occupational Therapy Education of the American Occupational Therapy Association, Inc. (2011). ACOTE Standards for an accredited educational program. Retrieved April 16, 2013, from www.aota.org/Educate/Accredit/Draft-Standards/50146.aspx?FT=.pdf

2. American Occupational Therapy Association, "Occupational therapy practice framework: Domain and process (2nd ed.)." *American Journal of Occupational Therapy* 62(2008): 625–683.

3. American Occupational Therapy Association, "Standards of practice for occupational therapy." *American Journal of Occupational Therapy* 64(Suppl.)(2010): S10 S11.

4. American Physical Therapy Association. APTA History. Accessed April 15, 2013, from www.apta.org/history

5. American Physical Therapy Association. APTA Chapters and Sections. Accessed April 15, 2013, from www.apta.org

6. American Physical Therapy Association, *Guide to physical therapist practice*, 2nd ed. American Physical Therapy Association; Physical Therapy 81(2001): 9–746.

7. American Physical Therapy Association. APTA PT Education. Accessed April 15, 2013, from www.apta.org/PTCareers

8. American Physical Therapy Association. APTA PT Education. Accessed April 15, 2013, from www.apta.org/PTEducation

9. Bent, M. A., P. A. Crist, L. Florey, and L. R. Strickland, "A practice analysis of occupational therapy and impact on certification examination." *OTJR: Occupation, Participation and Health* 25(3)(2005): 105–118.

10. Bureau of Labor Statistics, *Physical Therapists: Occupational Outlook Handbook*. Accessed April 15, 2013, from www.bls.gov/ooh/healthcare/physical-therapists.htm

11. Dunton, W. R., Jr., *Reconstruction Therapy*. Philadelphia: W.B. Saunders Co, 1919.

12. Dunton, W. R., Jr., and S. Licht, eds., *Occupational therapy: Principles and practice*. Springfield, IL: Charles C. Thomas Publisher, 1950.

13. Quiroga, V. A. M., *Occupational Therapy: The First 30 Years, 1900 to 1930*. Bethesda, MD: The American Occupational Therapy Association, 1995.

14. Scully, R. M., and M. R. Barnes, Eds., *Physical Therapy*. Philadelphia: J.B. Lippincott Company, 1989.

15. Spear, M. R., *Keeping Idle Hands Busy: Occupational Therapy*. Minneapolis: Burgess Publishing Co., 1950.

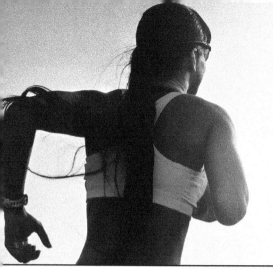

Chapter 16

CLINICAL EXERCISE PHYSIOLOGY

OUTLINE

OBJECTIVES

1. Describe the profession of clinical exercise physiology.
2. Define the role of a clinical exercise physiologist in a health care environment.
3. Identify the educational requirements and available professional certifications for clinical exercise physiologists.
4. Identify and explain the job duties of the clinical exercise physiologist.
5. Differentiate between diagnostic and functional capacity exercise testing.
6. Describe the various measurements taken during graded exercise testing.
7. Describe health-related physical fitness assessment as performed by the clinical exercise physiologist.
8. Describe some common clinical conditions and the role exercise can have in helping to prevent, treat, and manage these conditions.

Physical activity and exercise play an important role in the prevention, treatment, and rehabilitation of individuals with chronic diseases, helping to improve their medical and functional status. The Clinical Exercise Physiology Association provides a succinct definition for this health care practice field:

> A clinical exercise physiologist is a healthcare professional who is trained to work with patients with chronic diseases where exercise training has been shown to be of therapeutic benefit, including but not limited to cardiovascular disease, pulmonary disease, and metabolic disorders. Clinical exercise physiologists work primarily in a medically supervised environment that provides a program or service that is directed by a licensed physician.

In short, the clinical exercise physiologist applies exercise to: (a) prevent, delay, or minimize the risk of chronic disease associated with physical inactivity in *apparently healthy* participants and (b) provide therapeutic or functional benefits to *patients* with underlying pathologies. The clinical exercise physiologist starts with the base knowledge of normal physiological responses to acute and chronic exercise, but must also understand pathophysiology and how functional capacity and responses to acute exercise may be affected by different disease states and their medical management.

As a professional working in health care, the clinical exercise physiologist may be employed by hospitals, rehabilitation centers, outpatient clinics, corporate and commercial facilities, university facilities, fitness and wellness centers, retirement communities, and senior centers. The scope of practice of the clinical exercise physiologist is the use of exercise as a therapeutic modality for individuals with no known medical problems (apparently healthy) to patients with documented cardiovascular, pulmonary, metabolic, rheumatologic, orthopedic, and/or neuromuscular diseases and conditions. Specifically, the job functions of the clinical exercise physiologist include (a) evaluating functional capacity, (b) assisting physicians in diagnostic testing, (c) prescribing exercise based on patient needs and abilities, (d) patient education, and (e) supervising and monitoring the exercise session (Figure 16.1).

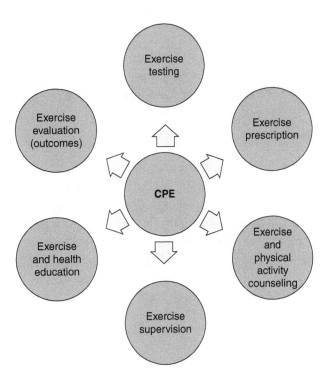

Figure 16.1.   *Job functions of a clinical exercise physiologist.*

Broadly, the clinical exercise physiologist improves the physical capabilities of individuals for the purpose of (a) chronic disease management, (b) reducing risks for early development or recurrence of chronic diseases, (c) creating lifestyle habits that promote enhancement of health, (d) facilitating the elimination of barriers to habitual lifestyle changes through goal-setting and prioritizing, (e) improving the ease of daily living activities, and (f) increasing the likelihood of long-term physical, social and economic independence.

It is important to note that exercise therapy may be altered by other concurrent treatments (drugs and medications, surgical procedures, radiation therapy, orthopedic bracing, casting or splinting, dialysis, and diet therapy). This requires the clinical exercise physiologist to understand individual and multiple effects of various treatments on people who are exercising. An example of this is seen in how heart rate and blood pressure response to exercise is blunted when the person is being treated simultaneously by beta adrenergic blocking agents typically used to manage angina or hypertension. These factors must be considered when developing exercise prescriptions for patients on these medications. Exercise may also alter a patient's medical therapy. Insulin dosages, for example, can be reduced in patients with Type 1 diabetes because exercise changes the pharmacokinetics of subcutaneously injected drugs.

Clinical exercise physiologists should have a solid education in basic exercise physiology and more advanced exercise science courses. This basic education should accompany advanced training in pathophysiology of chronic diseases, basic pharmacology, medical terminology, electrocardiographic interpretation, exercise testing for clinical populations, basic nutrition, and health promotion techniques.

In addition to their educational background and professional training, clinical exercise physiologists may choose to pursue professional certification. In fact, today many jobs require clinical exercise physiologists to be certified. Two well-respected organizations that offer certification for clinical exercise physiologists are the American College of Sports Medicine (ACSM) and the American Council on Exercise (ACE).

JOB DUTIES

As illustrated in Figure 16.1, a clinical exercise physiologist has several important responsibilities in helping healthy individuals and those with chronic disease find success with physical activity and exercise programs. Clinical exercise physiologists must have an understanding of how the human body responds to exercise and how various disease conditions can influence exercise responses. One essential responsibility of a clinical exercise physiologist is to ensure the safe participation of a patient or client during an exercise program. Thus, the clinical exercise physiologist must have a thorough understanding of the components of a pre-participation health screening.

Pre-Participation Health Screening

Physical activity and exercise stresses the human body. Because of the nature of this physical stressor, abnormal responses are possible, especially in people with various chronic and/or acute illnesses. Because of this, it is important that participants undergo a pre-participation health screening process. This process may include various levels of screening using self-administered questionnaires and/or risk stratification tools. Medical evaluations involving a physical examination and/or laboratory tests are also considered in the pre-participation health screening. The purposes of performing a screening are to (a) identify individuals with medical contraindications, (b) identify individuals with an increased risk for disease, (c) identify individuals with clinically significant disease, and (d) identify individuals with special needs.

Health History

Gathering health histories on potential participants is typically the first part of the screening process. Although a health history questionnaire may come in many forms and can be created to fit the needs of a particular facility, there are some instruments that have previously been created and may be used. One such instrument is the

Physical Activity Readiness Questionnaire for Everyone or PAR-Q+. This questionnaire is a more comprehensive form than the original PAR-Q and includes a section with questions pertaining to chronic medical conditions. Another questionnaire available is the AHA/ACSM Health/Fitness Facility Preparticipation Screening Questionnaire. Since a health history questionnaire may be tailored to meet the needs of individual facilities, additional information not addressed in either of these questionnaires may be required.

Risk Stratification

Risk stratification is a process through which an individual is placed in a classification schema according to the risks of abnormal responses during exercise participation and is based on various risk factors associated with atherosclerotic cardiovascular disease. Atherosclerotic cardiovascular disease (CVD) risk factors and their defining criteria are available (1). Individuals are placed into one of three categories based on the presence of these CVD risk factors and symptoms associated with cardiovascular disease (Figure 16.2).

Physical Examination

A physical examination is recommended prior to beginning an exercise program for an individual who falls into a moderate or high risk stratification group. Components of a physical examination include measurements of body weight/height, resting heart rate and blood pressure, auscultation of the heart and lungs, checks for edema (especially in the lower limbs), and neurological tests involving reflexes. Additionally, a physical examination may include laboratory tests for cholesterol, triglycerides, and blood glucose. Other tests that may be done for cardiac and pulmonary patients include chest x-rays, comprehensive blood analyses, and pulmonary function assessments. After a physical examination is completed, a physician may see the need to have the individual undergo an exercise test for the purpose of diagnosing disease. Especially for patients entering a rehabilitation program involving exercise, an exercise test is needed for determining the functional status of the individual prior to exercise participation. The test serves as the basis from which to write the initial exercise prescription.

Informed Consent

Informed consent is a process through which an individual is made aware of the purposes, risks, and benefits associated with an exercise test or exercise program. Through this process, the individual is given the opportunity to ask questions and have each of those questions answered. A signed informed consent demonstrates that an individual has agreed to the test or program and is satisfied with the information that has been provided. Safety of the participant is a priority and the informed consent process helps to ensure this.

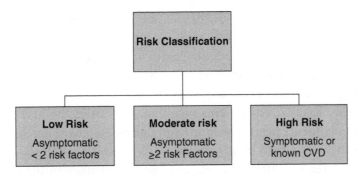

Figure 16.2.   *Risk stratification according to risk factors and symptoms associated with cardiovascular disease.*

Clinical Exercise Testing

As part of their duties, clinical exercise physiologists are usually responsible for conducting exercise testing to clear individuals for safe participation in physical activity and exercise and to design appropriate exercise prescriptions. Although the purposes and protocols of testing may vary, some common physiological measurements assessed during the testing procedure include heart rate, blood pressure, subjective ratings of intensity, oxygen consumption, and cardiac function data obtained through electrocardiography and echocardiography.

Diagnostic and Functional Capacity Testing

The two broad classifications of exercise testing are diagnostic and functional capacity testing, although exercise testing may have some prognostic value as well.

Diagnostic testing is performed for the purpose of detecting underlying disease, usually the presence or absence of heart or pulmonary disease. Indications for this category of testing include (a) symptomology of heart disease, (b) history of a cardiac event (or the possibility that one has occurred), (c) resting electrocardiographic (ECG) abnormalities, and (d) a high probability of underlying disease due to risk factors.

Functional capacity testing is performed to document an individual's physical fitness and provides information about a person's capacity for exercise. This is vital information if an appropriate exercise prescription is to be written. Functional capacity can be determined in two ways during exercise: a direct measurement of maximum oxygen consumption ($\dot{V}O_{2max}$) and an estimated measurement of $\dot{V}O_{2max}$.

> vo_2 is a common symbol in exercise physiology and merely stands for the volume of oxygen consumed, usually expressed in liters per minute ($L \cdot min^{-1}$) or in milliliters per kilogram of body mass per minute ($ml \cdot kg^{-1} \cdot min^{-1}$). The dot above the volume symbol signifies per unit of time (minute).

Regardless of the reason for their being performed, exercise tests are often referred to as graded exercise tests or GXTs, as these tests typically involve a stepwise progression from a light intensity to a maximal or near maximal effort. Exercise tests are performed on an ergometer, usually a treadmill or stationary cycle ergometer, and follow some set *protocol*. Thus, the progressive steps or stages in exercise intensity of a particular exercise test are measurable and repeatable. Although many protocols for exercise testing exist, the protocol chosen is determined by the purpose of the test and the health status of the individual being tested.

Heart Rate

Heart rate should be measured prior to, during, and following a GXT and is generally expressed as beats per minute. It is recommended that resting heart rate be measured after an individual has been sitting quietly for at least five minutes. Resting heart rate is usually measured through auscultation or palpation. *Auscultation* involves the use of a stethoscope placed on the individual's chest, while *palpation* is usually done at the radial pulse. During exercise, the measurement of heart rate is more difficult to obtain and is usually measured using electrocardiography. Heart rate is influenced by several factors and a clinical exercise physiologist needs to be aware of these. Tobacco use, caffeine ingestion, fever, stress, food digestion, medications, and prior physical activity can influence heart rate at rest and during exercise. Therefore, it is important that an individual follow pretesting instructions of no tobacco use, caffeine ingestion, and food consumption within three hours of the exercise test (1). Heart rate increases as the intensity of the exercise test increases and should be measured during each stage of the test to ensure the individual is having a normal response. Also, the clinical exercise physiologist can use the heart rate data from the exercise test in developing an appropriate exercise prescription.

Blood Pressure

Blood pressure represents the force exerted against the walls of arteries and is determined by the volume of blood pumped out of the heart per minute (cardiac output) and the resistance to the flow of this blood through the vasculature (peripheral resistance). During blood pressure assessment, there are actually two pressures recorded. The highest pressure recorded is called systolic blood pressure. This pressure occurs during the contraction or systolic phase of the cardiac cycle and represents the pressure within the arteries during ventricular contraction. The lower pressure recorded is referred to as diastolic blood pressure and occurs during the relaxation or diastolic phase of the cardiac cycle. The diastolic pressure represents the pressure within the arteries during ventricular relaxation.

Blood pressure is an important indicator of one's health and may be measured with an automated unit or manually using a stethoscope and sphygmomanometer (blood pressure cuff). Blood pressure is recorded in millimeters of mercury (mm Hg), with systolic over diastolic. A chronically elevated resting blood pressure is a condition known as hypertension. Hypertension is referred to as the "silent killer" because it often exists without any noticeable symptoms. Those who are hypertensive have an increased risk for stroke and cardiovascular disease. Categories for resting blood pressure are established by Joint National Committee on the Prevention, Detection, Evaluation, and Treatment of High Blood Pressure (26). The latest categories appear in Table 16.1.

Like heart rate, resting blood pressure should be measured after a minimum of five minutes of quiet sitting. During exercise testing, blood pressure is typically recorded during each stage of the test. A normal response in blood pressure during incremental exercise is a linear increase in systolic pressure with little or no change in diastolic pressure. It is not uncommon for systolic pressure to increase to about 200 mm Hg in healthy men and women during maximal exercise (1).

A physiological measurement of interest in cardiac patients is rate pressure product. Rate pressure product is determined by multiplying systolic blood pressure by heart rate and is used as an indicator of the workload on the heart (myocardial workload). The calculation of this measurement in cardiac patients is useful because many times symptoms in cardiac patients occur at a particular rate pressure product.

Rating of Perceived Exertion

During a GXT it is common to assess the individual's psychological perception of how hard he is working, in other words, how he perceives the exercise intensity. A widely used scale for this assessment is the rating of perceived exertion (RPE) scale (Figure 16.3) created by Gunnar Borg (2). The traditional scale runs from 6 to 20 and generally relates to heart rate from rest to maximal exercise when multiplied by a factor of 10. A revised RPE system has been created that provides a category-ratio scale of values ranging from 0 to 11. When used during a GXT, the RPE scale indicates to the clinical exercise physiologist how difficult the testing subject perceives her exercise and when the subject is nearing her maximal effort. RPE scales may also be used as a means of gauging intensity during exercise programming.

Table 16.1. Classifications for Resting Blood Pressure.

Classification	Systolic Blood Pressure (mm Hg)	Diastolic Blood Pressure (mm Hg)
Normal	< 120	And < 80
Prehypertension	120 – 139	Or 80 – 89
Stage 1 Hypertension	140 – 159	Or 90 – 99
Stage 2 Hypertension	≥ 160	Or ≥ 100

Category Scale		Category-Ratio Scale		
6		0	Nothing at all	"No P"
7	Very, very light	0.3		
8		0.5	Extremely weak	Just noticeable
9	Very light	0.7		
10		1	Very weak	
11	Fairly light	1.5		
12		2	Weak	Light
13	Somewhat hard	2.5		
14		3	Moderate	
15	Hard	4		
16		5	Strong	Heavy
17	Very hard	6		
18		7	Very strong	
19	Very, very hard	8		
20		9		
		10	Extremely strong	"Max P"
		11		
		•	Absolute maximum	Highest Possible

Figure 16.3. *The Borg Rating of Perceived Exertion Scales.*

Electrocardiogram

Another common measurement during a GXT is an electrocardiogram or ECG. An ECG is a recording of the electrical activity of the heart and may be used to determine heart rate during a GXT, but more importantly, the ECG is used to determine heart functioning during the physical stress of exercise. An individual may have a normal resting ECG. However, during a GXT when the heart encounters more stress, abnormalities may present. An abnormal ECG during testing may indicate an electrical conductivity problem within the heart, insufficient supply of oxygen to the heart muscle, or damage to the myocardium.

Echocardiography

Although not as often utilized during exercise testing as the other measurements previously discussed, the use of echocardiography can be extremely important during diagnostic testing. Echocardiography is a technique used to assess cardiac function by creating a real-time image of the heart as it is beating. Performed by a cardiologist or trained health care professional, an echocardiogram uses sound waves to create an image that allows for assessment of valvular function and blood flow through the heart chambers. In some cases a contrast dye may be used to enhance the images produced through echocardiography. When an echocardiogram is combined with a GXT, it is referred to as a stress echocardiogram, and can be an important tool in diagnosing cardiovascular disease.

Assessment of Health-Related Physical Fitness

Health-related physical fitness is physical fitness as it pertains to disease prevention and health promotion. It is characterized by an ability to perform daily activities with vigor and to demonstrate traits and capacities that are associated with low risk of premature development of hypokinetic diseases (11). Health-related physical fitness typically includes components in four areas: (a) body composition, (b) cardiorespiratory fitness, (c) muscular strength and endurance, and (d) flexibility. See Chapter 22 for an expansion of these traits to account for the prevalence of obesity, metabolic syndrome and diabetes, and osteoporosis today.

The assessment of health-related physical fitness is commonly performed in a clinical setting and thus, the clinical exercise physiologist needs to have the knowledge, skills, and abilities to conduct tests in each of the four components listed. The purposes of health-related physical fitness testing include the following:

- Educating participants
- Providing data for prescribing exercise
- Collecting baseline and follow-up data that can be compared to normative values
- Setting goals and motivating participants
- Stratifying risk and exposing underlying problems

When all four health-related physical fitness components are assessed in one session, it is recommended that an order is established—body composition, cardiorespiratory fitness, muscle strength and endurance, and flexibility (1).

Body Composition

Body composition refers to the relative percent of body weight that is composed of fat (adipose) tissue and fat-free tissue. Body composition is considered a health-related component because excess body fat is associated with chronic conditions such as hypertension, diabetes, metabolic syndrome, and hyperlipidemia. Additionally, too little body fat is associated with health problems as well. Fat tissue in the body can be classified as essential and nonessential fat. Essential body fat is necessary for normal functioning, whereas nonessential body fat is extra fat stored within the viscera or just below the skin. The body fat stored just below the skin is called subcutaneous fat.

Cardiorespiratory Fitness

Cardiorespiratory fitness is considered health-related because (a) low levels of cardiorespiratory fitness are associated with an increased risk of premature death (especially due to cardiac disease), (b) improvements in cardiorespiratory fitness are associated with a reduction in death from all causes, and (c) high levels of cardio-respiratory fitness are associated with many health benefits. The criterion measure for cardiorespiratory fitness is maximal oxygen consumption or $\dot{V}O_{2max}$. Maximal oxygen consumption can be assessed using submaximal and maximal exercise testing procedures.

Submaximal exercise testing is common in health-fitness environments and is based on heart rate response to submaximal workloads. Submaximal testing may be conducted using a treadmill or cycle ergometer. Additionally, there are various step test protocols that may be used. A submaximal test provides a way of esti-mating an individual's $\dot{V}O_{2max}$ and is generally safer for the participant and less expensive to perform. Because submaximal testing is used to estimate $\dot{V}O_{2max}$, there are a number of assumptions associated with this type of testing: (a) a steady heart rate is obtained for each exercise work rate, (b) a linear relationship exists between heart rate and work rate, (c) maximal heart rate for a given age is uniform, and (d) oxygen uptake at a given work rate is the same for everyone (1).

Unlike submaximal testing, which estimates, maximal exercise testing can be used to measure $\dot{V}O_{2max}$ through a process called indirect calorimetry. Treadmill and cycle ergometry are common modalities of this type of testing. With maximal testing, an individual is pushed to the point of volitional fatigue unless an abnor-mal physiological response worthy of stopping the test occurs prior to fatigue. Maximal exercise testing for the purpose of measuring $\dot{V}O_{2max}$ requires the use of an expensive metabolic system that is not always available in a clinical setting. Nevertheless, it is very important that the clinical exercise physiologist be trained on how to operate this equipment and on how to conduct this type of test.

When comparing submaximal and maximal testing and deciding which to use for a given situation, the clinical exercise physiologist needs to address the following questions:

- What is the reason for the test?
- Who is the subject to be tested?
- What equipment is available for the test?

Muscular Strength and Endurance

Muscular strength and muscular endurance are sometimes referred to together as muscular fitness. Activities of daily living require a certain level of muscular strength and endurance, and especially for individuals who are older, having adequate strength and endurance to allow them to live independently. Additionally, muscle strength and bone health are positively associated with each other.

Muscular strength is defined as the maximal force that can be generated by a specific muscle or muscle group. Muscular strength is usually measured by having a participant perform a one-repetition maximum (1-RM). Sometimes a 1-RM can be predicted using a multiple repetition protocol with a prediction equation.

Muscular endurance refers to a muscle or muscle group's ability to perform repeated contractions without fatigue. Muscular endurance may also be defined as a muscle or muscle group's ability to sustain a submaximal contraction over a period of time. Most tests for muscular endurance involve repeated contractions with a set amount of weight.

One important note is that both muscular strength and muscular endurance of an individual are specific to each muscle or muscle group. Because of this, when assessing muscular fitness, it is ideal to include measurements for upper, middle, and lower body muscles. This allows for a more complete assessment of this health-related physical fitness component. Some purposes of muscle fitness assessment include (a) identification of weak areas, (b) monitoring progress in rehabilitation, and (c) measuring the effectiveness of training.

Flexibility

Flexibility refers to the ability to move a joint through its full range of motion. Flexibility of a joint is dependent on several factors, some being internal factors while others are external. Some internal factors include the type of joint, the elasticity of muscle tissue around the joint, the elasticity of the tendons and ligaments that compose the joint, and the temperature of the joint itself. External factors consist of age and gender of the individual, viscosity of muscle tissue around the joint, environmental temperature, and restriction due to clothing or equipment.

Flexibility is joint specific. Thus, no single flexibility test can be used to assess total body flexibility. Because flexibility is joint specific, its assessment should involve tests of multiple joints. One of the most used assessments of flexibility is the sit-and-reach test. This test uses a specially designed box to measure flexibility of the low back area and hamstring muscles of the participant. Additional devices (goniometers, inclinometers, and tape measures) are available to assess flexibility of the various joints of the body, and the clinical exercise physiologist should be familiar with the use of these.

Exercise Prescription

Following pre-participation health screening and testing, the clinical exercise physiologist becomes involved in designing an exercise prescription for the individual. An exercise prescription is a plan for physical activity and exercise developed to enhance physical fitness, promote health by reducing risk factors for disease, and ensure safety during exercise participation. Exercise prescription is based in scientific principles, but there is an art to prescribing exercise. Exercise prescriptions typically require modification because physiologic and perceptual responses and adaptations and progression vary between individuals. The ability of the clinical exercise physiologist to prescribe exercise improves with experience in working with individuals with various conditions.

There are five basic components addressed by the exercise prescription: (a) mode or type of exercise, (b) intensity or degree of difficulty of exercise, (c) duration of exercise, (d) frequency of exercise, and (e) progression. The final design of an exercise prescription should be individualized, so how the clinical exercise physiologist addresses these five components within the exercise prescription will vary depending on the health status, risk factor profile, behavioral characteristics, personal goals, exercise preferences, and health and fitness needs of the participant. The following box contains a sample case study involving exercise prescription.

CASE STUDY: Exercise Prescription

A 45-year-old female client is referred to you with a five-year history of non-insulin dependent (Type 2) diabetes and a strong family history of cardiovascular disease. She is currently taking 5 mg of Glucotrol (glipizide) one time daily prior to breakfast. She is currently active, but her physician would like her to receive professional exercise advice and supervision that would allow her to become more regular with her exercise routine. Medical information from her recent visit to her physician includes a body height of 66 inches and a body weight of 145 pounds. Her resting heart rate is 82 beats per minute and she has a resting blood pressure of 122/76 mmHg. A lipid profile performed four weeks ago indicated a total cholesterol of 190 mg/dl, HDL cholesterol of 52 mg/dl, and triglycerides of 140mg/dl. She completed a graded exercise test (GXT) three weeks ago utilizing the Naughton protocol. Peak exercise recorded for your client was 6.0 METs (1 MET = rest oxygen consumption or 3.5 mlO$_2$/kg/min). She reached a peak heart rate of 165 beats per minute. Her maximal blood pressure was recorded at 176/82 mmHg. No ECG abnormalities were noted and the physician concluded that the test was normal.

This client has two risk factors for cardiovascular disease, a positive family history and Type 2 diabetes, for which she is receiving medical therapy. Because of her two cardiovascular risk factors, she is placed into a moderate risk group. She has a normal resting blood pressure and lipid profile, and her body mass index (BMI) is normal at 23.4. The results from her recent GXT were good with a normal response in heart rate and blood pressure and no ECG abnormalities reported. Her exercise program will focus on aerobic exercise training to help her manage her diabetic condition, thereby reducing the risk of complications associated with this type of disease. The program will also help her maintain her normal readings for resting blood pressure, lipids, and BMI. Her exercise prescription is below:

Mode of exercise: Different modalities of aerobic exercise including treadmill walking, recumbent cycling, and elliptical exercise. Resistance training and flexibility exercise will be infused into the program as she progresses.

Intensity of exercise: Aerobic exercise will be performed at a moderate intensity of 60 to 75% VO$_{2max}$ of and RPE of 12 to 14. Using her information above, her target heart rate for exercise is 131 to 144 beats per minute.

Duration of exercise: Initially, her exercise session will last approximately 45 minutes. This will include approximately 35 minutes of a stimulus phase and 10 minutes for warm up and cool down.

Frequency of exercise: She will exercise three times per week, once daily on Monday, Wednesday, and Friday. This will provide a rest day between exercise sessions.

CLINICAL CONDITIONS

One important distinction between clinical exercise physiologists and other exercise professionals is their knowledge and understanding of diseases. Clinical exercise physiologists use exercise as a means of improving the physiological functioning of individuals with various chronic illnesses. During the process of rehabilitation they must have an understanding of how a particular disease affects the exercise response and how exercise can be of benefit to the individual and his condition.

Because medications are often prescribed to individuals with clinical conditions, a clinical exercise physiologist must be familiar with medications commonly used to treat and manage such conditions. This section of the chapter briefly discusses some of the common pathologies to which the clinical exercise physiologist may be exposed in working with patients. The clinical conditions addressed include cardiovascular disease, pulmonary disease, metabolic disorders, orthopedic diseases, and neuromuscular disorders.

Cardiovascular Disease

Cardiovascular disease is an umbrella term that encompasses many specific diseases and conditions of the heart and vasculature. Some common cardiovascular diseases include ischemic cardiovascular disease, chronic heart failure, cardiac valvular disease, peripheral vascular disease, and hypertension. Cardiovascular disease is the leading cause of death in the United States, accounting for over 600,000 deaths annually (26). The death rate due to cardiovascular disease has declined since 1968, while the incidence rate has continued to increase (26). This indicates that individuals with cardiovascular disease are living longer, and this increased longevity may be attributed to the advancements made in medical therapy, surgical interventions, and rehabilitative programs for cardiac patients.

Ischemic Cardiovascular Disease

Ischemic cardiovascular disease is caused by atherosclerosis, a process that begins in early life and develops as a person ages. Atherosclerosis is defined as the accumulation of plaque (cholesterol, lipids, fibrous tissue) on and within the inner lining of a blood vessel, resulting in a narrowing of the vessel's lumen (Figure 16.4). When

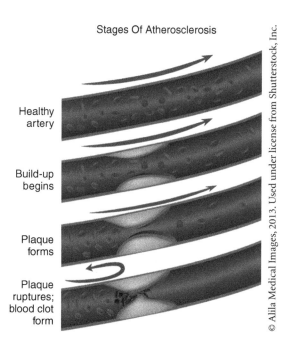

Stages Of Atherosclerosis

Healthy artery

Build-up begins

Plaque forms

Plaque ruptures; blood clot form

© Alila Medical Images, 2013. Used under license from Shutterstock, Inc.

Figure 16.4. *Progression of atherosclerosis of an artery.*

significant plaque develops in arteries that supply blood flow to the heart, it results in coronary artery disease (CAD). CAD causes a reduction in blood flow and oxygen to the myocardium (heart muscle), especially during times of physical stress. This deficiency in oxygen supply to the myocardium is termed myocardial ischemia.

Myocardial ischemia causes chest pain known as angina pectoris. Angina is one symptom of ischemic cardiovascular disease and typically accompanies a heart attack or myocardial infarction. Angina in a cardiac patient may be classified as stable or unstable. Stable angina is chest pain that presents at a certain level or intensity of physical exertion. Unstable angina is a more life-threatening situation as it is chest pain that occurs unpredictably.

In some cases, myocardial ischemia is associated with an absence of symptoms. This type of ischemia is referred to as silent ischemia and is more common in diabetics due to their gradual loss of nerve sensitivity (neuropathy) associated with their diabetic condition. Because silent ischemia is asymptomatic (without symptoms), it is usually detected with the use of electrocardiography. A physician can detect silent ischemia by looking for specific changes to an electrocardiogram (ECG) of the patient. One common ECG abnormality indicative of myocardial ischemia is ST-segment depression (Figure 16.5).

Exercise therapy is beneficial for the ischemic heart disease patient. A regular exercise routine may help prevent the progression of atherosclerosis and control cardiac risk factors such as hypertension and hyperlipidemia, diabetes, and overweight. Specific for the patient with stable angina, exercise training can increase the ischemic threshold through a reduction in myocardial oxygen demand. This means that a stable angina patient would require a greater intensity of exercise to cause angina symptoms.

Chronic Heart Failure

Chronic heart failure (CHF) is a condition characterized by an inability of the heart to adequately pump blood to body tissues. CHF resulting from direct myocardial damage due to a myocardial infarction or prolonged ischemic event is called ischemic cardiomyopathy. CHF resulting from nonischemic damage is called idiopathic dilated cardiomyopathy and may be due to long-standing high blood pressure or diabetes, alcohol abuse, valvular disease, or an autoimmune response to a viral infection.

With CHF, an individual may demonstrate a depressed systolic function, a depressed diastolic function, or a combination of both. A depressed systolic function occurs with a loss of heart muscle due to myocardial infarction and/or a decline in the contractile force of the myocardium. Diastolic function suffers from an increased resistance to ventricular filling and a decrease in ventricular compliance. It has been estimated that diastolic dysfunction may account for up to 40% of all CHF cases (18). Secondary organ changes associated with CHF include derangements in skeletal muscle, impaired vasodilation, and renal insufficiency resulting in retention of sodium and water.

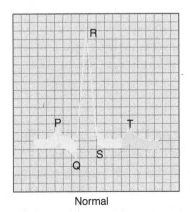
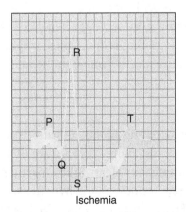

Figure 16.5. *A normal electrocardiogram on the left and an abnormal electrocardiogram on the right showing a depressed ST-segment.*

During exercise, CHF patients will demonstrate an impaired rise in cardiac output and an increase in left ventricular filling pressure. These hemodynamic changes result in an increased sympathetic discharge, greater peripheral constriction, and an increased heart rate for a given workload (18). Additionally, there is an increased likelihood of cardiac arrhythmias. These hemodynamic changes underlie the symptoms of CHF, which include fatigue, shortness of breath (dyspnea), and reduced exercise tolerance.

Prior to the mid-1980s, exercise programs for patients with CHF were discouraged with concerns over safety and effects of exercise on the diseased heart (18). Today, it is generally believed that exercise training neither harms nor significantly benefits the heart muscle in CHF. However, exercise therapy can improve functional capacity in CHF patients through peripheral adaptations such as improved skeletal muscle metabolism and improved dilation of vessels and distribution of blood flow.

Cardiac Valvular Disease

The heart has four valves that regulate blood flow through the heart chambers during the cardiac cycle. Appropriate cardiac output is dependent on the proper functioning of these valves. Any of the four valves are susceptible to some form of cardiac valvular disease; however, left-side abnormalities are most responsible for morbidity and mortality and present more risk for the patient during exercise.

There are two forms of valvular dysfunction—regurgitation and stenosis. Regurgitation occurs when the leaflets of a valve fail to coapt or close properly or the valve prolapses. This leads to movement of blood in the wrong direction; if severe enough, this may negatively impact stroke volume and cardiac output. Stenosis of a valve causes a valve to not open properly and significantly increases the resistance to flow through the valve. This condition also adversely affects cardiac output. The primary causes of valvular disease are rheumatic fever, congenital abnormalities, infection, and aging. The symptoms and limitations of a patient with valvular disease are dependent on the heart valves involved, the severity of the condition, and presence of comorbidities. The mechanical function of a valve will not improve with exercise training; however, training can result in peripheral (skeletal muscle) adaptations that improve functional capacity of the patient (9).

Peripheral Artery Disease

Peripheral artery disease (PAD) is a vascular condition caused by atherosclerosis of arteries of the lower extremities. The primary effect of PAD is claudication. Claudication is a cramping sensation in the lower legs (calves) that occurs during physical activity such as walking and is relieved with the cessation of activity. Claudication is the symptom associated with an inadequate supply of blood and oxygen to the working muscles of the lower legs. Because PAD is due to atherosclerosis, the risk factors associated with the condition are similar to those for ischemic heart disease. In fact, individuals with PAD are at a much greater risk for a myocardial infarction (28).Exercise training can serve as a beneficial means of therapy for PAD patients by reducing intermittent claudication. Exercise training reduces this symptom by increasing leg blood flow, reducing blood viscosity, and improving oxidative metabolism with the muscle of the lower legs (30).

Hypertension

A chronically elevated resting blood pressure is a condition known as hypertension. Hypertension affects over 76 million Americans, many of whom are unaware they have the condition (11). According to data from the well-known Framingham Heart Study, participants in the study with normal blood pressure at age 55 had a 90% lifetime risk for developing hypertension (27). This indicates that the prevalence of hypertension increases with age. Hypertension is categorized as either primary or secondary hypertension. Primary hypertension accounts for 90 to 95% of cases, and its direct cause is unknown (8). Secondary hypertension has a direct cause and is typically one of the following: kidney disease, pregnancy, adrenal gland disease, hyper- or hypothyroidism, or use of medications (birth control, diet pills, steroids).

Blood pressure in the body is determined by cardiac output and peripheral resistance. An increase in one or both of these variables will result in an increase in blood pressure with a corresponding rise in myocardial workload. Hypertensive individuals usually see an exaggerated rise in systolic blood pressure during exercise. Exercise tolerance may be impaired in untreated hypertension or by the use of hypertensive drugs. Longitudinal studies have shown benefits from aerobic training in hypertensive individuals with decreases of 5 to 7 mm Hg in both resting systolic blood pressure and diastolic blood pressure (10). Being physically active or having a high cardiorespiratory fitness is associated with lower mortality rates due to hypertension.

Pulmonary Disease

Pulmonary diseases significantly impair the body's ability to ventilate (breathe) and in some cases absorb oxygen into the blood. Ventilation involves the movement of air into (inhalation) and out of (exhalation) the lungs. Pulmonary disease may disrupt both processes, but for many with pulmonary disease, it is the exhalation part of breathing that suffers the most. Common treatments for pulmonary patients include medical therapy, supplemental oxygen, and breathing exercises. Physical activity and exercise are also extremely important means of treatment and can improve the overall functioning of pulmonary patients. Some of the common pulmonary diseases addressed in this section are chronic obstructive pulmonary disease (COPD), asthma, and cystic fibrosis.

Chronic Obstructive Pulmonary Disease

COPD includes conditions such as chronic bronchitis and emphysema characterized by chronic, typically irreversible, airway obstruction resulting in a slower rate of exhalation. Affecting an estimated 24 million Americans, COPD is the most common respiratory disease, and overall, is the fourth leading cause of death in the United States (7). As much as 80 to 90% of COPD cases are due to cigarette smoking (4).

Chronic bronchitis, a type of COPD, involves a chronic inflammation of the bronchial tubes, associated with an excessive mucous production from cells lining the bronchi and a persistent cough. Another type of COPD, emphysema, is a local or generalized condition of the lung marked by distension, progressive loss of elasticity, and eventual rupture of the alveoli. These changes to lung tissue are accompanied by labored breathing and a husky cough. Such changes associated with these types of COPD significantly impede lung function, causing a patient to experience dyspnea. Individuals with lung disease are typically deconditioned due to a lack of physical activity. Exercise can be an important means of therapy for pulmonary patients by improving ventilatory efficiency (breathing patterns) and overall cardiorespiratory fitness. Additionally, regular exercise may help these patients become less sensitive to dyspnea.

Asthma

Asthma is a respiratory condition that affects over 20 million Americans, including children and adults (5). Asthma most often presents during early childhood, and there is a broad range between individuals in the severity of the disease. Asthma is characterized by three factors: (a) airway obstruction, (b) airway inflammation, and (c) airway hyperreactivity. Asthmatics have an increased sensitivity to certain stimuli, called triggers, that initiate an asthmatic attack. There are many possible triggers for an attack, and not all triggers affect asthmatics the same way. Possible triggers include animal allergens, tobacco smoke, dust mites, molds and pollens, exposure to cold air, and air pollution. Exercise can actually be a trigger for some individuals. When attacks are triggered by physical activity, it is called exercise induced bronchoconstriction (EIB). EIB exists in 50 to 90% of asthmatics (23), but also can occur in those without diagnosed asthma.

Symptoms of asthma, such as dyspnea and difficulty in breathing, present during an asthmatic attack. The lungs of an asthmatic are chronically inflamed (23). Therefore, it is extremely important that an asthmatic properly care for her condition. Medical therapy can help control the disease and reduce asthmatic attacks. Although most asthmatics find physical activity to be a trigger for an attack, well-controlled asthma does not usually limit exercise performance and adaptations with exercise training should mirror the adaptations seen in those without asthma.

Cystic Fibrosis

Cystic fibrosis is a multi-organ disease that affects the lungs, pancreas, intestines, and sweat glands. It is an inherited condition that occurs in one of every 3,500 live births (20). Generally, cystic fibrosis results in thick mucus that clogs ducts, tubes, and tubules of the affected organs. In lung tissue, the thick mucus clogs the airways and leads to inflammation, infection, and fibrosis. These changes in lung tissue result in an irreversible loss of pulmonary function (20). Those with cystic fibrosis typically have a shortened lifespan.

Treatment for the cystic fibrosis patient is carried out to prevent or slow down the decline in lung function. Regular exercise is generally recommended for patients with cystic fibrosis because studies have shown benefits in those of all ages and disease states (13). However, it is worthy to note that exercise responses and adaptations will vary depending on the severity of the disease. Exercise programs should follow general recommendations for mode, intensity, frequency, and duration.

Metabolic Disorders

Metabolism is defined as all energy and material transformations that occur within living cells and involves the breakdown (catabolism) and building up (anabolism) of compounds to provide energy, growth, and repair for body tissues. A metabolic disorder is a condition that causes a disruption in the normal metabolic processes of the body and can lead to serious health issues. Exercise is beneficial in helping patients manage their metabolic conditions. Three common metabolic disorders discussed in this section are diabetes mellitus, hyperlipidemia, and obesity.

Diabetes Mellitus

Diabetes mellitus is a metabolic disease due to either an insulin deficiency or a resistance to insulin action or both, resulting in an inability to control blood glucose levels. Insulin is an important hormone for the body because it enables tissues to uptake glucose. Without adequate insulin production or improper insulin action, blood glucose levels can rise, resulting in hyperglycemia. Diabetes affects an estimated 25.8 million Americans with approximately 27% of cases undiagnosed (3).

A diabetic condition may be one of two major types (Type I and Type II), although there is a temporary diabetic state that may occur during pregnancy called gestational diabetes. Type I diabetes is characterized by a lack of insulin production, and for that reason, this type is commonly referred to as insulin-dependent diabetes. The cause of Type I diabetes is thought to involve an autoimmune response that destroys the beta cells of the pancreas. The beta cells are responsible for producing insulin, but with their destruction, the body is unable to regulate blood glucose. Type I diabetes typically develops early in life, with the onset usually occurring prior to age 30 (12). Type II diabetes occurs later in life as a person develops a resistance to the insulin being produced in the body. The pathophysiology of this type of diabetes is most likely due to multiple factors. Obesity is strongly associated with Type II diabetes. In fact, about 80% of patients with Type II diabetes are also obese (8).

The long-term health complications of diabetes are many and include heart disease, stroke, hypertension, eye disease, kidney disease, and nerve damage. Keys to controlling a diabetic situation are proper medical therapy through the use of insulin or glucose-lowering drugs (see case study), frequent monitoring of blood glucose levels, proper dietary habits, and regular exercise.

Exercise is an extremely beneficial means of therapy for the diabetic patient who has his or her disease under control. Exercise has an insulin-like effect on the body, and when properly scheduled around a patient's medical therapy and meals, can be instrumental in helping to regulate blood glucose levels and decrease risks of complications associated with the disease.

Hyperlipidemia

Hyperlipidemia is a condition characterized by elevated levels of cholesterol and/or triglycerides in the blood. Although necessary for normal functioning with cholesterol serving a precursor for several hormones and triglycerides as a fuel source, excessive amounts in the blood contribute to an individual's risk of cardiovascular disease by contributing to the process of atherosclerosis. Lipids are not soluble in water and must combine with proteins in order to be transported in the blood. The spherical structures formed are called lipoproteins and consist of proteins surrounding a lipid core. There are four principal classifications of lipoproteins, including chylomicrons, very low density lipoprotein (VLDL), low-density lipoprotein (LDL), and high-density lipoprotein (HDL). Chylomicrons, VLDL, and LDL are involved with forward cholesterol transport and move lipids from the intestine and liver to peripheral tissues. HDL is involved with reverse cholesterol transport and moves lipids from peripheral tissues back to the liver. Forward cholesterol transport is linked with the process of atherosclerosis.

The standards for lipid levels in the blood are established by the National Cholesterol Education Program. Simply put, it is recommended that an individual have a total cholesterol level of less than 200 mg/dl, an LDL level of less than 100 mg/dl, an HDL level of greater than 40 mg/dl, and a triglyceride level of less than 150 mg/dl (28). Hyperlipidemia is a common condition with approximately 17% of the U.S. population affected (19). Factors that contribute to the development of this condition are genetic influences, cigarette smoking, poor dietary habits, excessive body weight, and physical inactivity. The use of cholesterol-lowering drugs is a common therapy for those with hyperlipidemia, but diet and exercise can be effective means of therapy as well. Physical activity in the form of regular aerobic exercise can alter lipoprotein transport in the body helping to lower triglyceride levels and increase HDL.

Obesity

Obesity is a chronic condition characterized by excessive body fat that results in a significant impairment of health and an increased risk of other morbidities. Considered a health epidemic by many, obesity rates have rapidly climbed in recent years and currently affect approximately 35% of U.S. adults (21). Obesity may be linked to genetic factors, but lifestyle behaviors involving high-calorie, high-fat diets and insufficient energy expenditure play a role as well.

Losing weight and maintaining that weight loss can be a difficult task for an obese patient. The primary goal of therapy should be to reduce fat weight while maintaining lean body mass. The most successful individuals are those who are slightly to moderately obese, have upper body fat distribution, have no history of weight cycling, become overweight as an adult, or have a sincere desire to lose weight (29).

Behavior modification is typically the first means of helping an obese individual treat his condition and involves modification of dietary and physical activity habits. A patient should attempt to create a negative daily caloric balance by reducing caloric intake through improved dietary habits and increasing caloric expenditure through greater physical activity. A regular exercise program is an important component in a weight loss program and is also important in helping a patient maintain weight loss. For patients who are unsuccessful in losing weight solely through attempts in behavior modification, medical therapy and surgical procedures are available. Still, even with these more extreme measures, lifestyle management involving diet and exercise are crucial for long-term success in the obese patient.

Orthopedic Diseases

Orthopedic diseases are those that affect the skeletal system of the body resulting in alterations to the normal anatomy of bone structure. Two of the most common orthopedic diseases are osteoporosis and arthritis.

Osteoporosis

During the life of an individual, bone undergoes remodeling. This constant building up and breaking down of bone takes place due to activity of two types of bone cells. Osteoblasts are bone forming cells and osteoclasts are cells that resorb or break down bone. Peak bone mass of an individual is reached between the years of 20 and 30 (19). From there remodeling remains in balance until a person reaches 45 to 50 years of age (19). After that point, the breakdown of bone predominates.

Osteoporosis is a condition characterized by a significant loss in bone mass, resulting in weaker and more brittle bones. The breakdown of bone occurs more rapidly in some individuals, making them more susceptible to bone fractures. Of course, advancing age is a risk factor for osteoporosis, but other factors include, gender, ethnicity, bone structure and body weight, early menopause, history of eating disorders, medication and disease, and family history. Other lifestyle factors that may increase one's risk for osteoporosis include smoking, excessive alcohol intake, high caffeine intake, and little weight-bearing activity and exercise (24).

Women are more susceptible to osteoporosis, with Caucasian and Asian women having an even greater risk for the disease. Women in their postmenopausal years are highly susceptible to an osteoporotic condition due to the loss of estrogen production and its protective effect on bone health. Therapies for the osteoporotic patient include medical therapy, hormone replacement therapy for postmenopausal woman, calcium and vitamin D supplementation, and exercise.

Exercise can be a very beneficial preventive treatment and a means of therapy for the osteoporotic patient, but exercise training should vary depending on the severity of the disease. Regularly performed exercise can slow the age-related decline in bone mass with weight-bearing exercise being most beneficial. Weight-bearing exercise provides stress to the skeleton resulting in a stimulation of osteoblast activity. A program of aerobic exercise and strength training is advised with the inclusion of balance-enhancing exercise to decrease risk of falls in patients. Also, aquatic exercise is appropriate for clients with a history of fracture or those at a high risk for fracture.

Arthritis

Arthritis is a chronic condition that affects the joints of the body, causing inflammation, pain, degeneration of joint tissues, and restriction in movement. One in every six Americans has some form of arthritis, and it is the leading cause of disability among individuals older than 55 years (16).

Two common types of arthritis are osteoarthritis and rheumatoid arthritis. Osteoarthritis is the most prevalent form of arthritis, affecting an estimated 46 million U.S. adults (17). Osteoarthritis causes a degeneration of articular cartilage and alterations of bone structure in and around joints. Common sites affected by osteoarthritis include the fingers, knees, hips, and feet. Rheumatoid arthritis is a systemic disease initiated as an auto-immune response, possibly due to bacteria or viruses. Rheumatoid arthritis may affect a variety of tissues, but its primary effect in joints is an inflammation of the synovial membrane (synovitis). Women are affected most by rheumatoid, comprising 75% of patients. Peak onset of rheumatoid arthritis is between 20 and 45 years (16) and is associated with a decreased lifespan of 10 to 15 years (19).

The main goals of therapy for arthritic patients are to ease pain, decrease inflammation, improve functioning, and lessen damage. Treatments may include patient education, medical therapy, exercise with proper rest, use of heat and cold therapy, joint protection, and surgery. Persons with arthritic conditions tend to be less active and less fit. Exercise training can be used to improve cardiorespiratory and muscular fitness. Additional benefits from regular exercise include an improved flexibility, decreased joint pain and swelling, and reduced depression (17).

Neuromuscular Disorders

Neuromuscular disorders include diseases and conditions that affect the normal function of muscle tissues either directly or indirectly through damage to nerve tissue that stimulates or controls muscle action. Of the three discussed in this section, muscular dystrophy is the only one that affects muscle tissue directly. The other two, stroke and multiple sclerosis, cause damage to nerve tissue, resulting in abnormal muscle functioning.

Stroke

A stroke, sometimes referred to as a cerebrovascular accident, occurs when blood flow to an area of the brain is restricted causing brain cell damage. A stroke may be classified as ischemic or hemorrhagic. Ischemic strokes account for 87% of all strokes and occur due to a blockage of an artery (22). Hemorrhagic strokes occur when a vessel in the brain ruptures, leading to an escape of blood into the brain tissue.

Stroke is the third leading cause of death (22); however, survival rate for stroke is very good at over 70% (15). Unfortunately, many stroke victims suffer neurological impairments such as paralysis, spasticity, and disuse muscle atrophy. The severity of the resulting neurological impairment is dependent on the size and location of the area in the brain affected, as well as collateral blood flow.

Participation in a comprehensive exercise program of endurance and strength training is important in helping the patient regain lost functioning. Endurance exercise can increase cardiorespiratory fitness and improve muscle functioning. Resistance training can lead to increased muscular strength in affected and non-affected muscle groups, resulting in improvement in balance and walking gait for the patient. Additionally, an exercise program may benefit the emotional and psychological health of a stroke victim because many suffer depression following a stroke.

Multiple Sclerosis

Multiple sclerosis is a neuromuscular disease that damages the myelin sheath surrounding the axons of nerve fibers of the central nervous system. Myelin provides insulation for nerve fibers that aids in the transmission of nerve impulses. The demyelination process that occurs in multiple sclerosis slows the speed of nerve impulse conduction and disrupts the communication between nerve fibers. Multiple sclerosis is generally believed to be an autoimmune disease that may be triggered by exposure to one or more viruses, but genetic and environmental factors may also play a role. The symptoms associated with multiple sclerosis can vary greatly between individuals, depending on the severity of the disease. Some common symptoms in patients include spasticity, incoordination, impaired balance, fatigue, muscle weakness, and sensory loss and numbness (14).

It appears that exercise training has no direct effect on the disease and its progression (14). However, exercise can be used to improve the overall fitness and functional status of the patient. The exercise prescription for an individual with multiple sclerosis should incorporate exercise for the purpose of maintaining or improving cardiorespiratory fitness, muscular strength, flexibility, and balance.

Muscular Dystrophy

Muscular dystrophy represents a group of genetic disorders characterized by the deterioration of muscle tissue. There are several types of muscular dystrophy, each associated with its own set of symptoms and rate of progression. Common symptoms include muscle weakness and fatigue. Most forms of muscular dystrophy begin with weakness in the proximal muscles that eventually spreads to more distal muscles. As the disease progresses, individuals lose strength in the affected muscles, experience functional disability, and develop alterations in walking gait. There is no known cure for any of the different forms of muscular dystrophy, although the genetic defects that cause them have been identified (6).

Exercise programs for those with muscular dystrophy should provide a combination of cardiorespiratory training and resistance exercise with daily stretching. Cardiorespiratory exercise is good for caloric expenditure and reducing cardiovascular disease risk factors, especially in patients with a type of muscular dystrophy where survival into adulthood is possible (25). Overall, an exercise program should focus on increasing strength, improving functional capacity, and enhancing a patient's ability to perform activities of daily living.

SUMMARY

Clinical exercise physiology is a young profession that has an increasingly important role in providing treatment and management to those with a variety of clinical conditions. Applying an expertise in exercise physiology to the clinical environment, the clinical exercise physiologist is a true health care professional responsible for pre-exercise screening and assessment, exercise testing, patient education, and the development and supervision of exercise programs. The clinical exercise physiologist works with patients who have a variety of diseases and conditions, many of which have been described in this chapter. However, it is important that the clinical exercise physiologist understand that rarely does a patient have just one disease, but usually has comorbidities. In order to provide proper care for patients, the clinical exercise physiologist must have a thorough understanding of how a disease develops, how the disease affects the body and its function, and how exercise may be used to the benefit of the patient.

REFERENCES

1. American College of Sports Medicine, *ACSM's Guidelines for Exercise Testing and Prescription,* 9th ed. Baltimore: Lippincott, Williams & Wilkins, 2014.

2. Borg, G. *Borg's perceived exertion and pain scales.* Champaign, IL: Human Kinetics, 1998.

3. Centers for Disease Control and Prevention, *National Diabetes Fact Sheet: National Estimates and General Information on Diabetes and Prediabetes in the United States, 2011.* Atlanta, GA: U.S. Department of Health and Human Services, Centers for Disease Control and Intervention, 2011 [accessed 2013 May 20]. Available from: www.cdc.gov/diabetes/pubs/pdf/ndfs_2011.pdf

4. Cerny, F. W., and S. Zhan, "Chronic obstructive pulmonary disease." In, *Clinical Exercise Physiology: Application and Physiological Principles,* L. M. LeMura & S. P. von Duvillard, eds.. Philadelphia: Lippincott, Williams & Wilkins, 2004, pp. 157–168.

5. Clark, C. J., and L. M. Cochrane, "Asthma." In *ACSM's Exercise Management for Persons with Chronic Diseases and Disabilities,* 3rd ed., J. L. Durstine, G. E. Moore, P. L. Painter, & S. O. Roberts, editors. Champaign (IL): Human Kinetics, 2009, pp. 143–149.

6. Cohen, B. J., *Memmler's the Human Body in Health and Disease,* 11th ed. Philadelphia: Lippincott, Williams & Wilkins, 2009.

7. Cooper, C. B., "Chronic obstructive pulmonary disease." In: *ACSM's Exercise Management for Persons with Chronic Diseases and Disabilities,* 3rd ed., J. L. Durstine, G. E. Moore, P. L. Painter, & S. O. Roberts, eds. Champaign, IL: Human Kinetics, 2009, pp. 129–135.

8. Dishman, R. K., R. A. Washburn, and G. W. Heath, *Physical Activity Epidemiology.* Champaign (IL): Human Kinetics, 2004.

9. Friedman, D., and S. O. Roberts, "Valvular heart disease." In *ACSM's Exercise Management for Persons with Chronic Diseases and Disabilities,* 3rd ed., J. L. Durstine, G. E. Moore, P. L. Painter, & S. O. Roberts, eds. Champaign, IL: Human Kinetics, 2009, pp. 85–91.

10. Gordon, N. F., "Hypertension." In *ACSM's Exercise Management for Persons with Chronic Diseases and Disabilities,* 3rd ed., J. L. Durstine, G. E. Moore, P. L. Painter, & S. O. Roberts, eds. Champaign, IL: Human Kinetics, 2009, pp. 107–113.

11. Hoeger, W. W. K., and S. A. Hoeger, *Principles and Labs for Fitness & Wellness*. Belmont, CA: Wadsworth, 2014.

12. Hornsby, W. G., and A. L., "Diabetes." In *ACSM's Exercise Management for Persons with Chronic Diseases and Disabilities*, 3rd ed., J. L. Durstine, G. E. Moore, P. L. Painter, & S. O. Roberts, eds. Champaign, IL: Human Kinetics, 2009, pp. 182–190.

13. Huetler, M., and R. Beneke, "Cystic fibrosis." In LeMura LM, von Duvillard SP, editors. *Clinical Exercise Physiology: Application and Physiological Principles*, L. M. LeMura & S. P. von Duvillard, eds. Philadelphia: Lippincott, Williams & Wilkins, 2004, pp. 169–182.

14. Jackson, K., and J. A. Mulcare, "Multiple sclerosis." In *ACSM's Exercise Management for Persons with Chronic Diseases and Disabilities*, 3rd ed., J. L. Durstine, G. E. Moore, P. L. Painter, & S. O. Roberts, eds. Champaign, IL: Human Kinetics, 2009, pp. 321–325.

15. McConnell, T. R., "Stroke." In *Clinical Exercise Physiology: Application and Physiological Principles*, L. M. LeMura & S.P. von Duvillard, eds. Philadelphia: Lippincott, Williams & Wilkins, 2004, pp. 207–218.

16. McIntosh, L. J., D. M. Jenkinson, and K. W. Rundell, "Osteoarthritis and rheumatoid arthritis." In *Clinical Exercise Physiology: Application and Physiological Principles*, L. M. LeMura & S. P. von Duvillard, eds. Philadelphia: Lippincott, Williams & Wilkins, 2004, pp. 503–516.

17. Minor, M. A., and D. R. Kay, "Arthritis." In *ACSM's Exercise Management for Persons with Chronic Diseases and Disabilities*, 3rd ed., J. L. Durstine, G. E. Moore, P. L. Painter, & S. O. Roberts, eds. Champaign, IL: Human Kinetics, 2009, pp. 259–265.

18. Myers, J. N., and P. H. Brubaker, "Chronic heart failure." In *ACSM's Exercise Management for Persons with Chronic Diseases and Disabilities*, 3rd ed., J. L. Durstine, G. E. Moore, P. L. Painter, & S. O. Roberts, eds. Champaign, IL: Human Kinetics, 2009, pp. 92–97.

19. Nieman, D. C., *Exercise Testing and Prescription: A Health-Related Approach*. New York: McGraw Hill, 2011.

20. Nixon, P. A., "Cystic fibrosis." In *ACSM's Exercise Management for Persons with Chronic Diseases and Disabilities*, 3rd ed., J. L. Durstine, G. E. Moore, P. L. Painter, & S. O. Roberts, eds. Champaign, IL: Human Kinetics, 2009, pp. 150–155.

21. Ogden, C.L., M. D. Carroll, B. K. Kit, and K. M. Flegal, *Prevalence of Obesity in the United States, 2009–2010*. NCHS data brief, no 82. Hyattsville, MD: National Center for Health Statistics, 2012.

22. Palmer-McLean, K., and K. B. Harbst, "Stroke and brain injury." In *ACSM's Exercise Management for Persons with Chronic Diseases and Disabilities*, 3rd ed., J. L. Durstine, G. E. Moore, P. L. Painter, & S. O. Roberts, eds. Champaign, IL: Human Kinetics, 2009, pp. 287–295.

23. Rundell, K. W., and D. A. Judelson, "Asthma and exercise-induced asthma." In *Clinical Exercise Physiology: Application and Physiological Principles*, L.L. LeMura & S. P. von Duvillard, eds. Philadelphia: Lippincott, Williams & Wilkins, 2004, pp. 183–204.

24. Smith, S. S., C. E. Wang, and S. A. Bloomfield, "Osteoporosis." In *ACSM's Exercise Management for Persons with Chronic Diseases and Disabilities*, 3rd ed., J. L. Durstine, G. E. Moore, P. L. Painter, & S. O. Roberts, eds. Champaign, IL: Human Kinetics, 2009, pp. 270–277.

25. Tarnopolsky, M. A., "Muscular dystrophy." In *ACSM's Exercise Management for Persons with Chronic Diseases and Disabilities*, 3rd ed., J. L. Durstine, G. E. Moore, P. L. Painter, & S. O. Roberts, eds. Champaign, IL: Human Kinetics, 2009, pp. 306–312.

26. U.S. Department of Health and Human Services, *Morbidity and Mortality: 2012 Chart Book on Cardiovascular, Lung, and Blood Diseases* [Internet]. National Heart, Blood, and Lung Institute, 2012 [accessed 2013 May 20]. Available from: www.nhlbi.nih.gov/resources/docs/2012_ChartBook_508.pdf

27. U.S. Department of Health and Human Services, *The Seventh Report of the Joint National Committee on Prevention, Detection, Evaluation, and Treatment of High Blood Pressure (JNC7)* [Internet]. National High Blood Pressure Education Program; 2004 [accessed 2013 May 20]. Available from: www.nhlbi.nih.gov/guidelines/hypertension/jnc7full.pdf

28. U.S. Department of Health and Human Services, *Third Report of the National Cholesterol Education Program (NCEP) Expert Panel on Detection, Evaluation, and Treatment of High Blood Cholesterol in Adults (Adult Treatment Panel III)* [Internet]. National Heart, Blood, and Lung Institute, 2002 [accessed 2013 May 20]. Available from: www.nhlbi.nih.gov/guidelines/cholesterol/atp3full.pdf

29. Wallace, J. P., and S. Ray, "Obesity." In *ACSM's Exercise Management for Persons with Chronic Diseases and Disabilities,* 3rd ed., J. L. Durstine, G. E. Moore, P. L. Painter, & S. O. Roberts, eds. Champaign, IL: Human Kinetics, 2009, pp. 192–199.

30. Womack, C. J., A. W. Gardner, and R. Nael, "Peripheral artery disease." In *ACSM's Exercise Management for Persons with Chronic Diseases and Disabilities,* 3rd ed., J. L. Durstine, G. E. Moore, P. L. Painter, & S. O. Roberts, eds. Champaign, IL: Human Kinetics, 2009, pp. 114–119.

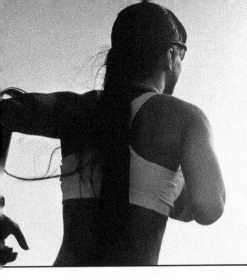

Chapter 17 ///

THERAPEUTIC RECREATION

OBJECTIVES

1. Discuss the historical development of therapeutic recreation as a health profession.
2. Explain the components of the therapeutic recreation process.
3. Discuss the role of therapeutic recreation specialists in different work settings.
4. Introduce the educational and training requirements of the profession.

Therapeutic recreation (TR) is an allied health profession in which recreation therapists purposefully implement recreation activities as interventions to help develop functional changes in individuals with physical, mental, or social disabilities. Like other health care professionals, recreation therapists are prepared with both theoretical knowledge and practical skills through academic preparation, clinical training, and the credentialing process. The purpose of this chapter is to provide a basic understanding of the field of therapeutic recreation by introducing the components of the therapeutic recreation process, some of the techniques utilized during the process, and potential service settings in which a therapeutic recreation professional might work.

WHAT IS THERAPEUTIC RECREATION?

Historical Development

Although professional organizations of therapeutic recreation were not developed until the early 20th century, the therapeutic value of leisure and recreation has been well-documented in healing practices for much of recorded history. For instance, priests in ancient Egypt and physicians in ancient Rome used dance, music, and games to help the sick relax the body and the mind (10). Health care leaders of the early 19th century—including Phillippe Pinel, William Tuke, Benjamin Rush, and Jean Itard—believed opportunities to experience leisure and recreation would benefit individuals with mental illnesses and therefore encouraged their patients to exercise, garden, and talk with attendants (12). Additionally, the therapeutic effects of recreation have been found to help soldiers cope with the horrors of war. When working in British hospitals during the Crimean War (1853–1856), Florence Nightingale established the Inkerman Café, which provided games, books, and other amusements for these soldiers to cope with their post-traumatic stress and to find friendships (8).

The Inkerman Café became the model of hospital recreation programs in the United States during World War I and World War II(12). The American Red Cross built recreation huts on military bases to provide books, music, movies, and games to keep convalescing soldiers entertained. In addition, the hospital recreation programs helped heal wounds by increasing circulation and to restoring wounded soldiers' self-confidence. Although most of the hospital recreation staff was eliminated after the war, the efficacy of recreational therapy had been recognized.

Later, the use of recreation as a therapeutic tool expanded beyond military hospitals. In the late 19th and early 20th centuries, the industrial revolution brought social problems to urban society, such as increasing rates of alcoholism and the numbers of prisons. Some people, Joseph Lee and Neva Boyd, for instance, believed that recreation could be a vehicle for promoting high morals and self-development and advocated the play and recreation movement. The most famous example of this movement was Hull House, a settlement house in a poor district of Chicago, where Jane Addams and others used recreation programs (e.g., creative writing, music, art, needlework, and games) to help immigrants adjust to the new culture, offered them a safe place to find friendship and escape their problems, and educated them to become better citizens (2). It is important to note that even though the therapeutic effect of recreation activities was found in these settings, the use of recreation activities was not *purposefully* delivered to achieve specific, pre-established treatment outcomes. Therefore, they cannot truly be considered "therapeutic recreation."

Definition of Therapeutic Recreation

Therapeutic recreation is actually a combination of two components: a leisure context and purposeful intervention (12). Recreation activities are purposefully chosen based on the client's interests in order to achieve specific treatment outcomes. For example, when working with older adults in a long-term care facility, gardening activities (such as planting seeds, positioning and watering plants, or pulling up weeds) can be a beneficial therapeutic activity to (a) improve flexibility and strength through lifting tools and shifting body weight from position to position during gardening tasks, (b) increase psychological well-being, as creating something beautiful often leads to feelings of contentment and a sense of achievement, and (c) promote socialization when interacting with other residents during the activity. In the leisure context, clients feel they are participating in something enjoyable, while therapeutic recreation specialists are able to further facilitate the process by guiding the clients in performing gardening tasks that will achieve specific treatment outcomes based on the results of the client's assessment. Although these residents all participate in the same activity, they might achieve different treatment goals through the therapist's deliberate effort. The intervention was purposefully chosen to meet pre-established goals based on each client's needs, and hence, it is called "therapeutic recreation."

The definition provided by the national professional organization for therapeutic recreation, the American Therapeutic Recreation Association (ATRA), further emphasized the uniqueness of TR services and defined TR as

> a treatment service designed to restore, remediate and rehabilitate a person's level of functioning and independence in life activities, to promote health and wellness as well as reduce or eliminate the activity limitations and restrictions to participation in life situations caused by an illness or disabling condition. (1)

This definition implies that TR services are specifically designed and delivered for an individual through a systematic process of (a) *assessing* the client's strengths and weaknesses, (b) *planning* appropriate recreation interventions to make functional changes, (c) *implementing* the interventions to achieve treatment goals, and (d) *evaluating* whether the client meets the pre-established treatment goals. This process of assessing, planning, implementing, and evaluating (or the mnemonic APIE) is commonly used in other forms of therapy; the unique feature of therapeutic recreation is that specialists design intervention strategies with the client's past, current, and future leisure interests in mind and purposefully develop recreational modalities (e.g., sports, games, crafts, and outdoor adventure activities) to help improve the client's functioning. How does the clinical TR process work in TR practice? The following case study illustrates how therapeutic recreation specialists use the APIE process to practice.

Role of Therapeutic Recreation in Health Promotion

Therapeutic recreation has been defined as more than mere leisure participation. Rather, TR is the use of recreation activity as an intervention to achieve specific therapeutic outcomes for individuals with an illness or disabling condition. Therapeutic recreation has a role in health promotion and disease prevention. Over 50 years ago, the World Health Organization defined health as "a state of complete physical, mental and social well-being and not merely the absence of disease or infirmity" (14). This definition of health shifted our view from a medical model focused on curing disease and illness to a holistic approach to one's health, a belief that physical, mental, social, emotional, spiritual, and environmental factors all play a part in one's well-being.

Leisure is often defined as enjoyable free time activities resulting from one's free choices (3, 7) and is considered to be an important part of our lives. It can also serve different functions in different life stages. Children are socialized into their culture and fulfill their curiosity about the world through play. Adolescents find their self-identity by interacting with peers. Young adults select their future spouse and develop their intimacy through social interaction. More importantly, research has found that active involvement in leisure and the social world leads to a happy and satisfied life (4).

However, individuals with disabilities often face constraints when participating in leisure activities due to lack of skills, inaccessible environments, and negative attitudes (11) and are therefore more likely to live a sedentary lifestyle than adults without disabilities (5). Therapeutic recreation specialists can help individuals with disabilities develop the necessary skills to be aware of and enjoy leisure experiences in integrated community-based programs. For example, through leisure education, TR specialists can promote a healthy, active lifestyle in this population by sharing the benefits of physical activity (e.g., reduced incidences of chronic diseases and secondary conditions). In

CASE STUDY: Ling

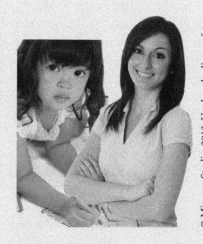

© Minerva Studio, 2013. Used under license from Shutterstock, Inc.
© Odua Images, 2013. Used under license from Shutterstock, Inc.

Background: Janelle is a therapeutic recreation specialist providing treatment services to children with a disability in a children's hospital in a metropolitan area. She works closely with other allied health professionals in the interdisciplinary treatment team. One of her recent clients, Ling, was admitted to the hospital due to a traumatic brain injury from a motor vehicle accident. Janelle has worked with Ling for the past four weeks aiming to improve her function through a variety of recreation interventions.

Assessment: In the assessment phase, Janelle learned Ling's leisure interests and current level of functioning through reviewing her medical chart, interviewing the client and her family, and her own observations. Janelle found that, as a result of her injury, Ling has decreased use and function of her right upper extremity (RUE) and has experienced memory impairments. Ling's language functioning was affected by the accident as well. She was having difficulty with verbal communication (only able to produce a few words) at the time of assessment, but was able to communicate with family and staff using body language, such as thumbs up/thumbs down, facial expressions, and eye contact. The client's family reported that Ling enjoys board games and crafts.

Planning Interventions: In the future, it will be important for Ling to use her RUE to complete activities of daily living and recreational activities. Based on the results of the assessment, Janelle determined one of the treatment goals was to improve Ling's upper extremity function, and therefore developed activities in which Ling would be able to integrate her RUE, focusing on fine and gross motor skills. In addition, Janelle planned to improve Ling's communication skills by using modalities that encourage Ling to use her communication board and/or verbalizations.

Implementation: Since Ling enjoys crafts, Janelle worked with her on these treatment goals through making cards. During the treatment session, Janelle consistently prompted Ling to use her RUE and to work on her fine and gross motor skills by asking her to peel and place stickers on a card. Throughout each session, Janelle encouraged Ling to socialize with her and other staff members.

Evaluation: After one month of participation in recreation interventions (30-minute sessions, three to four times a week), Ling increased her RUE functioning level and improved her verbalizations. In addition, Ling reported that she enjoyed having opportunities to play or engage in activities that she likes.

Case Summary: Janelle identified the client's treatment needs through assessment and established treatment goals based on the results of that assessment. She then developed the therapeutic recreation interventions based on the client's leisure interests and purposefully designed the program to increase social interaction opportunities and the use of the client's upper extremity in order to achieve the treatment goals (i.e., promote the client's social skills, as well as fine and gross motor skills). Within the leisure context, the client could practice these skills as part of her hospital stay, while having fun and relaxing. As Ling begins to re-enter the community and return to school, these skills will be important in helping her interact with peers and others in the community and in performing the activities of daily living as well as participating in recreational activities.

Points to Ponder

1. How is a TR approach different from other therapies?
2. How does providing treatment in the leisure context benefit an individual?
3. What other goals can be achieved in an arts and crafts activity?

addition, as these individuals may experience impairments, therapeutic recreation specialists can discuss adaptations and modifications for performing various activities with their clients. Recreation and leisure involvement not only enhance health and prevent secondary conditions (6), but also promote engagement to all areas of life. Therefore, therapeutic recreation services should be considered part of a health promotion program.

WORK SETTINGS

Therapeutic recreation specialists provide treatment services to individuals with a wide range of abilities and needs in both clinical and community settings. Most TR specialists work in inpatient healthcare facilities. Examples include (a) rehabilitation centers where TR specialists serve people with traumatic brain injuries or strokes, (b) mental health facilities where specialists work with people experiencing psychiatric disabilities or substance abuse issues, and (c) inpatient hospitals where specialists provide treatments to geriatric or pediatric clients. In addition, many TR specialists work in community settings, such as nursing homes, retirement centers, adult day care programs, residential facilities, schools, prisons, and halfway houses. It is important to note that while, based on the role of the professional in the setting, TR specialists may have varying job titles (including recreation therapist, recreational therapist, activity director, or inclusion specialist) their major goal is to promote positive changes in wellbeing through leisure engagement. Finally, the U.S. Bureau of Labor Statistics predicted the growth rate of TR to be comparable to other health occupations. With the expectation of a rapidly growing aging population, the need for TR is expected to continue growing. Refer to the professional portraits for a look at currently practicing TR specialists.

EDUCATION AND TRAINING

Therapeutic recreation is often situated in Departments of Leisure Studies, Recreation, or other such academic unit. Currently, there are over 100 colleges in the United States offering a therapeutic recreation specialty at the undergraduate level. Therapeutic recreation students acquire theoretical knowledge systematically through class preparation (9) and enhance their clinical skills in a professional practice environment through internships in a clinical setting (13). As recreation therapists can work in a variety of settings, students contemplating a career in the field are encouraged to assess their interests and the role of TR in various settings through hands-on volunteer experiences. In addition, students should develop a respectful attitude toward the clients with which they interact, as a therapist's ability to relate to his or her clients and be sensitive to their needs is crucial to successful treatment.

Individuals who are interested in the field of TR can seek certification through the National Council for Therapeutic Recreation Certification (NCTRC). Detailed information regarding the certification process can be found on the website of NCTRC: www.nctrc.org. In short, persons who meet the current standards of NCTRC (i.e., completion of the required TR-related coursework in an accredited program and 570 hours of practice experience) can then sit for the national certification exam. As with other similar professions, there are recertification standards in place to encourage a Certified Therapeutic Recreational Specialist to continue the development of their professional competence via education or alternative paths. CTRS certification is active for five years; hence, every five years these certified specialists are reviewed for their competence and experience in therapeutic recreation. The specialists may also choose to pass the national exam to obtain the certification.

ADDITIONAL RESOURCES

The reader is encouraged to seek more information related to careers and academic development in therapeutic recreation at:

- The American Therapeutic Recreation Association (ATRA), 629 North Main Street, Hattiesburg, MS 39401. Website: www.atra-online.com

TR Professional Portrait

Jason works in a physical rehabilitation facility where he helps individuals with acquired spinal cord injuries or other physical impairments regain their leisure ability and develop self-identity through adapted sports.

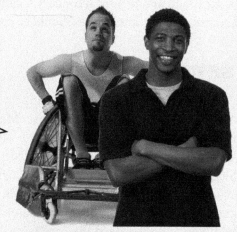

Anna works in a retirement center where she helps senior residents maintain their physical and cognitive functioning through yoga and meditation.

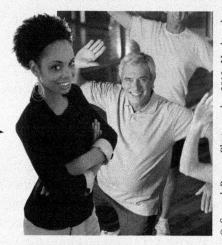

Jorge works in a community recreation program where he involves youths at risk in competitive sports to relegate their excess energy and to develop positive leisure interests.

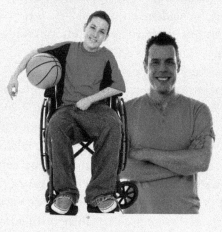

- The National Council for Therapeutic Recreation Certification, 7 Elmwood Drive, New City, NY 10956. Website: www.nctrc.org
- To find colleges in the United States offer that a therapeutic recreation specialty at the undergraduate and/or graduate levels, visit the website of the I Am A Recreational Therapist: www.iamarecreationaltherapist.com

SUMMARY

In health care settings, recreation therapists often work collaboratively with other therapists and social workers to improve or maintain the well-being of their clients. In TR practice, recreation-based interventions are purposefully chosen and designed to help each individual client achieve his or her treatment goals. While the majority of recreation therapists work in a clinical setting, a growing number of therapeutic recreation professionals provide services in a community setting. As the "graying" of society continues, it can be expected that recreation therapists will work with more senior clients.

REFERENCES

1. American Therapeutic Recreation Association, *What is TR?*, 2009 [cited 2013 June 4th]; Available from: www.atra-online.com/displaycommon.cfm?an = 12.

2. Bedini, L.A., "The 'Play Ladies'—the first therapeutic recreation specialists." *Journal of Physical Education, Recreation and Dance* 66(8)(1995): 32–35.

3. Cassidy, T., "All work and no play: A focus on leisure time as a means for promoting health." *Counselling Psychology Quarterly* 9(1)(1996): 77.

4. Godbey, G., *Leisure and leisure services in the 21st century*. State College, PA: Venture Publishing, 1997.

5. Havercamp, S.M., D. Scandlin, and M. Roth, "Health disparities among adults with developmental disabilities, adults with other disabilities, and adults not reporting disability in North Carolina." *Public Health Report* 119(4)(2004): 418–426.

6. Heller, T., et al., "Physical activity and nutrition health promotion interventions: What is working for people with intellectual disabilities?" *Intellectual and Developmental Disabilities* 49(1)(2011): 26–36.

7. Hutchinson, S.L., et al., "Leisure as a coping resource: Variations in coping with traumatic injury and illness." *Leisure Sciences* 25(2/3)(2003): 143.

8. James, A., "The conceptual development of recreational therapy," in *Perspectives in recreational therapy*, F.M. Brasile, T.K. Skalko, and J. Burlingame, eds. Idyll Arbor, Inc: Ravensdale, WA: Idyll Arbor, Inc., 1998, pp. 7–38.

9. Navar, N., "Keynote: Thoughts on therapeutic recreation education," in *Professional issues in therapeutic recreation:* On competence and outcomes, N.J. Stumbo, ed. Sagamore: Champaign, IL: Sagamore, 2001, pp. 23–35.

10. Reynolds, R.P., and G.S. O'Morrow, *Problems, Issues and Concepts in Therapeutic Recreation*. Englewood Cliffs, NJ: Prentice-Hall, 1985.

11. Rimmer, J.H., et al., "Physical activity participation among persons with disabilities: Barriers and facilitators." *American Journal of Preventive Medicine* 26(5)(2004): 419–425.

12. Robertson, T., and T. Long, *Foundations of Therapeutic Recreation*. Champaign, IL: Human Kinetics, 2008.

13. Skalko, T.K., Y. Lee, and R. Goldenberg, "Seeking active collaboration in a comprehensive fieldwork system for therapeutic recreation: a case example." *Schole: A Journal of Leisure Studies & Recreation Education* 13(1998): 63–72.

14. World Health Organization, WHO *Definition of Health*. 1948 [cited 2013; Available from: www.who.int/about/definition/en/print.html.

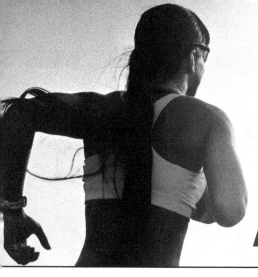

Chapter 18

ATHLETIC TRAINING

OBJECTIVES

1. Describe how athletic training is integrated into the health care delivery system in the United States.
2. Cite the basic principles related to the competency matrix of athletic training.
3. Describe the principles of injury evaluation, emergency care, and treatment of athletic injuries.
4. Explain the integration of rehabilitative exercise and therapeutic modalities to return an athlete to competition.
5. Describe common athletic injuries, their basic treatments, and expected outcomes.
6. Describe the education process for becoming an athletic trainer.

A thletic training is a health care profession specializing in injuries to physically active individuals. Athletic training works cooperatively within its scope of practice with sports medicine. Narrowly defined, sports medicine deals with the assessment, emergency care, treatment, and rehabilitation of sports-related neuromuscular injuries. Over the years this area has expanded greatly to include other physical pursuits as well as neurologic problems related to physical performance. Athletic training is an interdisciplinary field utilizing medicine, anatomy, physiology, pathomechanics, biomechanics, exercise physiology, nutrition, pharmacology, psychosocial strategies, and health care administration.

Athletic training traces its earliest beginnings to ancient Greece where athletic competition was revered (4). From after the fall of Rome until the 19th century, most physical activity was about war. In 1869 Rutgers and Princeton, each fielding a team of 25 men, introduced what became football. Athletic training began evolving in the United States when Harvard University hired James Robinson in 1881 (4). Athletic training spread as a service to athletes on men's sports teams between 1913 and 1925. The first athletic training text (*The Trainer's Bible*) was published in 1917 by a physician, S.E. Bilik, who served as a part-time athletic trainer while in college at the University of Illinois (1).

From these origins, athletic training has evolved into a profession encompassing multiple clinical environments: (a) individual and team sports in educational and professional settings, (b) sports medicine and orthopedic clinics, (c) industrial settings, (d) performing arts and dance, (e) military, law enforcement, and government, (f) recreational, amateur, and youth sports, among other settings. As a profession, athletic training is still evolving and redefining its scope of patient coverage and educational standards. Athletic trainers have a limited scope of medical practice, supervised by allopathic (M.D.) and osteopathic (D.O.) physicians. In most jurisdictions athletic training is defined by state practice acts within state law.

SCOPE OF PRACTICE

The term *athletic trainer* is often confusing. It has been an ongoing struggle for the profession to teach the media and public that the term is *athletic trainer*, not *trainer*. In other areas of physical activity, the word *trainer* has numerous meanings not affiliated with medicine. A trainer could be a boxer's coach, designer of fitness workouts for Hollywood celebrities, an instructor in techniques of physical conditioning at the local gym, or even a race horse's coach. In other parts of the world, a trainer is a coach of team and individual sports, although the term *coach* is becoming more accepted. In contrast, athletic training defines a health care profession. The term is unrelated to "training" athletes in strength or technique.

Athletic Medicine

The sports medicine team is headed by the physician. The athletic trainer is the on-site representative of the physician. Athletic trainers are most often the initial person to see and interact with injured physically active individuals. They triage injuries and provide initial first aid and care leading to referral to another member of the sports medicine team or return to participation. Providing effective health services will require a group of professionals led by a physician. The physician may be a team physician hired by the institution to supervise all aspects of health care to the institution's athletes, or in some cases the athlete's primary care (family) physician.

This team approach utilizes a number of specialists who provide immediate support services. These include orthopedic surgeons, physician assistants, physical therapists, dentists, ophthalmologists, neurologists, and equipment managers (10). Related support specialists include emergency medical technicians/paramedics, exercise physiologists, nutritionists, sport psychologists, and substance abuse counselors. Additionally, the team must work in conjunction with position coaches, athletic directors, administrators, and strength coaches, keeping them apprised of the status of the injured athlete (Figure 18.1).

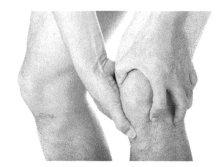

Figure 18.1. *Injury to the knee.*

Job Placements

Athletic trainers practice at a variety of job sites. The largest areas for jobs are high schools and in sports medicine clinics. In the sports medicine clinic setting, athletic trainers may be involved with outreach placement to high schools and other job sites in the area that contract athletic training services from the clinic, or in the care and rehabilitation of injuries to physically active individuals who may or may not be part of organized sports. Many athletic trainers in clinics work in conjunction with physical therapists, orthopedic surgeons, and other medical personnel. In some states athletic trainers in the clinical setting work with worker's compensation claims when the referring physician specifies athletic training services. Additional roles for clinical athletic trainers include work as a physician extender, marketing, health care administration, and clinic owner. Parts of this market are becoming more difficult because athletic training services are still not authorized by Medicare.

With the realization that a teacher in a school setting who is also the athletic trainer for that institution is really covering two full-time positions, fewer and fewer of these positions are available or desirable. The profession of athletic training began in colleges of education, but today most athletic training education programs are housed in colleges of health sciences. A teaching certificate is an additional credential requiring one to three more years of study after the athletic training education program is completed. Most high schools today either hire athletic trainers as full-time or part-time non-teaching employees or they contract with sports medicine clinics for services. With the current emphasis on concussion management as a major area of concern, the high school venue is an ever-expanding market.

Slightly less than 10% of athletic training positions are found in the college and university setting. A master's degree is the preferred entry-level credential for this setting. There are many practical reasons why entry-level athletic trainers prefer this setting: (a) similar social interests with the athletes, (b) fast-healing bodies in excellent physical condition, and (c) the athlete's compliance with physician's orders and rehabilitation programs. The job market for employment with college and university athletics has been stagnant for a considerable time, with little or no creation of new jobs. The job market is limited in professional sports, with only 1% of all athletic trainers hired by professional teams. The route to practice in a major league setting is varied, usually requiring minor league or summer camp experience. Networking is also a very valuable skill in obtaining a professional sports position. Surprisingly, until the advent of the WNBA in the 1990s, few women worked at any level of professional sport. In December 2011, the Los Angeles Dodgers hired Susan Falsone, ATC, PT, as their head athletic trainer, the first female head athletic trainer in any men's team professional sports. The Pittsburgh Steelers hired a female assistant athletic trainer, Ariko Iso, in 2002. There are women in assistant athletic trainer positions in the NBA. There is limited opportunity for athletic trainers on both the men's and women's professional tennis and golf tours.

Most of the involvement of athletic trainers with the Olympic movement and U.S. national teams is on a volunteer basis. The USOC employs athletic trainers at the USOC training centers, but major event coverage requires far more athletic trainers than are employed by the USOC. Often, athletic trainers will volunteer for three to five years before being asked to participate in various international games.

The job market is expanding in the performing arts area with athletic trainers working with Broadway shows and dance companies such as American Ballet Theater. Athletic trainers have been hired by the U.S.

Army to work at basic training sites and other branches of the military to work with elite units. Athletic trainers also work with law enforcement personnel at various sites.

Job placement in industrial settings is continuing to expand through, work in manufacturing settings, with baggage handlers at airports, and in many other physically demanding jobs. The athletic trainer in the corporate/industrial setting is the go-between for employees (athletes), supervisors (coaches), and plant physicians (team physicians). Businesses and corporations are adding athletic trainers to their work site because it is cost effective to treat and rehabilitate workers within the facility, decreasing lost time and lost productivity.

DOMAINS OF REQUIRED KNOWLEDGE

The body of knowledge comprising the core of athletic training has been divided into five domains by the Board of Certification. These domains include Injury/Illness Prevention and Wellness Protection, Clinical Evaluation and Diagnosis, Immediate and Emergency Care, Treatment and Rehabilitation, Organizational and Professional Health and Well-Being (10).

The domains have been broken down to individual statements specifying the knowledge required of an entry-level professional by the Commission on Accreditation of Athletic Training Education. These content areas include Evidence-based Practice, Prevention and Health Promotion, Clinical Examination and Diagnosis, Acute Care of Injuries/Illnesses, Therapeutic Interventions, Psychosocial Strategies, Healthcare Administration, and Professional Development (8)

Evidence-Based Practice

Evidence-based practice for athletic training evolved out of current practice in the medical community over the past 20 years. Insurance companies are demanding that treatments applied to patients can demonstrate efficacy. Research has shown that some commonly used treatment protocols could not demonstrate significant improvement in the patient's condition. The combination of input from clinical research and the expertise of the clinician give rise to best practice. For example, research on injuries to a specific body area may show different results in a pediatric population, a geriatric population, an adolescent population, and a young adult population.

Evidence in clinical presentation is divided into a number of areas. Initially, inter-rater reliability and intra-rater reliability is calculated. Test results are then applied to a diagnostic gold standard to establish a true positive (test positive, patient has the condition), false positive (test positive, patient does not have the condition), true negative (test negative, patient does not have the condition), and false negative (test negative, patient does have the condition) (8). While sensitivity can show positive results, it also can have too many false positives. Similarly, specificity may show too many false negatives. The answer to this problem has been the use of likelihood ratios.

Likelihood ratios explain the shift in expectation that a patient has a condition after a test is administered. Pre-test probabilities are population specific and derived from the available data. Often, however, data are not available due to lack of research so that the probabilities must be estimated on the basis of clinical expertise (8). With the use of evidence-based practice, some commonly used tests have been found to lack the necessary sensitivity and specificity to be clinically useful.

Prevention and Health Promotion

Injury can happen during physical activity at any time. The one thing that no one can predict is who will be injured and when. One of the main duties of an athletic trainer is to ensure that the competitive environment is as safe as is humanly possible. A major factor in injury prevention is for the participant to be fit and able to withstand the rigors of the competition prior to engaging in the sport or activity. Pre-participation physical examinations are used to qualify individuals for the physical demands of the activity. These examinations have a medical component, an orthopedic component, patient information, and possibly baseline neurologic testing in sports where concussion may be prevalent. Often these exams will uncover pre-existing conditions from previous untreated injury.

Athletic trainers need to take the time to educate patients that injury can happen at any time and in any place. Prevention is the responsibility of the athlete (or worker), just as much as it is the coach's, supervisor's, and athletic training staff's. After a person sustains an injury, it is necessary that the patient and anyone close to her or him know what signs and symptoms signify a deteriorating condition or knowledge that the healing process is proceeding as expected.

Risk management is a critical element in prevention of injury. Unsafe conditions are caused when pieces of equipment not in use are lying on a playing surface or in a work area; broken safety equipment can injure the user as can broken competitive equipment. Simply having two separate groups of athletes work in opposite directions on the field instead of toward each other will decrease the potential for injury. Requiring that active people wear mandated safety equipment will significantly minimize injury. In some sports, like soccer or wrestling, athletes will frequently attempt to practice without mandatory equipment.

In the athletic environment, some coaches teach improper techniques in an attempt to punish an opponent. Lowering the head just before impact is more punishing than hitting with the front of the helmet, but it also straightens out the cervical curve in the vertebrae and exposes the athlete to significantly greater likelihood of fracture or dislocation, possibly leading to quadriplegia. When an athletic trainer witnesses these errors, he or she must consult with the coach. If this does not resolve the situation, the athletic trainer must notify the head coach or supervisor, team physician, athletic director, or other administrator.

In the industrial setting, athletic trainers may spend significant time on job-specific training to correct ergonomic deficiencies before a worker becomes part of the production team. Workers are instructed in proper body movements, like bending and lifting techniques that help minimize risk of injury. Athletic trainers may also devote significant time to work site fitness centers, assessing body mechanics, and implementing lifetime fitness programming.

Environmental conditions are an extremely important risk that must be accommodated. Hyperthermia, hypothermia, lightning safety, altitude sickness, severe weather, sun overexposure, air pollution, and circadian dysrhythmia are all very real problems. Every year, between five and 10 U.S. high school football players die from heat stroke during August practices in a hot environment. Heat stroke is a preventable situation when reasonable care is shown. Those most at risk are overfat, underconditioned, young males in areas of the country where both high temperatures and high humidity are a problem. Cold injury can run the gamut from frostbite to exposure to cold, to wet playing conditions leading to hypothermia. Lightning injures a significant number of outdoor participants in physical activity each year. When lightning is detected, everyone must leave the area and seek shelter. Participation should not resume for 30 minutes after the last strike.

Altitude effects on physical performance play a much greater role in winter sports than in warm weather sports. The first extensive study of the effects of altitude on track and field took place leading up to the Mexico City Olympics in 1968, which were conducted at an altitude of 7,800 feet. Since that time most endurance athletes in the United States attempt to train significant portions of the year at altitude. Altitude pulmonary edema occurs in some at between 9,000 and 10,000 feet. The best treatment is to move the athlete to a lower altitude and provide oxygen.

Circadian dysrhythmia or jet lag occurs when traveling across three or more time zones. It is more difficult to adjust when traveling from west to east because it is harder to force yourself to sleep when your internal clock indicates that you are not tired.

Clinical Examination and Diagnosis

In most team and individual sports settings, athletic trainers are the eyes and ears of physicians. Often at practice athletic trainers must sit and wait for the injury to happen without losing focus on the job at hand. It is not practical to employ a physician to attend all practices and competitions for all sports. When an injury occurs, the athletic trainer most likely will be the first person to intervene. A planned systematic approach to evaluation is critical to a successful outcome. When a method of proceeding is planned and practiced, the small things are not forgotten. The primary survey for life-threatening situations is followed by the secondary survey, taking of history, observation, palpation, and special tests. Assessing and maintaining cardiac function is the main goal of the primary survey. The taking of the history, if well done, can lead a clinician about 80% of the way to a working diagnosis. Confirming suspicions throughout the secondary survey gives an initial plan of action. The athletic trainer then communicates the results of the evaluation to the supervising physician who will incorporate this information into a definitive diagnosis.

Athletic trainers act as the bridge between physicians and athletes (or workers), coaches (or supervisors), families, and often between the athletic program and the media concerning the extent of injury to a particular athlete. There are even times when the athletic trainer must attempt to protect the athlete from himself/herself. Athletic trainers must possess current certification in cardiopulmonary resuscitation (CPR) from the American Red Cross, the American Heart Association, or the National Safety Council (9). In addition, first aid certification is strongly encouraged.

There are a number of different injury evaluation systems in use that all have certain elements in common. All first aid texts start with primary survey, either formal or informal. If the patient is unresponsive, the athletic trainer has a plan to assess the situation and maintain life. The emergency medical service needs to be activated and notified of the level of emergency. Cardiopulmonary resuscitation, rescue breathing, or careful monitoring of an unconscious individual is initiated, depending on the circumstances. If the patient is alert and speaking, yelling, crying, etc., then he or she is breathing and has a heartbeat. The primary survey is informal yet completed. If an athletic trainer always thinks primary survey first, no mistakes will be made in the method.

This is followed by a secondary survey, which evaluates the specific complaint of the athlete. Care must be taken at all times to avoid exposure to bloodborne pathogens due to contact with blood and other bodily fluids when performing an evaluation and/or first aid procedures (10). OSHA guidelines require that all medical professionals use proper barriers, material disposal, and cleanup procedures any time blood or other fluids are present. Athletic trainers are considered by OSHA to be in Category I for risk of exposure to Hepatitis-B and HIV. This means they are required to have been immunized against Hepatitis-B or provide a signed waiver declining the protection. Depending upon the injury, careful monitoring of an athlete's level of consciousness may still be an important consideration in overall management.

The most important step in the secondary survey is taking an accurate injury history. What the athlete felt and heard, what exactly the athlete was doing when pain set in and what type, and how extensive is the disability are important clues to obtain an accurate diagnosis from the physician at a later time. Often by the time an athlete has been seen by a physician, acute muscle spasm will prevent accurate structural testing; however, an on-site athletic trainer can accomplish the musculoskeletal structural testing before spasm sets in. The athletic trainer needs to know if the athlete has ever injured the body part (or contralateral body part) before and the outcome of that injury. Those outcomes will have a bearing on structural and functional testing done on this new injury site. If at any point the results indicate an unfavorable outcome from further testing, the evaluation should be terminated, and transportation of the athlete to an appropriate medical facility should be initiated. At all times during the history, the athlete's body language is observed. This will give a better indication of pain than the athlete's words ,since most athletes believe they will return to play at once.

History is followed by a more formal observation of the injured area, seeking out obvious deformities, changes in skin color, shape and size of various structures. During the observation, the athletic trainer will note how the body is carried, self-protected, gait abnormalities, and other external signs to internal problems.

Once the area of injury has been observed, the next step is to palpate the area, both bone and soft tissue. A good approach is to first ask the athlete to identify the most painful area with a pointed finger. Then the athletic trainer begins to touch the body part away from the most painful area, arriving last at the site of greatest pain. Touching the skin without causing pain establishes a rapport with the person and suggests to the athlete that the athletic trainer is not attempting to hurt her or him. Circulation beyond the injury site, response to touch, and ability to activate muscle are assessed. When these tests are normal, the range of motion (ROM)

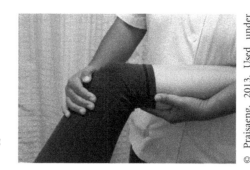

Figure 18.2. *Testing for ligaments in the knee.*

of the injured body part is established in order: (a) active range of motion, (b) passive range of motion, and (c) resistive range of motion. In active range of motion testing the athlete moves the body part in response to the athletic trainer's commands. Next the athletic trainer moves the body part, comparing what the person will do willingly and what the athletic trainer can do when antagonistic muscles are relaxed (passive ROM). Finally, the athlete attempts to move in the middle of the range of motion against resistance applied by the athletic trainer (resistive ROM), essentially a breakdown test.

Once the injured area has been isolated, specific structural tests designed to identify the presence of injury at that body part are completed. The tests used will be based on all previous information obtained during the evaluation and the clinical experience of the athletic trainer. Should these tests be normal, the injured person is put through specific functional tests that are activity specific to the skills the patient is attempting to resume. This determines if the person may safely return to full activity. For these (and all other musculoskeletal tests), bilateral comparisons are made to account for the variability found in individual people (Figure 18.2). When an injury evaluation is complete, the athletic trainer must (a) release the person to return to activity (mild injuries), (b) remove the athlete and refer the individual to a physician (moderate injuries to severe injuries), or (c) activate the emergency medical service and transport the athlete to the nearest appropriate facility (some severe and all potentially catastrophic injuries).

Once the evaluation and diagnosis are complete, a written record is constructed from the notes taken during the evaluation and the test results. All results must be recorded for use by the physician and other personnel for diagnosis, treatment, and rehabilitation of the injury. A properly executed injury evaluation and therapy record will allow other athletic trainers and medical professionals to supervise ongoing rehabilitation and continue and expand upon the rehabilitation plans developed by the original athletic trainer and physician.

When constructing a written record, it is of paramount importance that everyone who will use the record has the same understanding of basic terminology. There are a number of record-keeping formats. Perhaps the most accepted format is known as the SOAP Note. SOAP stands for Subjective, Objective, Assessment, and Plan (6).

Subjective information is what the athlete tells you. The quality, intensity, duration, and character of pain are all subjective. Mild sprains may feel like the end of the world to one individual while fractured bones are not enough to stop others from competing. Much of history taking is subjective.

Objective information can be measured by objective means. Signs, observation, palpation, and special tests all give objective information. Body temperature, heart rate, respiratory rate, blood pressure, limb circumference, limb volume, blood tests, MRIs, and x-ray are all objective.

Assessment is the professional opinion of the athletic trainer or other health care professional about the nature and extent of the injury.

Plan includes all goals, treatments rendered and disposition of the injury, whether referral or continued local intervention and rehabilitation. Accuracy is paramount. Any errors must be dealt with as soon as they come to light. The athletic trainer should make corrections by drawing a single line through the information to be eliminated and the new information entered. The change must be signed and dated by the athletic trainer making the change. Care must be exercised that all removed information is readable in case the patient record becomes part of a lawsuit.

Acute Care

Acute injuries to athletes and many other physically active individuals are most often seen by an athletic trainer before any other health care professional. The most common first aid treatment for acute musculoskeletal injuries is the RICE method (rest, ice, compression, elevation).

Rest may mean removal from physical activity for a time or resting a particular body part by utilizing crutches and slings. Rest may also mean decreasing the intensity and duration of physical activity, such as having a 400 m runner jog lightly. If an athletic trainer wants decreased activity, he or she must be very specific about to how to establish what happens. In extreme cases physicians will enforce rest by placing the joint or bones in a functional brace or cast.

Ice is the most common form of cold applied to injury sites. Wrapping ice packs onto the body using elastic wraps adds the dimension of compression and helps limit swelling. The goal of cold application is to decrease metabolic rate of the injured area and blood flow thereby limiting the accumulation of swelling. After the application of cold, the person should be sent home in a compression wrap and with instructions to repeat the cold application at regular intervals.

The extremities should be elevated to allow gravity to assist in lymphatic drainage. Four to six inches of elevation is usually enough and can be accomplished by placing a bed pillow under a sprained ankle while sitting on a couch or in bed.

Any athletic training setting must have an emergency action plan. The purpose of the plan is to minimize response time of EMS personnel and prevent secondary injury caused by inappropriate movement or treatment. The emergency action plan must be a written document, clearly displayed at any site of danger, emphasizing the roles, personnel, and equipment required to triage an injury and begin emergency first aid. The plan must include contact information and map directions to the site for use when calling 911 to activate the EMS.

Emergency medical system personnel are not often at sporting events in a stand-by mode to assume responsibility over life threatening injuries. Usually the athletic trainer is the first qualified person to respond. In situations where there is an on-field injury and the athletic trainer responds, the first evaluation is made immediately by the athletic trainer, even if EMS personnel are at the site. Once the athletic trainer makes the decision to involve the EMS in the case, EMS personnel then take charge of the care of the injured athlete.

Former NATA President Bobby Barton once stated that if an athletic trainer practices at the college or university setting for over five years, he or she will see at least one potentially catastrophic, life-threatening situation. When such an injury happens, the emergency action plan must be activated. The team physician or senior ranking athletic trainer or designate should take charge and assess the patient. Other persons will be assigned roles as needed. These roles should be practiced at least monthly, with each involved party able to function comfortably in more than one role.

It is important to consult with an emergency medical service professional, along with the team physician, local police, and the institution's legal counsel while creating the plan to find out the best traffic flow plan for each area and for overall advice on the emergency procedures.

Therapeutic Interventions

The immediate effects of injury include redness, swelling, heat, pain, and loss of function. These cause a period of inactivity that can lead to disuse atrophy and decreased strength, endurance, and neuromuscular coordination. One can think of swelling as nature's way of placing the body part in a cast to stop movement.

Joints, ligaments, and bone all need *intermittently* applied stresses to maintain or expand their tissue content and the efficiency of their function. When body parts are restricted cardiovascular impairments may ensue (10). To control these problems, systematic rehabilitation involving various forms of active, passive, and resistive exercise combined with therapeutic modalities are utilized. To maintain cardiorespiratory function, exercises incorporating upper body ergometers, cycling, or a swimming pool are all excellent. The choice of exercise is designed to minimize stress on the injured body part while providing a cardiovascular workout.

Traditional voluntary or physiological movements are known as *osteokinematics*. Accessory movements are small movements not under voluntary control that reposition the bones for maximum efficiency of voluntary movement. Restoration of the normal range of motion incorporates both osteokinematics and accessory movements about a joint (5). For example, flexion and extension are movements at the knee, while anterior or posterior tibial translation and tibial rotation are accessory accompaniments. *Joint play* is a term used to describe how the shape of the joint surfaces controls movement. The use of free weights during an exercise program will emphasize all of these movements while machine weights limit the activity to only the osteokinematic movements.

Athletic trainers assess whether range of motion is adversely affected by forces or pathology altering voluntary or accessory movements. The two are intimately related and must be properly integrated for normal function about a joint. To increase voluntary movements, large muscles must move a body part utilizing active, passive, and resistive range of motion throughout the full range of motion, stressing the endpoints of the range to increase function. Accessory movements are more often restored with joint mobilization techniques.

Exercise comes in a variety of forms. Isometric exercise involves muscle contraction without joint motion. Strength is increased, but only for about 20 degrees around the joint position angle (5). Range of motion about the knee for flexion (normal range 0 to 140–150 degrees) would require seven or eight separate exercises, one in each 20-degree arc. For some joints and activities this is practical, but for many others it is extremely inefficient.

Isotonic exercises move a joint through a range of motion and has been subdivided into two areas: concentric and eccentric. Concentric muscle actions involve actual shortening of the muscle and generating enough force to overcome an external resistance. A typical bench press or arm curl with the arm down at the side is a concentric activity. Eccentric muscle actions attempt to shorten the muscle, but the contractile elements are broken apart by the superior combination of the exterior force and the force of gravity, so the body simply controls the rate of moving the mass. In a bench press, with the arm fully extended, the weight is then returned toward the body in an eccentric action. The same muscles that pushed the weight up concentrically now lengthen to control the effect of gravity and return the weight to the starting position.

Both concentric and eccentric muscle actions can be performed using a variety of methods including manual resistance, elastic tubing, elastic bands, free weights, or machines. Often in rehabilitation, a weight will be moved to a position by contracting muscles in both limbs. The weight is controlled back to the starting position by eccentric action. In this way, greater weights can be moved eccentrically than concentrically. However, there is greater residual muscle soreness from eccentric muscle action.

One type of isotonic exercise is isokinetic. This allows movements at functional speeds due to the principle of accommodating resistance. The speed of the contraction is preset electrically by a machine and the force generated is variable at the preset speed. An advantage of isokinetic exercise is the capability to maximize workload throughout a full range of motion while concentric movements are limited by the weakest part of the range of motion.

In closed kinetic chain activity compressive forces are applied to the terminal segment, usually the foot or hand. Forces are then transmitted up the chain of joints to the trunk. Proximal motions are influenced by succeeding distal segments. An example of a closed chain activity is using a slide board to simulate speed skating motions during the rehabilitation of anterior cruciate ligament injuries. Proprioceptive input from the foot helps to sequence motor units at appropriate forces and times. Closed chain activities have gained great popularity in athletic training and physical therapy rehabilitation programming in recent years.

Open kinetic chain activity does not have the terminal segments in contact with external surfaces, thereby decreasing or eliminating the effect of proprioception in the terminal segment from the sensory input side of restoring function. An example of an open chain activity is using a knee extension bench where the arm is fixed to the tibia above the ankle. Proprioceptive input from the foot does not affect contraction sequences.

The recovery of proprioception, normal range of motion, and neuromuscular coordination are primary goals of the rehabilitation process. Functional progression is the movement from the acute inflammation phase to the repair phase to the remodeling phase and may take days to months to complete depending on the extent and severity of an injury. The restoration of normal range of motion controlled by normal strength/power relationships is facilitated by a proper mixture of therapeutic modalities and therapeutic exercise.

Therapeutic modalities are used in combinations (physical agents, machines, massage, manual and therapeutic exercise) to modify an inflammatory response, restore tissue, or increase strength and range of motion. Cold has been the treatment of choice for over 40 years in athletic medicine when dealing with acute inflammation. Cold minimizes the accumulation of edema and decreases hemorrhage by decreasing the metabolic demands of the injured tissue, thus reducing blood flow. Cold also provides a strong analgesic effect. Depending on the treatment parameters, superficial cold can penetrate to a depth of up to 10 cm (3). However, it is important to realize that cold will not decrease edema that is already present.

There is still some confusion in the scientific literature as to when it is permissible to switch from cold to heat. Some suggests that after 48 to 72 hours heat should replace cold (10). This appears to be beneficial in tissue that is at rest for a few days during early rehabilitation. In an athletic population, however, switching to heat too early may cause problems. Most athletes continue to perform some form of activity when injured, which may lead to increased edema formation. Knight has suggested that it is not safe to switch to heat in an active population until about day 14, and then only when rehabilitative exercise does not induce any further pain (7).

Cold treatments average 20 minutes in length (with variation for relative body fatness). Methods of application include crushed ice packs (bags), ice cups in a massaging action, slush buckets, cold whirlpools, chemical gel packs, and single use chemical packs. For acute musculoskeletal trauma where rest, ice, compression, and elevation are the treatment of choice, ice packs wrapped against the body with a compression wrap appear to work the best.

A major effect of cold was thought to be a decrease in the secondary injury caused by decreased blood flow due to swelling in an area. When distressed tissues were deprived of oxygen, required nutrients, and suffered waste buildup, surviving normal cells would be injured. Since cold lowers metabolic rate, the nutritional

CASE STUDY: Wrist Injury

A 5' 10" basketball player is offended that the other team's backup center, an offensive tackle on the football team, is attempting to dunk. He jumps into the air, lands on the taller player's shoulder and proceeds to fall over the shoulder and straight down to the floor. He puts out his hand to break his fall, causing severe pain in his right wrist.

What are possible injuries in this case? Sprained wrist, dislocated carpal bone in the wrist, fractured carpal bone in the wrist, Colles' fracture of the distal end of the radius at the wrist.

What would the initial first aid be in this case? Splint the wrist in a rigid splint and apply cold. Refer to a medical facility for an x-ray.

Diagnosis: the athlete has sustained a Colles' fracture. What happens next?

The wrist is placed in a cast for approximately six weeks. A follow-up x-ray to demonstrate healing will precede cast removal and the beginning of rehabilitation.

How will you begin the rehabilitation program?

Have the athlete work on range of motion and preliminary strength. Utilization of orthopedic putty (or even a tennis ball with the covering removed) and warm whirlpool range of motion activity will be helpful.

requirements of damaged tissues decrease as well and cells suffer less damage from impaired blood flow. Cold has also been shown to have a positive influence on muscle spasm, possibly due to decreasing pain breaking the pain/spasm cycle.

Heating modalities have been utilized most successfully on post acute and chronic inflammation. Superficial heat is produced by moist heat packs, paraffin baths, warm whirlpools, and fluidotherapy. The penetrating level of these forms of heat is usually not into skeletal muscle. Their actions then, to relieve pain and muscle spasm, must be mediated through the nervous system to some degree. Deep heat comes in the form of ultrasound, diathermy, and therapeutic laser. Ultrasound is the treatment of choice over small areas, while diathermy may be more effective over larger treatment areas. These modalities heat tissues within the body through convection, targeting especially muscle. They will increase blood flow, increase metabolic rate, decrease pain and muscle spasm, and assist in the resolution of posttraumatic edema.

Athletic trainers need to first develop a written plan with both short-term and long-term goals of the rehabilitation process, the methodology that will be used to reach the goals, and the outcomes that signify passage to the next stage of the process. An athlete may be returned to competition before the completion of the rehabilitation program. This does not release the athlete from further exercise to finish the progression to full recovery. See the case study for a typical treatment plan developed by an athletic trainer.

Correctly used, modalities will help limit the inflammatory response to the injury and increase the rate of repair and remodeling, minimizing the time lost by the athlete. Incorrectly used, modalities may lengthen healing time, or lead to further medical complications having a negative impact on the athlete.

Psychosocial Strategies

Athletic trainers must constantly watch for at-risk athletes with mental illness. Initially, the athlete may report problems with sleep and/or appetite. These may be a precursor to anxiety disorders, depression, bipolar disorder, attention deficit/ hyperactivity disorder, eating disorder, substance abuse, or overtraining.

When an athlete is injured and unable to perform for any appreciable length of time, generalized anxiety disorder or post-traumatic stress disorder are possibilities. These may require cognitive therapy or medications. Having a strong social network and activities and a social identity away from sports are good steps in dealing with anxiety. Injured athletes need to remain a part of the team. If they fail to respond appropriately, athletic trainers should look for secondary gains (if they are injured, they cannot fail in competition) or they may be malingering (pretending to have symptoms to avoid returning to play).

Depression is an altered mood affecting feelings and behavior. Symptoms unique to athletic competition include sustained poor performance, failure to complete rehabilitation, and withdrawal from team functions and involvement. If this persists for two or more weeks, referral to an appropriate medical professional is warranted. This should not be ignored, because athletes have committed suicide when depression is improperly treated.

Bipolar disorder is characterized by sequential bouts of depression and mania. When in the manic state, excessive involvement of pleasure activities is frequently observed. Treatment is difficult because an athlete during a manic episode sees no reason to be on medication. The most common medication is lithium under a physician's care.

Eating disorders (most commonly anorexia nervosa and bulimia) are a response to a disturbance in body perception. Most of the patients are women. However, any athlete who must make weight is a potential sufferer. Women have an especially deadly combination called the *female athlete triad*: disordered eating, amenorrhea, and osteoporosis. In the female adolescent and young adult age range, stress fractures are often linked to the triad. All eating disorders should be referred to a physician.

Substance abuse consists of utilization of prescription drugs, nonprescription drugs, illicit drugs, or performance-enhancing drugs to the detriment of the patient. Addiction is a maladaptive pattern of substance use over 12 or more months leading to impairment, development of tolerance, or withdrawal. This needs referral to a physician.

Health Care Administration

The area of health care administration encompasses personnel management, emergency action plans, facility management and design, budgeting, record keeping, insurance, third party reimbursement and public relations (11). Personnel management functions include the hiring and utilization of personnel. Decisions must first be made on the scope of coverage for a particular athletic training setting, hours of operation, and patient load before deciding how to equip and staff the facility. Basic policies and procedures at a site may or may not be the same at all other sites in a system. Working with a budget to purchase expendable supplies and permanent equipment sometimes requires advanced imagination to cover an athletic trainer's needs.

Medical record keeping is a critical area in any health care setting. Complete, accurate, and legible records inform others about the initial impression of the injury, decisions regarding referral and emergency treatment, follow-up care, and rehabilitation programs implemented. The information is used to communicate with physicians, other athletic trainers and allied medical personnel, lawyers, and insurance companies. The information is confidential without the express permission of the athlete.

Professional Development and Responsibility

The athletic trainer has a duty to maintain his or her knowledge and skills at the current standard of practice. Since this standard may change over time, it is important that athletic trainers continue to upgrade their skills through continuing education programs offered through a variety of outlets. Athletic trainers have a duty to help educate the athletic training students who work with them, acting as mentors and clinical preceptors. Athletic training is a profession in which classroom knowledge must be placed into practice frequently during the learning process to implant it firmly in long-term memory.

Concern for and control of exposure to the legal system is an extremely important health care administration function. Negligence is certainly a consideration in any health care setting. Negligence is a branch of tort law that excludes contracts but recognizes legal responsibility for harm done to others. Juries usually award damages to the injured party, most often in the form of money. The elements of negligence include: duty, breach of duty, causation, and damage.

All four of elements of negligence must exist for a negligence claim to be successful. Most often breach of duty is defined as an act of commission in which the accused does something that a reasonable and prudent person would not do, or an act of omission in which the accused fails to do something that a reasonable and prudent person would do. An example of doing something that should not be done would be moving a seriously injured athlete off the playing field at the request of the officials who wish to restart the competition while the emergency medical service is in route. An example of failing to do what is required would be allowing an athlete to return to play with only a superficial examination, missing a potentially life threatening closed head injury such as clear signs of an epidural hematoma.

Defenses against negligence include (a) the assumption of risk by the athlete for common injuries that occur within a sport, (b) statutes of limitation, which specify a time limit to the filing of negligence actions, and (c) waivers, which are contracts between the athlete and the administration whereby the athlete receives the right to participate in return for agreeing to hold the athletic administration blameless for injury incurred during practice and competition. Unfortunately, waivers are only as binding as the court agrees that they are. They can be found to be not in the best public interest and therefore declared null and void.

COMMON ATHLETIC INJURIES

Athletic injuries are usually either from out-of-control internal or external forces or from repetitive motion leading to overuse. To classify injuries, the symptoms, signs, and functional significance of the trauma must be evaluated. A symptom is subjective information described by the athlete. Pain is a symptom, as are nausea, lightheadedness, and dizziness. A sign is information gathered through objective assessment, such as heart rate, blood pressure, and body temperature.

Injuries lead to a loss of function or the inability to move a body part throughout a normal range of motion and against normal resistance. When someone sprains an ankle, swelling inhibits the range of motion. Signs, symptoms, and loss of function increase as the severity of the injury increases.

Contusions (bruises) are compression injuries ranging from superficial damage to deep muscle or bone bruising with significant hematoma. They are caused by a direct blow to a body part and result in pain and swelling. Skin discoloration (ecchymosis) may follow the contusion and is often characterized by a dark purple color that turns into a greenish-yellow color as healing occurs.

Strains are a stretch or twist of a muscle, a tendon, or muscle-tendon unit beyond normal physiological limits. The cause of muscle strains is debatable. Certainly absorbing the outside forces generated by a collision or inappropriate placement of body parts causes some strains, but most strains are attributed to abnormal muscle contraction, often when antagonist muscles work against each other in a fatigue situation. Strains result in pain on movement, pain on stretch, and loss of function.

Strains are graded according to severity. First-degree strains involve minimal stretching or microtrauma, minimal pain, and loss of function. Second-degree strains are more extensive, with partial tearing of some tissue, moderate pain, loss of function, hematoma formation, muscle spasm, and inflammation. Third-degree strains are severe injuries, with a complete tearing of a muscle, tendon, or musculotendinous interface accompanied by a severe loss of function, significant pain, severe loss of strength, hematoma formation, possible calcium formation during the healing process, and a possible palpable defect in the muscle (10).

Overuse injuries are common in athletics and are due to repetitive microtrauma. Most injuries that contain the suffix *itis* are overuse. Before an original injury has been allowed to heal, the mechanism of injury is repeated again and again. Without visible or palpable defects, there is pain on movement and passive stretch, some swelling, loss of function, and inflammation (10). Tendinitis, an inflamed tendon, is a common overuse injury.

Sprains are a stretch or a twist beyond normal anatomical limits of a ligament in the same way that strains involve muscle or tendon. A person cannot strain ligaments, just as a person cannot sprain tendons. Sprains are characterized by pain, point tenderness, mild loss of function to complete joint instability, swelling, hemorrhage, and inflammation.

Sprains are graded in a similar fashion to strains. A first-degree sprain stretches a ligament without tearing fibers and without deformity. It is accompanied by mild pain, minimal swelling, point tenderness, inflammation, and loss of function. First-degree sprains respond readily to treatment, and athletes usually may return to competition in a few days. Second-degree sprains are more significant, with partial tearing of the ligament, moderate to strong pain, moderate swelling, inflammation, and loss of function. They may result in substantial lost time and rehabilitation. Third-degree sprains involve a severe loss of joint function, often with complete tearing of the ligament. There is severe pain, swelling, joint instability and inflammation (10). This injury often requires surgical intervention or extensive rehabilitation and time away from sports activity.

Many of the special tests athletic trainers utilize assess joint laxity and ligament stability. When moving a joint through its full range of motion, a sharply defined end point (called the end feel) to this range is good, while a soft mushy ending is usually indicative of a third-degree injury.

Dislocations involve complete disruption of articulating joint surfaces with tearing of most, if not all, ligaments surrounding a joint. Common sites for dislocations include the interphalangeal joints of the fingers, elbow, glenohumeral (shoulder) joint, and the patella. A dislocated acromioclavicular joint is termed a shoulder (or A-C) separation rather than a dislocation. Dislocations should be treated as fractures, splinted in the position they are found, and referred to a physician or emergency room for treatment. In a subluxation (partial dislocation), the joint surfaces have become disassociated, but spontaneous reduction (moving back into the normal position) of the deformity has taken place.

Fractures are a disruption in the continuity of a bone caused by stress, either tension, torsion, compression or bending. Stress is consolidated at points where bones change their shape or direction (10). The forces adversely affecting bone can operate independently or in conjunction with each other. While spiral fractures are caused by twisting forces, oblique fractures are caused by compression, bending, and twisting. Transverse fractures are caused by bending forces.

Open fractures present more of a challenge to the athletic trainer for immediate management because outside pathogens enter the open wound. Closed fractures remain under the skin. Any fracture that is displaced does collateral damage to surrounding tissues (muscle, nerve, blood vessels). Fractures should be splinted in the position that they are found, and the patient transported to a physician or emergency room for reduction and fixation.

Neurological injuries are also a part of sport participation. When body parts are injured, the displacement of body elements can stretch or tear peripheral nerves. Closed head injuries include concussions and vascular damage. A concussion, also known as mild traumatic brain injury, is a trauma-induced alteration in brain function. It is functional, not structural, and may or may not involve loss of consciousness. This can come from something striking a stationary head, a moving head striking a stationary object, or from a severe rotation leading the brain to strike the inside of skull with no outside impact. Refer to the case study on concussion.

As of the Zurich Statement in 2008, there is no grading system for concussion. There is no severe or mild, simple or complex, or having one's bell rung. Return to play decisions are based on functional recovery. Step 1 involves complete physical and cognitive rest. Step 2 progresses when there are no symptoms in step 1 and consists of light aerobic exercise at less than 70% of predicted maximal heart rate. Step 3 begins sport-specific exercise. Step 4 involves non-contact training drills that are sport specific. Step 5 is full contact practice. Step 6 is full return to play. The minimum duration of each step is 24 hours. If any symptoms return, the patient backs up one step and begins that level 24 hours later (Figure 18.3).

With the awareness of the effects of concussion on long-term functioning today, especially in retired professional athletes (which should include college and high school athletes), attention must also be paid to post-traumatic stress disorder. There is a study ongoing in Massachusetts examining the brains of deceased former players. Preliminary findings have shown the same type of twisted structural proteins as are seen in Alzheimer's patients. There is currently a lawsuit against the National Football League by over 3,000 former players alleging the league did not inform the players of the effects of concussion and did little to minimize exposure.

A fractured cervical vertebra can have fragments penetrate the spinal cord damaging nervous transmission below the level of the injury. A bulging lumbar disk can put pressure on spinal nerve roots, leading to atrophy of musculature, abnormal pain sensations, and gait problems.

An athletic trainer's worst nightmare is to be confronted with an acute injury where the athlete is unconscious and face-down. All unconscious athletes should be assumed to have a closed head injury and severe cervical trauma until proven otherwise. With the individual face down, it is paramount to assess airway, breathing, and circulation. Should it be necessary to begin CPR, the athlete must be properly positioned using the correct technique. One of the worst decisions an athletic trainer may face is keep the athlete alive at the expense of producing quadriplegia due to his/her actions to save a life.

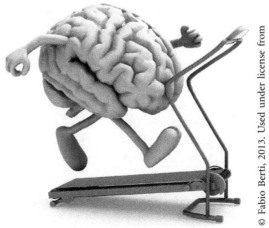

Figure 18.3. *Functional recovery from concussion.*

Inflammatory Response

Inflammation is a complex process to vascular tissue from the effects of trauma, bacterial and viral invasion, chemical irritants and decreased blood supply (3). The classic signs and symptoms include pain, redness, temperature, swelling, and loss of function.

The acute phase of inflammation begins immediately after injury and lasts as long as three days. For the first few seconds the arteries constrict, which allows white blood cells in the capillaries to line the walls. Following this there is a more general dilation of blood vessels with increased blood flow. The capillaries then begin to leak (increased vascular permeability). White blood cells and proteins move outside into the tissues. This attracts water from plasma and swelling occurs. In later stages of acute inflammation, a protein system in the blood, becomes activated which increases the development of the inflammatory process, attracts more white blood cells, and increases phagocytosis and vascular permeability. Along the edge of the traumatic damage, cells do not function normally. Each cell has enzymes that destroy that cell when it becomes damaged beyond repair. These enzymes digest cell membranes and then attach to structures on the cell membranes of uninjured cells, causing additional cell death. This is a secondary injury due to enzymes.

The swelling decreases blood flow through an area. This swelling is compounded by the shutting down of the lymphatic system. The additional pressure on the vascular system leads to a decrease in the availability of oxygen and glucose to normal cells on the periphery of the injury site, leading to a secondary injury due to hypoxia (lack of oxygen).

The factors that limit the size of the damage include blood clotting and accumulation of blood into a hematoma. Blood clotting is a complex process that begins with the exposure of platelets to molecules that are not normally found in the vascular system. The platelets begin to get sticky and clump together, which is sometimes enough to seal capillaries. Larger vascular injury requires the process to continue. Chemicals from the platelets travel through the blood to the liver, leading to the production of a chemical that helps the clot to form. With this chemical at the injury site one of the proteins in the blood binds to the platelet plug. If the bleeding is in a local internal area, a hematoma forms, which limits range of motion.

Tissue Repair

Beginning at the third day after the injury and continuing for about three weeks is the process of repair. The first week involves scar formation, especially synthesis of collagen, a protein molecule. With collagen formation, developing capillaries bud from intact capillaries on the outer edge of the wound and a scar takes on

---

CASE STUDY: Concussion

A receiver on a football team must lean forward to catch a pass. The defender lowers his helmet and contacts the receiver helmet to helmet, knocking the receiver on his back. He is groggy and disoriented when the official calls for the athletic trainer to assist. The player has no awareness of his surroundings. The team physician is summoned from the sideline and he determines the player has suffered a concussion. What is the next step in treating this athlete?

If there has been pre-competition cognitive screening, a repeat test is warranted. If not, the athlete is transported to the sideline and observed. The athletic trainer periodically checks with the athlete to determine cognitive status. Such questions as "Where are you? What time is left in the game? How many people hit you? What was the play before you were injured? Please count backwards from 100 by 7," and others will be helpful.

The athlete is removed for the rest of this game. Upon clearance from the physician, the athlete will be placed in the Zurich protocol, at minimum a six-day recovery period.

a reddish granular appearance. Then the scar begins to contract. Some individuals will scar more than others, a process that can limit function and requires therapeutic intervention. Muscle and nerve tissue have little or no ability to reform the original tissue, hence collagen scar repairs these tissues.

Beginning at day nine the maturation phase takes place. Collagen is initially laid down in random directions. In maturation the collagen molecules are reordered along stress lines through an injury site. When this is complete, the scar is still only 70% of the strength of the original tissue and has fewer blood vessels. Further, as the collagen is replaced, capillaries will be removed. The final scar has few blood vessels and a white appearance. Maturation can go on for a year or more.

Several factors modify the inflammatory and repair process. Drugs have been utilized by physicians to inhibit the process. Nonsteroidal anti-inflammatory drugs such as aspirin or ibuprofen and corticosteroids such as prednisone inhibit the development of inflammation. Placing an injured body part in a rigid splint or cast while clearly beneficial in early inflammation, if used for prolonged periods of time has been shown to lead to tissue atrophy and the development of adhesions. Some therapeutic agents including electrical stimulation, hyperbaric oxygen, and therapeutic ultrasound have been shown to have positive effects on repair and remodeling (7).

HOW TO BECOME AN ATHLETIC TRAINER

Athletic training is still a developing profession. The original method of educating an athletic trainer was for that person to obtain a degree in physical education and work in an apprenticeship arrangement with an athletic trainer. In 1959 a list of formal course work in athletic training was proposed. The apprenticeship evolved into an internship, with some additional course work and fine tuning of the clinical requirements.

In 1970 Certified Athletic Trainer (ATC) became the entry-level credential. Formal education programs were developed at a number of universities under guidelines from the NATA Professional Education Committee. Completion of an approved program was one route to certification, as was completion of an apprenticeship program, completion of a physical therapy program, or being actively engaged in the practice of athletic training for a minimum of five years. On January 1, 2004, to sit for the BOC Examination students had to be a graduate of an accredited athletic training education program.

The 1983 *Guidelines for Development and Implementation of NATA-approved Undergraduate Athletic Training Education Programs* introduced competency-based education (2). The competencies were divided into the six domains identified by the Board of Certification in the Role Delineation Study. Currently, the competency matrix is in its sixth edition (8). The latest edition has added the competency area of evidence-based practice and took from the combined other competency areas to conclude with a clinical integration area.

In the 1980s it became apparent that state credentialing of athletic trainers would become a necessity. To accomplish this goal accreditation of athletic training education programs was necessary. A major step toward accreditation came in 1990 when athletic training was formally recognized as an allied health profession by the American Medical Association.

In 1994 the first accredited athletic training education programs were endorsed by the Committee on Allied Health and Accreditation (CAHEA), which was shortly thereafter replaced by the Commission on Accreditation of Allied Health Education Programs (CAAHEP) to accredit entry-level athletic training education programs. This body was replaced by a discipline specific accrediting body, the Commission on Accreditation of Athletic Training Education (CAATE) in 2006.

The National Athletic Trainers Association created the Education Task Force in June 1994 to look at all aspects of athletic training education and propose reforms leading to standardization of education programming. In 1996 the NATA Board of Directors adopted 18 reforms for educating athletic trainers, among which was the recommendation that the NATA and the NATABOC, Inc., work to initiate regulations that take effect in 2004 that only graduates of accredited athletic training education programs would be eligible to take the certification examination (9). This led to a major increase in accredited education programs between the years 2000 and 2004. Currently, there are over 350 accredited entry-level athletic training education programs.

During the 1990s, there was an explosive growth in the credentialing of athletic trainers by state governments. Much of the reform movement within NATA was prompted by the interaction of state credentialing bodies with other allied health professions and state legislatures. Athletic trainers are now credentialed in one form or another in 48 of the 50 states, either by licensure, registration, or certification. Credentialing by state governments has led to a tightening of educational standards, and, through state practice acts, to control in some states over who can be served by athletic trainers and what those services may be.

The advent of licensure also heralded change in clinical education. The current accreditation standards specify that a student may practice skills in a clinical setting only when under direct observation by a licensed or certified professional. Constant visual and auditory supervision allows the supervisor to step in to protect the student and patient from untoward consequences. At one point the accrediting agencies allowed, but did not condone, a student acting as a first aider. That is no longer the case.

Students must be introduced to new material in a classroom setting, refine the skills in a laboratory setting, and then practice those skills in a clinical setting. The accrediting body, CAATE, calls this learning over time, a model developed from the nursing profession. Students must obtain clinical experience with individual and team sports, equipment-intensive sports (helmets and shoulder pads in football, ice hockey, or men's lacrosse), patients of different sexes, non-sport patient populations (e.g., outpatient clinic, emergency room, primary care office, industrial, performing arts, military), and a variety of conditions other than orthopedics (e.g., primary care, internal medicine, dermatology). Frequently, state licensure requirements specify standards that expand or limit the accreditation standards such as a minimal number of hours of clinical education to obtain a license. The state practice act always supersedes other requirements.

There is considerable discussion in athletic training at the present on the appropriate entry-level degree credential. Currently, athletic training requires at the minimum a bachelor's degree with a major in athletic training. The discussion centers around the concept that since athletic trainers hold themselves to be peers to other professions with a practitioner doctoral degree, the difference between a bachelor's degree and a doctoral degree is too great. Those individuals supporting this line of thought believe a master's degree should be the entry-level credential. This leads to a myriad of other problems including the fact that some colleges with accredited entry-level athletic training education programs are not allowed by law to have graduate programs. Another concern is the status of the graduate assistant in college-university athletic departments.

Athletic training is a health care practice field that works cooperatively with physicians and other health professionals in all aspects of health care delivery to athletes. Specifically, athletic training deals with the prevention, care, and rehabilitation of injuries to active individuals. The domains described by the NATA Board of Certification describe the body of knowledge required to practice athletic training. Prevention of athletic injuries is a vast underrated area, encompassing pre-participation physical examinations, physical conditioning for specific sport activities, and ensuring a safe competitive site from both physical and environmental aspects. Recognition, evaluation, and emergency care of athletic injuries is part of the basic job of the athletic trainer.

REFERENCES

1. Bilik, S. E., *The Trainer's Bible*. New York: Reed, 1956. (Originally published in 1917)

2. Board of Certification, Inc., *6th Role Delineation Study/Practice Analysis*. (Online)

3. Denegar C. R., E. Saliba, and S. F. Saliba, *Therapeutic Modalities for Musculoskeletal Injuries*, 3rd ed. Champaign, IL: Human Kinetics, 2010.

4. Ebel, R. G., *Far Beyond the Shoebox: Fifty Years of the National Athletic Trainers' Association*. New York: Forbes, 1999.

5. Higgins, M., *Therapeutic Exercise: From Theory to Practice*. Philadelphia: F. A. Davis Company, 2011.

6. Kettenbach, G., *Writing SOAP Notes*, 3rd ed. Philadelphia: F. A. Davis Company, 2004.

7. Knight, K. L., *Cryotherapy in Sports Injury Management*. Champaign, IL: Human Kinetics, 1995.

8. NATA Professional Education Council, *Athletic Training Education Competencies,* 5th ed.

9. NATABOC, *BOC Exam Candidate Handbook.* Omaha: Board of Certification, 2014.

10. Prentice, W. E., *Principles of Athletic Training: A Competency-Based Approach,* 15th ed. New York: McGraw-Hill, 2014.

11. Rankin, J. M., and C. D. Ingersoll, *Athletic Training Management: Concepts and Applications,* 3rd ed. New York: McGraw-Hill, 2005.

12. Starkey, C., S. D. Brown, and J. L. Ryan, *Examination of Orthopedic and Athletic Injuries,* 3rd ed. Philadelphia: F. A. Davis Company, 2010.

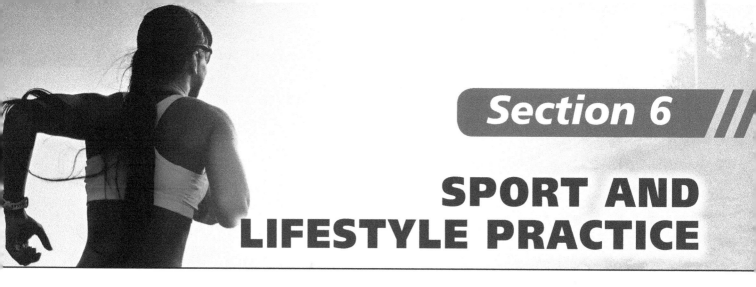

Section 6

SPORT AND LIFESTYLE PRACTICE

The five chapters in this section present the more traditional professional fields that were aligned to the "old" discipline field of physical education. As you can see, sport pedagogy (physical education) is now just one aspect of the umbrella that kinesiology has become. As is the case with the health care practice fields of kinesiology, the sport and lifestyle fields, while diverse, nevertheless remain connected through their common tie—the practice of exercise, physical activity, and sport.

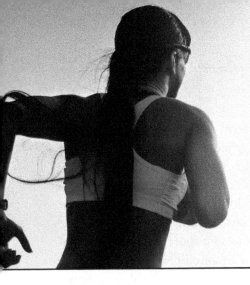

Chapter 19 ////

SPORT PEDAGOGY

OUTLINE

OBJECTIVES

After reading the chapter, students should be able to:

1. Understand the description and meaning of the term *sport pedagogy*.
2. Understand the importance of the field of sport pedagogy.
3. Understand the difference between physical education and physical activity.
4. Understand why people choose to enter the field of sport pedagogy.
5. Understand the motives behind agencies that support the field of sport pedagogy.
6. Understand educational strategies designed to promote physical activity in the school curriculum.
7. Understand the differences and similarities in teaching elementary and secondary physical education.

SPORT PEDAGOGY DEFINED

According to the National Board for Professional Teaching Standards, the term *pedagogy* refers to the skills teachers use to impart the specialized content of their specific subject or discipline area (6). There are many organizations that further define, debate, and dissect the meaning of what teachers must do to demonstrate the skills and abilities necessary to promote student learning, but there is controversy surrounding what these skills and abilities might be. Everyone agrees, however, that creating a learning environment where all students feel comfortable, safe, and able to succeed academically and personally is the goal of teaching.

Sport is not as easily defined as pedagogy. For elementary physical education, sport is defined as organized games that have established, accepted, and published rules of play with an emphasis on having fun (3). Coakley (2) defines sport based on a sociological point of view as being "institutionalized competitive activities that involve rigorous physical exertion or the use of relatively complex physical skills by participants motivated by internal and external rewards." The sociological definition is much more complex and not only begs for greater clarification, but it is not as easily applied in an attempt to define sport for inclusion in pedagogical reference.

However, the sociological definition is more appealing based on the exclusionary composition of the terms. That is, not all games are included as sport and would consequently be excluded by definition. Checkers is a game, but using Coakley's definition, it would be excluded as a sport because it does not require rigorous physical exertion. Using the elementary physical education definition, games and fun are stressed in the place of rigorous physical exertion and relatively complex physical skills. It would stand to reason that in an elementary setting the motivational aspect of fun would preempt the physical complexity aspects of sport. Although, with the physical requirements removed, cards and board games become sport, and anyone teaching these skills become simply supervisors and scorekeepers. This is not to say that sports cannot be fun to be considered sport, but there are numerous things a child can gain from sport participation that involves rigorous physical exertion. For the purpose of this chapter, sport will be defined as a physically demanding activity that requires a defined motor skill set and has an established set of rules that is played for competition. The reason for this particular definition is its ease of use with the term *pedagogy*.

Putting the two words together, *pedagogy* refers to the whole, including instruction in every discipline or content area, and *sport* refers to the part, that is, the specific content area. If sport is considered, the content area used in pedagogical practices, defined as the instructional skills necessary for the specific content area of sport, then sport pedagogy would be defined as the instructional skills teachers use to impart the specialized knowledge to motivate and enable students to participate in physically demanding activities that require a defined motor skill set and have an established set of rules and is participated in for competition.

According to the National Association for Sport and Physical Education (NASPE), *physical education* is a discipline that uses pedagogical practices that are based on state and/or national physical education standards, which result in all students developing the knowledge, skills, and confidence needed to participate in a physically active lifestyle (5). The greatest distinction between the two definitions is that the NASPE definition of physical education identifies state and national educational standards as being used to promote the pedagogical practices. The definition of *sport pedagogy*, however, provides a better sense for the discipline as a profession. The differences between the two definitions are primarily technical; hence, the two titles are essentially interchangeable. Since the two titles are so closely related, why not just use physical education?

Many institutions of higher education have used various terms, phrases, and labels to identify the physical education teacher education program. There has been a nationwide push to change the name to provide greater support and respect, or to more clearly state the exact nature of the program. The profession itself has undergone several changes, so why not a name change?

There is a greater emphasis on developing motor skills to enhance participation in lifetime fitness to enhance overall health at every grade level than ever before. There is greater respect for the profession from educational leaders than before, although change has been slow and has required many pieces of federal legislation to mandate such change. The label—*physical education*—itself provides a barrier to the change in attitude regarding the pedagogical field. It provokes negative thoughts of potentially bad experiences that current educators and administrators might have had during their mandatory school "PE" class.

Although the definition of sport pedagogy for use as a label for the profession provides a better definition, it is often met with controversy by those in the educational community. When the educational standards are not included as a part of the definition, although they are implied, it produces an artificial and apparent reduction in the level of importance in state and national standards. This artificial reduction of importance in standards is incorrect, but is not seen as favorable in the eyes of the educational community. Physical Education as a profession has been fighting an uphill battle for respect within the educational system from the onset. Even a name change that dictates greater respect in and of itself is frowned upon, as if the profession was not worthy of such respect. Some claim there is a lack of respect given to physical education by members of the school community (4). This is also true of colleges of education within institutions of higher learning. That is, other content areas in higher education fail to see the importance of physical education. To be viewed as "good" for a physical educator, you must be "exceptional," or as many educational rubrics would depict, "target."

WHY CHOOSE SPORT PEDAGOGY AS A PROFESSION?

Why would anyone want to choose a profession that is not respected by other people in the profession? To offer a simple explanation, it is chosen for the love of the game. To expand upon this statement, individuals who choose sport pedagogy as a career are passionate about the field and understand the importance of being physically active to a person's overall health and the future health of the nation. They also understand how students must be taught skills to be able to take advantage of available activities, and they must be able to participate in regular physical activity to benefit their self-esteem and cognitive development and to help their overall social adjustment.

To teach in any subject area, mentoring is a major aspect. It is a continually evolving entity that should always motivate students to have the desire to pursue their goals. The best motivation a teacher/mentor can provide comes from a passion and the in-depth understanding of the subject area. That is why many individuals choose sport pedagogy, because they simply love the field, they love to be physically active, they understand the importance of physical activity, and they love to share their passion of sports and activities with others to motivate them to pursue their own personal goals.

For any teacher to be effective, he or she must know the material inside and out and be involved in their chosen field of study. In addition to knowledge and involvement, a teacher must have the belief that students can learn and that what they are teaching will make a difference in their students' lives. Any sport pedagogist knows the importance of physical activity and the outcome for inactivity including the impact it has on national health.

Teaching is stimulating. It contributes to personal growth and development while assisting the growth and development of students. Many true to life stories similar to the following can be told.

> I was once a tutor for undergraduate athletes, and asked one of the football players what he was in college to pursue. He replied that he wanted to be a teacher and a coach. He said that he wanted to give back to society and the youth in the community what his physical education teacher and coach had given to him. He claimed that if it had not been for the potential his coach saw in him, he would be dead or living on the streets.

Teachers touch lives every day and have the opportunity to help their students aspire to greatness instead of settling for mediocrity or worse. Sport pedagogists have the opportunity to find the potential in all students, no matter what their situation, and provide them with appropriate outlets to physically express themselves through a variety of activities.

Teaching is also modeling and provides opportunities to show concern for students. It is imperative for educators to provide the most up-to-date and practical information available. With this in mind, a teacher needs to stay current in the topics they are responsible for teaching, and needs to know the content area in great depth. In order to motivate students' learning, teachers are required to provide coursework that is practical and applicable for their future. A wide variety of teaching strategies should be used to maintain the interest of students, and they should be provided as many practical opportunities as possible. Teaching physical education lends itself to a greater variety of teaching formats and a greater opportunity to interact with the students. Modeling skills necessary to be physically active and leading a healthy lifestyle, as well as mentoring students to develop socially and emotionally, is the main goal of sport pedagogy.

Overall, teaching is a dynamic phenomenon that requires knowledge, creativity, discipline, and patience. A teacher must provide the most current information in a variety of ways to stimulate the interest and enthusiasm of students. A teacher should not only provide information during class, but demonstrate this information outside of the classroom. Therefore, a teacher is a role model and it is imperative that each one lives what he or she teaches. In doing so, it teaches the student respect for the teacher and for the chosen profession. The most successful teachers mentor for direction and guidance and model for greatness and success.

NATIONAL PUBLIC HEALTH CAMPAIGNS AND THE IMPACT ON SPORT PEDAGOGY

There are numerous public health initiatives attempting to bring sport pedagogy to the educational forefront. Underlying this effort is the premise that educating the physical provides a positive impact on academic and intellectual performance. A few of these initiatives include the National Physical Activity Plan (NPAP), White House Task Force on Childhood Obesity Report to the President, and Healthy People 2020 Objectives.

The National Physical Activity Plan (NPAP) is a comprehensive set of policies, programs, and initiatives that aim to increase physical activity in all segments of the American population (7). The NPAP has identified eight societal sectors: (a) business and industry; (b) education; (c) health care; (d) mass media; (e) parks, recreation, fitness, and sports; (f) public health; (g) transportation, land use, and community design; and (h) volunteer and nonprofit.

Within the education sector, the NPAP has identified seven strategies that are listed in Table 19.1 for teachers, coaches, school administrators, and school district officials to help them in their leadership roles to implement physically active lifestyles.

All of the strategies listed in Table 19.1 are focused on the development and implementation of educational programs that emphasize physical activity for all ages. They are excellent suggestions, but probably more theoretical than applied. The development of policies, training, facilities, and programs provides excellent ideas, but without appropriate funding or the ability to enforce program plans or promote changes they are merely suggestions. An important aspect of the strategies developed by the NPAP is that they provide support for physical education leaders attempting to obtain funding for continued training, programs, or facilities.

The White House Task Force on Childhood Obesity Report to the President is part of "Let's Move," which was initiated by the First Lady as a comprehensive initiative attempting to help solve the problem of childhood obesity (11). As part of this effort, President Barack Obama established the first-ever Task Force on Childhood Obesity to develop and implement an interagency plan that details a coordinated strategy, identifies key benchmarks, and outlines an action plan to end the problem of childhood obesity within a generation. State and local education agencies are challenged to increase the quality and quantity of sequential, age- and developmentally appropriate physical education for all students, taught by certified physical education teachers. The entire report may be found and downloaded from their website:

www.letsmove.gov/white-house-task-force-childhood-obesity-report-president The strategies listed in this report are as follows:

- Creating infrastructure and policies within schools that increase access to and encourage physical activity for all students.

Table 19.1.   Strategies for Educators to Promote Physical Activity Lifestyles

STRATEGY 1	Provide access to and opportunities for high-quality, comprehensive physical activity programs, anchored by physical education, in pre-kindergarten through grade 12 educational settings. Ensure that the programs are physically active, inclusive, safe, and developmentally and culturally appropriate.
STRATEGY 2	Develop and implement state and school district policies requiring school accountability for the quality and quantity of physical education and physical activity programs.
STRATEGY 3	Develop partnerships with other sectors for the purpose of linking youth with physical activity opportunities in schools and communities.
STRATEGY 4	Ensure that early childhood education settings for children ages 0 to 5 years promote and facilitate physical activity.
STRATEGY 5	Provide access to and opportunities for physical activity before and after school.
STRATEGY 6	Encourage post-secondary institutions to provide access to physical activity opportunities, including physical activity courses, robust club and intramural programs, and adequate physical activity and recreation facilities.
STRATEGY 7	Encourage post-secondary institutions to incorporate population-focused physical activity promotion training in a range of disciplinary degree and certificate programs.

Source: (7)

- Maintaining strong physical education (PE) programs that engage students in moderate to vigorous physical activity for at least 50% of PE class time.
- Providing a variety of activities and specific skills so that students can be physically active not just during PE class but throughout the day and year.
- Providing qualified school professionals who are trained in teaching methods to engage students in PE, including for students who face greater barriers to activity.

Similar to the NPAP strategies, "Let's Move" has excellent suggestions and provides excellent support for sport pedagogy programs in the public schools.

Healthy People 2020 Objective on Physical Activity is a national initiative that originated from the U.S. Department of Health and Human Services and the Centers for Disease Control and Prevention (1). The Physical Activity Guidelines for Americans (PAG) is a publication released in 2008 to serve as national guidelines for physical activity. Included in the guidelines are the physical activity objectives for Healthy People 2020 that are supported by the science basis regarding the health benefits for regular physical activity for youth and adults. The goal for the physical activity objective of Healthy People 2020 is to improve the health, fitness, and quality of life through daily physical activity. Some of the means to reach this goal include:

- Increase the proportion of the nation's public and private schools that require daily physical education for all students.
- Increase the proportion of adolescents who participate in daily school physical education.
- Increase the proportion of adolescents who meet current federal physical activity guidelines for aerobic physical activity and for muscle-strengthening activity.

More information may be found on the website www.healthypeople.gov/2020/topicsobjectives2020/overview.aspx?topicid=33

PHYSICAL EDUCATION AND PHYSICAL ACTIVITY

The majority of public agencies that help promote sport pedagogy and stress the impact fitness has on public health discuss the importance of physical activity and physically active lifestyles, but merely mention education as a component within the strategically designed system. Sport pedagogy and physical education are used in this chapter interchangeably, but what about physical education and physical activity?

The National Association for Sport and Physical Education (NASPE) believes every child in the United States deserves both a quality physical education and a physical activity program. Physical education programs within the school system provide the venue for students to participate in physical activity by offering the skills and knowledge students need to develop and maintain an active, healthy lifestyle. According to NASPE, A quality physical education program provides learning opportunities, appropriate instruction, with meaningful and challenging content for all children (5). Within a quality *physical education* program, students have the opportunity to participate in regular *physical activity*. The U.S. Department of Health and Human Services (USDHHS) suggests the benefits of regular physical activity include (9):

- Reducing the risk for overweight, diabetes, and other chronic diseases
- Assisting in improved academic performance
- Helping children feel better about themselves
- Reducing the risk for depression and the effects of stress
- Helping children prepare to be productive, healthy members of society
- Improving overall quality of life.

One of the main ideas within any sport pedagogy curriculum is that all children should have the opportunity to be taught skills necessary to participate in daily physical activity. As demonstrated in Figure 19.1, the percentage of children classified as obese continues to increase at an alarming rate.

All physical education programs should provide the skills, motivation, and concepts at developmentally appropriate levels so all children can learn about and participate in active lifestyles to avoid becoming sedentary. Physical education is the only avenue whereby children can be provided with the opportunity to make appropriate activity choices and set goals. Many organizations, like NPAP and Let's Move, advocate for children to be more active during the day and claim that recess is a good avenue to increase the amount of physical activity children can accumulate during the day. The problem with that is free time, exploratory activity, and recess do not provide skill assessment, structured activity promoting national objectives, motivation to participate in activity, or physical self-efficacy. Physical education is designed to meet the needs of every student in regard to his or her personal developmental motor skill level.

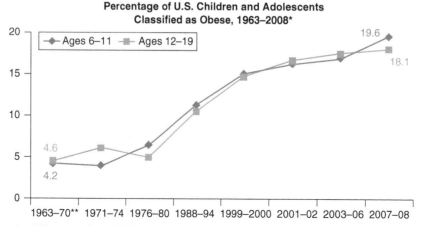

Percentage of U.S. Children and Adolescents Classified as Obese, 1963–2008*

* ≥95th percentile for BMI by age and sex based on 2000 CDC BMI-for-age growth charts.
**1963–1970 data are from 1963–1965 for children 6–11 years of age and from 1966–1970 for adolescents 12–17 years of age.

SPORT PEDAGOGY AS A PROFESSION

Within any profession, there must be a governing body. NASPE is the governing body for sport pedagogy. NASPE (5) is one of the five associations that combined make up the American Alliance of Health Physical Education Recreation and Dance (AAHPERD). The five national associations are:

1. American Association for Health Education (AAHE): Serves health educators and others in the health profession to promote health for all individuals including those in the public schools, public health agencies, medical care settings, and business and industry.

2. American Association for Physical Activity and Recreation (AAPAR): Links professionals in education with community and agency-based programs to encourage fitness programs across the lifespan. Many of the programs supported by AAPAR include aquatics, adapted physical activity, outdoor recreation, facility design and management, fitness for older adults, and safety and risk management,

3. National Association for Girls and Women in Sport (NAGWS): Concerned with equity issues in sports and provide information for administrators and teachers working with girls and women and are the main proponent for Title IX.

4. National Association for Sport and Physical Education (NASPE): Sets the standards for physical education and is the basic governing body for the teaching profession in physical education (sport pedagogy),

5. National Dance Association (NDA): Advocates dance in the arts and physical education programs.

In addition to the five associations within AAHPERD, there is also the Research Consortium. The Research Consortium serves as the coordinating organization to support research across the disciplines and the professions served by AAHPERD.

According to NASPE, recess, after-school recreation programs, or free play are not substitutes for quality physical education. Sport pedagogists are movement specialists trained to assess, identify, demonstrate, provide appropriate feedback, and motivate students at every level. They are required to develop teaching and learning objectives in three domain areas:

1. Affective – interests, attitudes, appreciations, and values
2. Cognitive – learning and application of knowledge
3. Psychomotor – learning physical skills

Sport pedagogists are required to know the different standards that identify what a physically educated person is able to do. Table 19.2 lists the NASPE standards for physical education teacher education programs that identify the competencies pre-service teachers must be able to understand and demonstrate prior to receiving certification in teaching.

NASPE also provides National Standards for K-12 physical education on what students should know and be able to do as a result of a quality physical education program. Table 19.3 lists what NASPE indicates as items a physically educated person should be able to demonstrate.

In addition to National Standards, there are state standards that are specific to each state regarding physical education requirements for K–12 students. According to NASPE, in response to the need for high-quality physical education and sport programs, many states have adopted physical education standards that closely align with NASPE's voluntary National Standards and provide a link to each state's standards from its web page. For more state specific information on standards for quality physical education, go to the following link: www.aahperd.org/naspe/standards/stateStandards/

NASPE's guidelines provide appropriate instructional practices for K-12 physical education. The appropriate and inappropriate practices are separated into five sections: (a) learning environment, (b) instruction strategies, (c) curriculum, (d) assessment, and (e) professionalism. Table 19.4 includes each of the five sections of appropriate practices guidelines broken down into subsections.

Table 19.2. Standards for Physical Education Teacher Education Programs

Standard 1: Scientific and Theoretical Knowledge	Physical education teacher candidates know and apply discipline-specific scientific and theoretical concepts critical to the development of physically educated individuals.
Standard 2: Skill-Based and Fitness-Based Competence	Physical education teacher candidates are physically educated individuals with the knowledge and skills necessary to demonstrate competent movement performance and health-enhancing fitness as delineated in NASPE's K-12 Standards
Standard 3: Planning and Implementation.	Physical education teacher candidates plan and implement developmentally appropriate learning experiences aligned with local, state, and national standards to address the diverse needs of all students.
Standard 4: Instructional Delivery and Management.	Physical education teacher candidates use effective communication and pedagogical skills and strategies to enhance student engagement and learning.
Standard 5: Impact on Student Learning	Physical education teacher candidates utilize assessments and reflection to foster student learning and to inform instructional decisions.
Standard 6: Professionalism	Physical education teacher candidates demonstrate dispositions essential to becoming effective professionals.

Each section is further broken down into subsections related to sport pedagogy and then broken down further for distinctions between elementary and secondary instructional practices. Sport pedagogy differentiates appropriate practices between educational levels, but all emphasize the same global outcome of *educating the physical* for every student. The school setting, and more specifically physical education within the school setting, may be the only place children of all ages have the opportunity to be active. Also, most teacher preparation programs certify pre-service teachers for K–12 physical education. Therefore, even though there is a difference between the physical and developmental needs of elementary school children as compared to secondary students, the sport pedagogist needs to be able to address the needs of all children K-12.

Figure 19.2 demonstrates an inappropriate use of a resistance activity for children. Although the figure is "cute," illustrating the family that lifts together is fit together, it is misleading. It is recommended that children participate in muscle-strengthening activities, but at the younger ages these activities should be things

Table 19.3. Physically Educated Person Competencies

Standard 1	Demonstrates competency in motor skills and movement patterns needed to perform a variety of physical activities.
Standard 2	Demonstrates understanding of movement concepts, principles, strategies, and tactics as they apply to the learning and performance of physical activities.
Standard 3	Participates regularly in physical activity.
Standard 4	Achieves and maintains a health-enhancing level of physical fitness.
Standard 5	Exhibits responsible personal and social behavior that respects self and others in physical activity settings.
Standard 6	Values physical activity for health, enjoyment, challenge, self-expression, and/or social interaction.

Table 19.4. NASPE Instructional Practices for Physical Education

Learning Environment	Instructional Strategies	Curriculum	Assessment	Professionalism
Establishing the Learning Environment	Expectations for Student Learning	Productive Motor Skill Learning Experiences	Assessment Use	Professional Growth
Exercise as Punishment	Class Organization	Concept Knowledge	Variety of Assessments	Professional Learning Community
Safety	Class Design	Regular Participation	Fitness Testing	Advocacy
Diversity	Learning Time	Developing Health-Related Fitness	Testing Procedures	
Equity	Maximum Participation	Self-Responsibility & Social Skills	Reporting Student Progress	
Inclusion	Teaching/Learning Styles	Valuing Physical Activity	Grading	
Competition & Cooperation	Teacher Enthusiasm	Interdisciplinary Instruction	Program Assessment	
	Success Rate	Special Events		
	Teacher Feedback			
	Technology Use			

like playing on playground equipment, playing tug-of-war, or resistance by activities that use their own body weight. Structured muscle-strengthening activities like resistance training with weights are suggested for adolescents, once they have matured into the higher intensity level of strength training.

As with resistance training and level of muscle-strengthening activities for children, aerobic activity needs are also different for children as compared to adolescents. Table 19.5 indicates the guidelines for aerobic activity for children and adolescents to be the same, but how they achieve the recommended guidelines are different. As indicated, most of the 60 or more minutes a day should be aerobic physical activity either of moderate

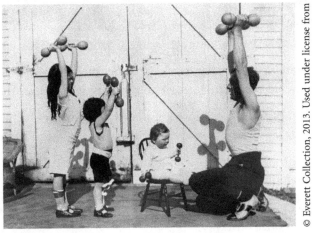

© Everett Collection, 2013. Used under license from Shutterstock, Inc.

Figure 19.2

or vigorous intensity. This does not mean that children should be active for a continual 60 minutes, but each period of activity throughout the day should add up to 60 minutes.

Children have different movement patterns and may produce short bouts of highly intense activity followed by periods of rest. That is their natural movement pattern. All of the intermittent activities are combined for their total of 60 minutes of aerobic activity. That is contradictory to the way many adults think about aerobic activity. As children mature, and mature into adulthood, the patterns of physical activity change. They are able to sustain longer periods of activity that help them to develop a stronger aerobic capacity that will allow them to participate in sports and leisure activities that require a sustained aerobic capacity.

SPORT PEDAGOGY AT THE ELEMENTARY SCHOOL LEVEL

As a part of normal maturation and development, children grow, move, play, and establish all the skills necessary for normal everyday activities. At least that is the belief by a vast majority of adults. The adults who support those beliefs were evidently not one of the children standing around either wanting to participate in activities but were rejected because of their motor skill insufficiencies, or the ones refusing to participate because of the fear of rejection.

Regardless of why this misconception has occurred, it has existed for years. Children need to be provided not only the opportunity to practice movement skills but to be guided with appropriate feedback to develop the movement skills necessary for successful participation in physical activities (10).

Similar to teaching math skills, movement skills must be taught to become useful in everyday life. Children who lack appropriate motor skills are often rejected from game play or refused the opportunity to participate (1). Furthermore, the likelihood of continued activity stems from successful participation in organized and structured activities. Although these are known facts, many school districts fail to employ certified physical educators at the elementary school level.

In addition to the importance of teaching sport skills at the elementary school level, the U.S. Department of Health and Human Services published physical activity guidelines for youth. The guidelines are included in Table 19.5.

The guidelines in Table 19.5 are all in reference to fitness. Consequently, at the elementary school level, it is necessary for children to obtain the developmental motor skills necessary to participate in various physical activities to achieve and maintain a healthy fitness level designed specifically for their age.

A sport pedagogy program at the elementary school level should be designed to equip children with the knowledge, skill, and abilities to motivate them to participate in daily activity. The appropriate program should

Table 19.5. Physical Activity Guidelines for Youth

Youth Physical Activity Guidelines
Children and adolescents should have 60 minutes (1 hour) or more of physical activity daily.
Aerobic: Most of the 60 or more minutes a day should be either moderate- or vigorous-intensity aerobic physical activity and should include vigorous-intensity physical activity at least three days a week.
Muscle-strengthening: As part of their 60 or more minutes of daily physical activity, children and adolescents should include muscle-strengthening physical activity on at least three days of the week.
Bone-strengthening: As part of their 60 or more minutes of daily physical activity, children and adolescents should include bone-strengthening physical activity on at least three days of the week.
It is important to encourage young people to participate in physical activities that are appropriate for their age, that are enjoyable, and that offer variety.

Source: (8).

also be designed to assist them in acquiring the self-confidence they need to participate in activity and instruct them in making choices to behave in appropriate social interaction. There are seven basic requirements for a successful elementary school program: (a) developmentally appropriate activities, (b) skill development, (c) development of fitness, (d) maximize active time, (e) cooperation and competition, (f) motivation and inclusion, and (g) assessment. There are other requirements that could be included in a sport pedagogy program designed for the elementary school age-child, however, the seven listed here are the minimum required.

Developmentally Appropriate Skills

This takes into consideration the level of maturity of the child to maximize enjoyment, success, and continued participation in movement activities. Children are not developmentally ready to follow sequential instruction or complex movement patterns until certain developmental milestones are met. Figure 19.3 shows a suitable environment for children to explore and to help guide them in developing movement skills at their own rate. If the task is too simple, children are not challenged, and if the task is at a level that is above the individual's level of development, it sets them up for failure. The sport pedagogist is trained to identify the developmental patterns and milestones for children at all ages to ensure maximum understanding and participation of the child.

Skill Development

Skill development takes into consideration the level of the child and the expectations for that particular level. All children develop at their own pace, but most motor skill development will occur at similar ages given similar environmental demands. Motor skills can be further broken down to basic movement skills (body awareness, spatial awareness, object control skills, locomotor skills), basic game skills (skills that lead up to participation in sports), and creative and rhythmic skills (movement to music and movement as a form of self expression).

Development of Fitness

As seen in the Table 19.5, physical activity has standards that are developed and suggested at every level. Elementary school requirements for physical activity are essential to the future health of the nation. Making a positive impact on young children to help them develop an active lifestyle can make the difference in the future success or failure of every child in the program. The sport pedagogist understands the importance of physical fitness and develops appropriate physically active goals for the children in their programs.

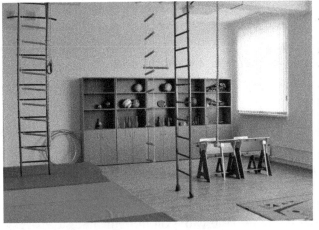

© Martynova Anna, 2013. Used under license from Shutterstock, Inc.

Figure 19.3

Maximize Active Time

Time on task is another way to express this concept. There is only a small portion of the day that allows for children to be physically active and practice movement skills in an attempt to become proficient at those skills. It is the responsibility of the sport pedagogist to teach the skills, make corrections, provide appropriate feedback, and keep the students active. Maximizing movement time requires planning and excellent classroom management by the teacher. There can be no waiting in lines, no elimination games, and no classmates as spectators. All activities need to be individual, partner, and small group activities unless the children "waiting" are performing another activity or another form of the same activity while they wait for equipment, space, or other accommodations to perform the task at hand.

Cooperation and Competition

At the elementary school level there are two different lines of thought on competition. Some believe that *indirect competition* is the only form of competition that should be encouraged at this level. Indirect competition is thought of as individual achievement by achieving self-set goals. On the other hand, *direct competition* for elementary children may be discouraged because it results in producing winners and losers. Proponents for indirect competition believe that children are not emotionally mature enough to properly understand the concept of winning and losing and believe indirect competition or cooperative games are the only useful form of instruction at the elementary level. Proponents of direct competition in elementary school believe that winning and losing is a part of life and should be taught early and that physical education is the best avenue for this form of instruction. Additionally, competition is by definition part of sport pedagogy. Within the definition there are no suggestions for appropriate ages to learn competition, but children by nature are going to be competitive. How to emotionally accept our humanistic competitive nature should be part of every sport pedagogy program, regardless of the competition as being direct or indirect.

Motivation and Inclusion

The belief that all children can learn and all children can learn to move is more than fundamental, it is the law. Title IX of the Educational Amendments Act of 1972 calls for equal educational opportunities for boys and girls. Therefore, all activity offerings must be coeducational except in some instances of contact sports. At the elementary school level, it is not generally an issue especially since girls generally mature and reach developmental milestones earlier than boys. Another law, PL 94-142, the Education for All Children Act of 1975 and its subsequent amendments, addresses the need for equal educational opportunities for children with and without disabilities. This has a great impact on every physical education program, since physical education is stated as a direct service by the law. It is at the elementary school level that children start to realize similarities and differences and start to compare themselves to others in their classes. No child should be singled out and not allowed to participate for any reason unless safety is a concern. The effect of singling a child out could cause ridicule and emotional harm, making any differences appear to be much greater than they actually are. Sport pedagogists are trained to adapt and include all children. The main concern is that all children should be encouraged and motivated to embrace physical activity.

Assessment

Assessment is the cornerstone of any quality sport pedagogy program. Without assessment no benchmarks are set, and without benchmarks there is no way to determine if the program is successful. Assessment in sport pedagogy is part of the daily program and comes in many forms. Some forms of assessment may be conducted through authentic means, such as activity logs, checklists, self-reports, and portfolios. Others may be done through the use of rubrics or scoring guides to determine student progress or changes in student skills, assessment to determine mastery or non-masterly of skill movement, or formal assessment that may be done as formative program or student evaluation. All assessments must be conducted with a direct purpose and are generally part of the daily sport pedagogy routine.

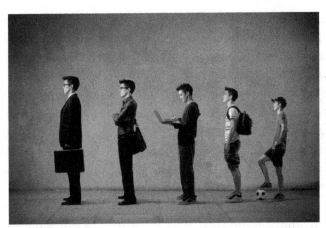

Figure 19.4

If all of the above program characteristics are appropriately addressed by the sport pedagogist at the elementary school level, children will transition into the secondary sport pedagogy setting with much greater ease as Figure 19.4 demonstrates. They will have mastered or have begun to master skills at the appropriate developmental level and will have gained confidence in their ability to learn movement skills. Children will have greater self-esteem and be more highly motivated to continue an active lifestyle. However, without the basic foundation, the transition to middle and high school sport pedagogy programs could prove to be a difficult task.

SPORT PEDAGOGY AT THE SECONDARY LEVEL

Educating the physical aspect of students at the secondary level poses different challenges for the sport pedagogist. These challenges have to do with the students themselves, state requirements for physical education, the secondary school environment, acceptance of physical education within the school environment, teaching style, and the interaction of all the challenges. Most of these challenges are evident at the elementary school level, but they are manifested at a greater intensity at the secondary level because of the interaction of these variables.

Some school systems understand the need for physical education while other schools see it as something that can be cut because of budgetary restraints and by administrators who do not realize the importance of the program. Some administrators believe it takes up valuable time students can use to participate in some of the primary academic programs like science, math, and English. The truth of the matter is that less than three out of every 10 high school students get at least 60 minutes of physical activity every day (9).

Some dynamic individuals involved in sport pedagogy realize that left to their own choice, adolescents are normally going to choose a more sedentary lifestyle. Successful sport pedagogists have been able to promote the discipline by having well-respected programs through an ability to motivate students to participate in an active lifestyle. Physically active adolescents will over time enhance the overall well-being of the community. This type of program is usually more innovative in its use of community resources. Other sport pedagogists inadequately reach out to students and fail to promote their physical education program, which generally results in the failure to meet state and national requirements, subsequently hurting the community and future generations.

At the elementary school level, children need to be guided to demonstrate functional motor skills appropriate to meet their developmental needs. That is, a child must first learn to step and then to hop before learning to skip. Children learn simple to complex movement skills and at different rates. At the secondary level, students should have already mastered the fundamental motor skills and should be ready to apply the basic skills to sports or lifetime activities. A problem is, not all secondary students have mastered the basic movement skills necessary to participate in age appropriate activities. This leads to embarrassment and an avoidance of physical activity. However, with both elementary and secondary programs, the ultimate goal is the participation in physical activities that help promote healthy lifestyles.

There are other special concerns specific to that of the adolescent student. These include the characteristics of stress and coping, alienation, drug use, abusive home environments, diverse cultural backgrounds, and adolescents with disabilities. Once again, it is not an issue that these concerns do not occur in the elementary grades, but they are experienced at a different level during the secondary educational experience.

The middle and high school student places a great deal of emphasis on their appearance. Not only is the student's physical appearance an issue, but their social appearance is an issue as well. Some students at this age have gone through puberty while others are still at the pre-pubertal level of development. Some students are demonstrating a great deal of talent in athletics while others have not yet mastered more basic motor skills. Because of the highly visible nature of physical education and physical activity, it is difficult for students that lag behind in the developmental process to have an opportunity to improve without taking the risk of being ridiculed. Consequently, those that fall short in the area of physical skills may continue to lag behind until they are left behind. Additionally, older students may not want to sweat before going to their next class, feeling equally embarrassed for not performing a skill properly and for "smelling bad" the rest of the day.

A topic at the secondary level that has recently received more attention is the adolescent student who appears to be a loner or bully. Some adolescents may not have developed a sense of identity or are confused about their identity. They may become frustrated, lack direction, and lack hope for the future in addition to a lack respect for others. They may subsequently act out in delinquent ways. In class they may appear as disrespectful, cynical, and unwilling to participate. Ignoring the issue tends to compound the matter. Teachers and counselors need to work together to address the issue, and often physical activity may be used as an appropriate outlet for unacceptable behaviors.

Adolescence is a time for rebellion and experimentation. Drug use in all forms may be an appealing outlet for adolescents regardless of the harmful effects it could have on the student's life and the lives of friends and family. Regardless of the reasons, physical activity can have a positive effect on healthy life choices. However, an alarming national trend is the increasing use of anabolic steroids by junior and senior high-school students. This is an issue sport pedagogists need to be aware of so they can have a direct impact on student's awareness of the harmful effects it can have on themselves, athletics, and society. Mentoring and being a positive role model in the lives of young adults is a powerful tool that sport pedagogists can use to their advantage to assist them in becoming healthy adults.

Most secondary schools only require one year of physical education in their school curriculum. Adolescents who have not had good past experiences in physical education, have been slower at developing movement skills, or lack self-confidence in their ability to move will not choose to participate in physical activity during school. Consequently, many students at the secondary level taking physical education as an elective are already competent in movement skills and athletics. Adolescents who need physical activity the most will be the ones least inclined to participate. Elective physical education classes at the secondary level should be designed to engage all students, especially those students who are the least active.

Adolescents with disabilities may find themselves with greater challenges than those without disabilities. Adolescence is already a time when appearance plays a key role in social acceptance. Children with disabilities often have an outward appearance that does not fit in. They may also be at a disadvantage for the development of physical skills because of not being included in games and activities outside the school environment. The lack of self-confidence and inadequate physical activity may also be a compounding factor in the development of obesity. With the combination of obesity and disability, adolescents will be ostracized to a greater extent, which becomes a cyclic phenomenon.

Just like the elementary school program, all good sport pedagogists know how to adapt their program so everyone can participate. Adolescent students with a disability, unlike those without a disabling condition, will have an Individual Education Program (IEP) designed to meet the specific needs of the student. All IEPs should include some type of physical education to assist them in the development a healthy lifestyle. Physical education may be their only opportunity to be active and to be included equal to their peers. All children and young adults need to have the opportunity to be active, to learn about activity, to be in a safe environment to learn movement skills, to have accomplishments through movement, to be motivated to participate in movement activities, and to embrace a physically active lifestyle.

SUMMARY

The physical education curriculum in the public schools has gone through several changes and developmental growing pains. The curricular emphasis now embraces the mind and body connection by educating the physical person as a whole and involves teaching lifetime fitness to enhance the overall well-being of students. In doing so, this provides a tremendous and positive impact on the future health of the nation.

Along with the change in the curriculum, the title is also changing to better reflect the impact and the serious nature of the discipline. Sport pedagogy truly captures the spirit of the discipline by definition as "the instructional skills teachers use to impart the specialized knowledge to motivate and enable students to participate in physically demanding activities that require a defined motor skill set and have an established set of rules and is participated in for competition."

Many national public health agencies and organizations have rallied in support of physical education in the public schools. These agencies realize the importance of physical activity and rely on sport pedagogy programs to provide adequate direction to the youth of the nation to reduce the rapid rate of morbidity and mortality caused by inactivity and obesity. The majority of these agencies provide strategies and ideas for sport pedagogy professionals in leadership roles to assist in the promotion of lifestyle physical activity. Three of these agencies include the National Physical Activity Plan, White House Task Force on Childhood Obesity Report to the President, and Healthy People 2020 Objectives conducted through the Centers for Disease Control and Prevention.

Sport pedagogy as a profession provides a curriculum designed to educate the physical for youth and young adults, grades pre-K through 12. Many pre-service teachers in domains other than sport pedagogy specialize in either elementary or secondary education, but pre-service teachers in sport pedagogy must be prepared to teach at the elementary and secondary level. There is a vast difference in the physical and developmental needs of elementary school children as compared to young adults at the secondary level. This, however, is just one of the many obstacles the sport pedagogist must overcome. The individual who chooses sport pedagogy as a career does so because he or she is passionate about the discipline. This person understands the importance of educating the physical aspect of every child, and that every child should have the opportunity to be physically active, to learn skills necessary to participate in activity, to grow socially and emotionally through participation in physical activity, and to have the opportunity to love the game.

REFERENCES

1. Centers for Disease Control and Prevention, *Guidelines for school and community programs to promote lifelong physical activity among young people.* Retrieved January 18, 2013, from: www.cdc.gov/healthyyouth/npao/strategies.htm

2. Coakley, J., *Sports in Society: Issues and controversies,* 8th ed. New York: McGraw-Hill, 2008.

3. Kovar, S., C. Combs, K. Campbell, G. Napper-Owen, and V. Worrell, *Elementary Classroom Teachers as Movement Educators, 2nd ed.* New York: McGraw-Hill, 2007.

4. McCormack, A., and K. Thomas, "You'll be OK: Induction experiences and reflections of NSW beginning teachers in physical education." *ACHPER Healthy Lifestyles Journal* 50 (2003): 7–11.

5. National Association for Sport and Physical Education, an association of the American Alliance for Health, Physical Education, Recreation and Dance (2012). Available: www.naspeinfo.org

6. National Board for Professional Teaching Standards, Washington, DC: Author, 1998. Available: www .nbpts.org

7. National Physical Activity Plan (2012). Available: www.physicalactivityplan.org/index.php

8. U.S. Department of Health and Human Services. *Physical Activity Guidelines for Americans*. Washington, DC: U.S. Department of Health and Human Services, 2008.

9. U.S. Department of Health and Human Services, Centers for Disease Control and Prevention. Healthy People 2020 Objectives. Available: www.healthypeople.gov/2020/topicsobjectives2020/overview .aspx?topicid=33

10. Wallhead, T. L., and J. Buckworth, "The role of physical education in the promotion of youth physical activity." *Quest*, 56(3)(2004): 285–301.

11. White House Task Force on Childhood Obesity Report to the President. (2013). www.letsmove.gov/ white-house-task-force-childhood-obesity-report-president

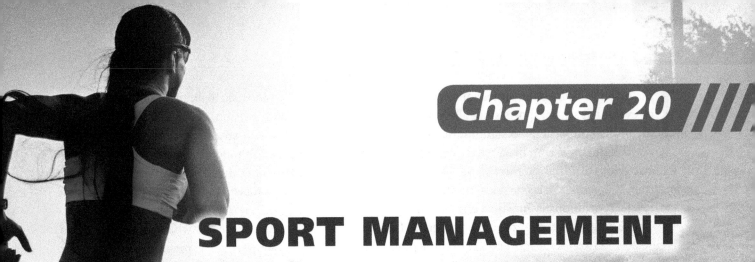

SPORT MANAGEMENT

 OUTLINE

 OBJECTIVES

1. Identify the key differences in managing people in entertainment sport organizations and participation sport organizations.
2. Describe the key marketing challenges facing sport managers in entertainment and participation sport organizations.
3. Explain the ways in which sector (for-profit, not-for-profit) impacts the financial management of sport organizations.
4. Discuss the ways in which cities and non-sport businesses use sport to advance their marketing efforts.
5. Describe the unique characteristics of sport for social development.
6. Identify potential business opportunities that flow from sport and explain their relationship to sport organizations.

It is easy to think about professional sports like football, baseball, and basketball, or to reflect on college or even high school sports since all these are commonly viewed on television, described in magazines, or mentioned on local radio stations. In truth, though, these are only a very small part of the sport industry. The sport industry is a bit like an iceberg; only a small portion is visible. Although the fundamental management activities of administering, marketing, and managing finances are common to nearly all parts of the sport industry, the necessary tasks, skills, or foci for managing sport can be somewhat different depending on the part of the sport industry in which one works.

The complexity of the sport industry derives from the many different purposes for which sport is intended. Figure 20.1 illustrates the most salient of those purposes. As Figure 20.1 shows, management may be concerned with delivering sport either as an entertainment or as an activity in which people participate, and sometimes it may be concerned with how sport is used to deliver desired or claimed social or economic benefits. The necessary requirements for effective management of sport depend on the particular objectives of the sport organization, which can be multifaceted. Sometimes one hears the phrase "sport business" as if that delimits the conversation to a particular segment of the sport industry, but as we will see, that is misleading insomuch as each element of the industry affects or relies upon the other. In other words, although the sport industry is multifaceted, no one segment is independent of the other. The remainder of this chapter considers the managerial concerns that are particularly salient in the presence of different objectives, and it considers the interdependence of each of those objectives, including the consequent implications for management.

DELIVERING SPORT

Sports that deliver entertainment, such as the professional or college sports one sees on television, rely to no small degree on sport as an activity in which people participate. The athletes who provide entertaining competitive events are created and selected from systems of sport participation (5). Thus, recreational sport and school sports provide a foundation for the elite sport that is the cornerstone of sport as an entertainment. The two are not separate; they are part of an integrated system.

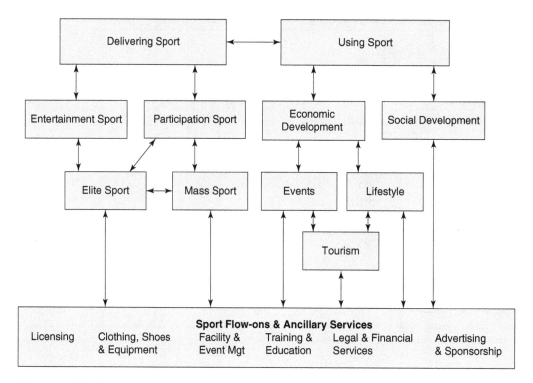

Figure 20.1. *The sport industry.*

Both aspects—entertainment and participation—must be managed. In both, it is necessary to recruit, train, and supervise personnel; in both, it is necessary to design appealing services and promote them to potential users; in both, it is necessary to have funds available to deliver the services and to enable the organization to sustain itself and grow. However, the tasks in each are somewhat different.

Human Resource Management

Professional sport and nearly all collegiate sport rely on employees who are hired and paid a salary for their work (see sidebar). In order to identify and hire the right personnel, it is necessary to determine which tasks each will perform, design a job description, and then screen applicants to find the best match. A system for training, evaluating, and supervising each employee must be in place (13).

Sidebar Sampling of Job Descriptions in Sport Management

Sales Manager—Texas Motor Speedway
Responsible for annual sales and profits quest and working in partnership with operations.

Director, International Sports
Assist with growth and development our International Sports to include building our recruitment of athletes in all sports in South America.

Sports Marketing
Marketing partner to assist with rapidly growing team travel, tickets, collectibles, and business opportunity markets.

Manager, Business Development & Operations
Grow and develop revenues, fan base, and consumption metrics via development and execution of strategic sales, marketing, and content distribution initiatives.

Manager, Basketball Operations
Scout and help recruit potential players by attending summer leagues, pre-draft camps, and college basketball games, evaluating tape, and providing scouting reports . . .

Course Manager—AUS
Looking for a smart and outgoing course manager to join the operations team to assist in organizing all logistics for events.

Swim Manager
Managers in training are responsible for assisting with the management of a swim school facility by supervising and executing corporate plans and actions.

Asst. Mgr., Paralympic Communications
Oversee the coordination, writing, editing, and production of all Paralympic publications, including, but not limited to, conference programs, games media guides, athlete biographies, etc.

Some of the personnel who deliver sport as a participative activity may also be employees, and the tasks for recruiting, screening, hiring, training, supervising, and evaluating may be similar for these employees. However, the job description is likely to look quite a bit different because the requisite skills are different. Whereas employees who are concerned with sport as an entertainment must focus on putting on the best possible show, employees who are concerned with sport participation must be capable of designing and implementing an array of sport programs suited to different ages, genders, and skill levels. In other words, although the fundamental principles of human resource management are pertinent in both settings, the particulars that must be applied are different because the jobs are different.

The same applies to volunteers. A great deal of sport is delivered by volunteers. That is true for both entertainment and participation. Nearly all events require a substantial number of volunteers, and more are required as events become larger. Consider, for example, that the London Olympics used over 70,000 volunteers (1). Nearly all local-level sport programs provided outside of school also rely heavily on volunteers to coach and to provide some or all of the necessary administration. As with employees, the tasks and consequent skills required in the two settings are clearly different. Thus, recruitment, selection, training, evaluation, and supervision must be designed differently in the two settings. When delivering sport as an entertainment, people who have skills in such things as event staging, customer service, or player management will be sought and trained to apply those skills for the particular organization that has hired them. Supervision and evaluation will reference those skills. On the other hand, when managing sport as a participative activity, people with the skills necessary to design, implement, and/or supervise sport programming will be required. Thus, the criteria for hiring, supervising, and evaluating an employee for sport participation services will be different than those for employees who deliver sport entertainment services.

It is also important to bear in mind that volunteers are not merely unpaid employees. Unlike employees who are doing a job, volunteers are choosing to use their free time to provide a service to sport. Volunteers thus see their experience as a leisure experience, not as work (7). Although it is tempting to place volunteers in roles that mimic their work experience, volunteers often seek experiences that are in no way related to their day-to-day jobs. Instead, they seek roles that allow them to do things they do not normally get a chance to do, to be an insider at events (go behind the scenes), to interact with athletes and professionals they would otherwise not have an opportunity to meet or to learn from, to give back to a sport they care about, or to support a person or cause dear to them.

The relationship between the two systems becomes particularly salient when one considers where the elite athletes who provide sport entertainment are developed. Nearly all begin in participative programs in their particular sport. Thus, sport organizations that seek to enhance development of the pool of elite athletes from which they can draw must have systems of relationships that enable them to identify and recruit (sometimes "draft") athletes as they transition from systems focusing on participation to elite systems where they provide sport entertainment to audiences.

Marketing

Whether sport is a passive entertainment or a participative activity, it must have customers to survive. After all, if no one wants the product, then it will cease to exist. Thus, both kinds of sport systems must find customers. However, since they offer different products and have different access to channels for communicating about their products, the marketing tasks differ.

Clearly, customers seeking sport as an entertainment would be attracted to very different elements of the sporting mix. Consequently, the products and services offered by entertainment sport are designed to appeal to distinctive markets and provide very different benefits to customers than are provided by participation sport (16). Consider your own sport experiences. It is likely that the reasons you seek out opportunities to participate in sport are different from the reasons you watch sport. The experience of participating in sport can provide a chance to socialize with friends, build or maintain fitness, master and display new skills, challenge oneself physically or mentally, and perhaps experience first hand the thrill of competition. The challenge for product design for participation sport is to design a sport setting that can deliver multiple benefits sought after by potential participants.

It is critical to understand the benefits a potential market values. For example, a sport program designed to provide the most sociable environment for young singles to meet and get to know one another could provide this environment by including large, co-ed teams for which people can register as individuals rather than as a team. This would encourage singles to join a team without requiring them to form a team themselves. This type of program could further the social experience by partnering with a local restaurant or bar to facilitate socializing after games, thereby expanding the potential social network beyond one team and to the entire league. Notice that other elements providing added benefits can also be included: (a) competition between teams, (b) coaches and training sessions to facilitate skill development, and (c) physical activity that can facilitate fitness development. This is just one example of product design for participation sport. Another program might cater to potential participants seeking to challenge themselves, enhance their fitness, or lose weight. Programs designed to train for endurance sports such as a triathlon, marathon, or cycling events are good examples. Although the main emphasis in these programs is often on the physical training, they can provide social support and build new friendships by having participants train in the same group over a period of time in order to enable members to get to know one another. The point is to provide the experience to participants they most value, which often requires more than just sport.

This is just as important for entertainment sport marketing, although the benefits that people seek from entertainment sport tend to differ from those sought from participation sport. Entertainment sport experiences are designed with the "show" in mind. The most extreme fans are the most easily entertained by merely seeing the game, whether live or on television. They are already highly connected to the team, its symbols, its personnel, and sometimes even the stadium or arena in which it plays. It is easy to forget that these fans also seek benefits that should be designed into the fan experience. Highly identified fans often seek experiences that provide ways to celebrate and share their fanship with others (2). Opportunities to extend the experience via tailgating, special fan sections in the stadium, fan-cams, and interactive websites for posting photos, comments and interactions with players, coaches, and other fans are prized elements of the fan experience for hard-core fans.

Yet the more challenging task for marketing entertainment sport is to design products and services that attract non-fans or fair weather fans (those who are fans only when the team is winning) and turn them into loyal fans. For these potential customers, the team and the competition are not enough. They require entertainment that is exciting and stimulating without requiring much previous knowledge or even interest in the sport, the team, or the competition. Professional minor league teams have become expert in creating entertaining sport experiences for non-fans. In addition to the game itself, minor league games often include other entertainment such as fireworks, concerts, play areas for children, and numerous contests throughout the game. These elements can be changed to attract specific groups by changing the contests, giveaways, and artists that appear as part of the game experience. For example, families could be attracted by bundling tickets and concessions into family-sized packs, offering a chance for children under 12 to run the bases, and including a family-friendly post-game show such as fireworks. Ballparks have recently sought to attract religious groups by including testimony by well-known athletes and a post-game concert featuring a contemporary Christian artist. The point is that the experience features more than just a sport competition and is tailored to provide elements designed to attract and entertain a particular target market.

Pricing is often an important element in designing a product to appeal to a target market. Both entertainment sport and participation sport prices are sensitive to changes in market demand, and both products are perishable in that they cannot be saved for later. If there is no demand for a ticket, that ticket cannot be sold later as the event has already happened. Similarly, a tennis league has opportunities to compete that cannot be stored, and a tee time on Saturday morning cannot be sold (or played) later that day. This is a common aspect of services, including sport services (11). A key task for sport marketers, then, is to create prices that appeal to the target market, signal value to customers, and balance demand with the perishability of the experience. Most entertainment sport pricing is designed to maximize income for the sport organization. However, participation sport prices are often set with a broader array of objectives in mind, such as the quality of life engendered for community residents.

When the sport organization is concerned with profits (as most entertainment sport organizations are), pricing will seek to optimize profits, but when the sport organization is not-for-profit (as most participation driven programs are), then pricing will depend on its effect on the organization's ability to deliver services as determined by its mission. For example, a for-profit fitness center will price in order to maximize revenue. However, a Boys and Girls Club fitness center or youth sport league may price to cover costs rather than maximize revenues. The difference derives from the mission of the organization. Youth sport clubs, for example, may provide alternative ways of paying for services that include non-monetary contributions such as volunteer time in lieu of cash payments. Although it is rare for entertainment sports to accept flexible payment for services, some are experimenting with pay-what-you-like pricing, albeit as a promotion. In 2010, Mansfield Town, a Football (Soccer) Club in the U.K., allowed fans to pay what they thought was appropriate for their match against Gateshead, more than doubling their attendance for the match (4). More recently, a team in the National Pro Fastpitch (NPF) League used this pricing effectively to promote a 2013 game. It is notable that both of the entertainment sport organizations using this pricing model were struggling to increase attendance and resorted to this method as a promotion rather than an ongoing pricing strategy. The promotion was intended to enhance future revenues, rather than to enhance any service-to-mission.

Promotions are part and parcel of the entertainment sport experience and are widely used by participation sport organizations as well. While promotions are clearly an important part of the marketing mix for all sport organizations, the types of promotions used vary considerably. The key differences are a result of variations in budget and access to communication channels. Large entertainment sport events, leagues, and organizations receive significant coverage by the media. The media coverage of events such as the Olympic Games, World Cup, and Super Bowl are unprecedented and not available to the majority of sport organizations, although major league teams in the most popular sports also receive significant media attention. In fact, these teams, leagues, and events receive a significant portion of their revenue from media rights to broadcast their competitions (12). This provides a way to communicate with customers and potential customers over a wide swath of the country and, for some, the world. As a result, a key task of major entertainment sport marketing is to manage the media attention, capitalize on partnerships with sponsors and other businesses, and maintain interest in the brand and the products and services the brand represents. Major sports and events also have a large budget for advertising. Advertising allows them to manage carefully the message sent to current and prospective customers, and to create an integrated set of images and messages directed at a desired set of consumers.

Sports that generate less media attention do not have this luxury. Like their more high-profile counterparts, they also seek to generate interest in their products and services. For these events, teams, and leagues, a key task is to promote their product to the media, as well as to consumers, while trying to assert and maintain a desirable brand image (14). Media relations in this case is more akin to selling the media on the interest and excitement in their sport competition, its players, and rivalries than is it to manage the media's existing focus on the sport. As a consequence, promotions such as advertising and public relations are even more important. Driving audience and media attention is a bit of a chicken-and-egg problem. Media coverage occurs when there is significant interest by the public in the event or sport competition, yet the media attention is often critical to develop interest and attention on the sport or event. Therefore, promotions are developed to reach both audiences—the media and the end consumer (the spectator). A combination of advertising, public relations, community relations events, and social media is necessary to reach these groups.

Although participation sports are almost never dependent on spectator audiences for their survival, they too benefit from media attention (see the following case study). Ideally, media coverage focuses on their products and services—the club, the facility, the league, and so on. However, media attention on the sport itself can raise awareness of the sport, which in turn can generate interest in participation. This routinely occurs around the Olympic Games, which bring a variety of sports not often seen on television into our living rooms once every four years. Perhaps an effect of inspiration, perhaps just novelty, but media attention on sports such as gymnastics and BMX in the Summer Games, and curling and women's ice hockey in the Winter Games has stimulated interest in participation (8). In this way, we see, once again, the interrelationship of entertainment and participation sport. Yet a caution is in order. There is often the expectation that participation in a sport automatically generates interest in watching that sport—either live or on television or the Internet. However, this relationship has never been clearly shown. One has only to consider the wide participation in soccer by most

CASE STUDY: Cavaliers Youth Hoops—Player Development, Social Development, or Marketing Tool?

The Cleveland Cavaliers, like many NBA teams, are investing in youth through their Youth Hoops Program. The official Cavaliers Youth Hoops Program provides camps, clinics, leagues, and individualized training for youth players in the community. The Cavaliers program claims that it teaches, "the fundamentals of the game in a very fun, exciting, and Cavaliers-packed environment (1)." The interesting question is, why? Why do professional teams like the Cavaliers—whose core product is clearly entertainment—create participation programs for children? To understand, let's examine the Cavaliers' youth camp.

The Cavaliers partner with an experienced camp provider, National Basketball Academy, to deliver weeklong camps throughout the summer. The camps are spread across northeastern Ohio and western Pennsylvania, the core fan base for the Cavaliers. The camps include boys and girls from 7 to 16. Camp activities are similar to other basketball camps and include skill development stations, contests, and competitions. Some of the camps (i.e., Player Camps) are associated with one of the Cav's current players. For example, the 2013 camps included Player Camps featuring Alonzo Gee, Marreese Speights, and Tristan Thompson. Although there are no specific promises made, participants may choose to attend the Cavaliers camp for the opportunity to interact with Cavaliers players and coaches.

The benefits of attending the camps are clearly identified on the website (www.) as follows:

1. Between the first day of camp and the last day, we want every camper to improve his or her basketball skill level.
2. We want all of our campers to walk away knowing what it will take for them to get better.
3. We want all of our campers to have fun and learn to truly enjoy the game of basketball.

So, this seems to be about player development. The camp activities emphasize skill development and competition. The objectives are to improve campers' skill levels, understand what it will take to get better, and enjoy sport. In fact, the camps use the marketing slogan, "Training the Players of Today and Tomorrow." Further, the other elements of the Cavaliers' Youth Program seem to also support player development. The clinics promise that, "our expert coaches will help you take your game to the next level!" Leagues and tournaments provide opportunities for continued skill development throughout the year, and specialized training can be obtained to, "help basketball athletes improve at every skill level: high school, jr. high school, community and travel team, college, and professional." Clearly there is a huge emphasis on player development. But why would the Cavs be in the player development business? Their players come from the collegiate ranks. Schools, AAU, recreation programs, and a host of other sport providers develop youth basketball players. Why would an NBA team feel the need to develop youth players?

Perhaps there is more than meets the eye. The description of training program on the National Basketball Academy website hints at a broader goal—social development—when it states: "We are the best basketball training company in the United States because we teach players how to be successful both on and off the court." Is this program, then, using basketball to better the lives of participants beyond sport? It is difficult to tell, yet the emphasis on broader social development adds credence to the Cavaliers' involvement. The Cavaliers, like most professional sports teams, work hard to be active in their home community. The organization (as well as many of its players) has created a foundation whose mission is to "support programs designed to positively impact young people in the areas of education, recreation and employment and life skills." In addition, the Cavaliers are heavily involved in community outreach programs such as the local food bank, Snack Like a Pro nutrition program, and the Wheelchair Cavaliers. So, perhaps the youth program is about social development. And yet, there is another possible explanation.

Could this be a marketing exercise? Consider the tangible take-aways from the youth camps. All campers receive the following: a Cavaliers' branded basketball, t-shirt, and wristband or headband, a ticket to a future Cavaliers game, and a chance to participate in a unique fan experience. Every one of these items is designed to increase fan involvement and create more loyal fans. Notice that the branded items identify the camper as a part of the Cavaliers family, a sentiment that can only be strengthened by meeting Cavaliers players and coaches, perhaps even playing with them at the camp. Positive interactions with the team and the brand have been shown to enhance fans' identification with, and loyalty to the team. But wait, there's more. Notice also, the free ticket and fan experience. These elements bring the participant *and his or her family* back for yet another interaction with the team. Children can't drive themselves to the game, so that single ticket provided now comes with additional ticket sales. Special recognition of campers at the game enhances the experience for the participant and the parents. Every positive interaction creates a more powerful bond with the team. In this way, youth camps would seem to be a powerful and efficient tool for long-term fan development.

So . . . is it player development? Social development? Fan development? You decide.

References

http://tnbabasketball.com/programs/cavaliers

www.nba.com/cavaliers/community

www.nba.com/cavaliers/kids/cavs_youth_camps.html

American children to see the fallacy in this argument. Far more people play or have played soccer than have played football, yet there is no comparison in the interest and consumption of the two sports—football is one of the most popular sports in terms of attendance and viewership in the United States. Soccer is not even close.

Promoting participation sport, then, is similar to promoting spectator sport in the overall use of advertising, public relations, community relations, and social media. However, they way in which each is used differs dramatically from the ways each is used for entertainment sport. Rather than relying on a professionally produced advertising campaign that integrates television, print, and radio ads, sport participation programs may instead rely on the word-of-mouth generated by participants and flyers distributed in the community. Public relations also occur on a reduced scale. Local sport clubs benefit by creating relationships with local media, rather than regional or national media. News releases and story ideas may focus on the community or human-interest side of participation. Coverage of participation events can be included in the community events calendar of the local paper and relevant websites. Even social media are typically focused more locally or regionally than nationally or internationally. In short, participant sport organizations focus on promotions that share the same label as the promotions used by major entertainment sport providers; yet the actual tasks are significantly different.

This is also true of marketing focused on product distribution (aka: place). Distributing the final product to the consumer is the final element of the marketing mix. Whereas sport products such as sporting goods are produced in a factory and then transported to distributors, then retailers, and finally are purchased by the end consumer, sport services are produced and consumed at the same time (11). With the exception of delayed media broadcasts and DVDs, nearly all sport services fit this mold. As a result, the place of production—stadium, field, court, etc.—is also the distribution channel. Not surprisingly, the key elements that consumers of entertainment sport use to evaluate place are very different from those used to evaluate the delivery sites of participation sport. Spectators at entertainment sport contests evaluate the experience in terms of the sportscape—the elements of the facility and its employees that provide comfort and ease of use (15). These include such elements as signage, seat comfort, sight lines, refreshments, parking, aesthetics, and customer service. The more one pays for a sport spectator experience, the higher are one's expectations for comfort, convenience, and customer service.

While increasingly luxurious spectator experiences are becoming more common, television coverage of professional, college, and even some high school sport is raising the expectations for even non-elite sport participants. Although participation sport is produced and delivered for a different purpose than entertainment sport, athletes are beginning to expect facilities that mimic those of major entertainment sport. This has spawned a new wave of facility design, such as ESPN's Wide World of Sports complex in Orlando, Florida. Here, amateur players can play on and in facilities built to mimic iconic entertainment sport facilities (3). Still, the focus of participants remains on the playing fields and courts rather than on the seating areas, concessions, and customer service elements of the facility.

At least on the surface, marketing sport seems consistent. It is necessary to design appropriate products and service to appeal to target markets. Those products and services must be priced to stimulate purchase. Promotions are designed to communicate messages intended to generate awareness, interest, and ultimately purchase. The delivery system (the place/facility) should create satisfaction and stimulate repeat purchase. These tasks are essential for both entertainment and participation sport. However, the materials needed to implement these tasks and the relative focus on each element varies dramatically. Differences in mission, objectives, and financial standing play an important role in the focus and ability to market and manage sport organizations for participation and entertainment, respectively.

Finance

All sport organizations rely on sound financial management to sustain themselves. However, there are distinct differences in the financial goals and strategies of sport organizations as a function of their sector. The majority of entertainment-based sport organizations are for-profit businesses. The purpose of these organizations is to maximize owners' equity—that is, to make a profit for the owners of the business. Consequently, the major task in managing a for-profit business is to build revenues while minimizing expenditures. Although no business wants to lose money, the goals of not-for-profit sport organizations are less about maximizing revenue than about service-to-mission. Indeed, this is the key difference between for-profit and not-for-profit organizations. For example, many youth sport programs are created for the purpose of providing sport opportunities to young people. Costs are kept low to allow children in low-income families to access sports activities. In this case, sponsorships may used to offset costs rather than to enhance the organization's the bottom line.

Two things are important to note. First, not-for-profit businesses are allowed to make money. Once the organization breaks even, further revenues are used to grow and sustain the organization. In other words any financial surplus is required (by law) to further the organization's service to its mission. Second, most (but not all) entertainment sport is for-profit, just as the majority of participation sport organizations are not-for-profit. However, participation sport is also provided on a for-profit basis, and entertainment sport can be delivered via a not-for-profit organization. For example, national governing bodies, such as the United States Tennis Association or USA Volleyball provide both elite sport competitions designed for a spectator audience, as well as participation opportunities for grassroots participation; both are not-for-profit organizations. Further, there are increasing numbers of youth sport providers incorporated as for-profit businesses. These distinctions do not neatly divide into participation and entertainment sport businesses, rather, they point to another key difference in the way sport organizations raise revenue.

Fundraising is a critical component of revenue generation strategies for not-for-profit sport organizations. Youth sport organizations hold fundraisers to send their teams to regional and national competitions; high school booster clubs solicit donations to buy uniforms; college athletics programs seek donations for facility improvements; and foundations seek to raise funds to provide programs to needy participants. The funds may be used for a variety of purposes, and the fundraising strategies may range from the sale of candy bars at the field to soliciting millions of dollars from donors, but fundraising is a central task for managers of not-for-profit sport organizations. For-profit sport organizations raise revenue in other ways—typically through ticket sales, media rights, sponsorships, and the sale of licensed products (12). Interestingly, revenue generation, including fundraising, requires skill in selling. It is only the object of the sale that changes.

Size and Scope

The final distinction between organizations delivering participation sport and those delivering entertainment sport is the size and scope of the organizations. As with the preceding discussion of differences, there is a great deal of variety in the size and scope of sport organizations both within and across categories. However, the size and scope of major entertainment sport businesses tends to be fairly large. As a result, jobs in entertainment sport are often more narrowly defined by functional area. For example, an NCAA Division I athletics program typically has jobs in event management, marketing, sponsorship procurement, development (i.e., fundraising), sports information, compliance, and a host of other areas. Professional sport teams hire in areas such as accounting, community relations, marketing, sales, player development, and operations. These organizations are large and support a highly differentiated mix of staff members.

It is also the case that large, national participation sport organizations such as the Boys and Girls Clubs of America or Lifetime Fitness have a similarly large and differentiated staff. However, most participation sport organizations are smaller in size and in scope. Jobs in these organizations tend to cross functional lines and require skills to plan and implement a wide variety of tasks, activities, and programs. For example, the Marketing Director of USA Football was responsible for overseeing the strategic marketing for the organization, obtaining sponsorships for the International Bowl and other events, entertaining visiting dignitaries, setting up signage at events, and assisting with event operations. Smaller organizations may combine tasks such as volunteer recruitment, website design, registration, fundraising, and even coaching or officiating.

USING SPORT

The previous section discussed the most recognizable parts of the sport industry—the delivery systems for sport. Sport managers take a direct and primary role in planning, implementation, and evaluation of sport delivery systems, programs, and activities, whether for entertainment or participation. Yet, sport managers are also needed to assist businesses, service providers, and government agencies whose primary purpose is not to provide sport, but to make use of sport. These organizations work with sport providers to incorporate sport into broader portfolios for economic development or social change.

Economic Development

The vast majority of sport organizations rely on some contribution from public (government) funds. Professional teams often play in facilities that were built using public monies, or in facilities that are government owned, but leased to them below market rates. Many college stadia use land that has a market value far beyond what the stadium generates. Sport events, ranging from running events to the Olympic Games, rely on public services (e.g., police, roads, sanitation) that are often provided at rates below their costs to the taxpayer. Similarly, participative sport programs often use facilities that are tax supported and may even rely on some personnel who are public employees.

Why would governments choose to invest in sport? After all, the investment requires tax revenues to sustain. The three most common arguments in support of government investment are (a) sport is good for the economy because it helps to attract other industry to the city, (b) sport retains a strong workforce (which is attractive to industry) by adding to the quality of life that residents obtain, and (c) sport draws tourists whose spending adds to the wealth of the local economy. Although these arguments continue to be advocated, the research evidence suggests that none of these benefits derives from sport per se, but depends on the ways that sport is designed, managed, and marketed.

Since sport (even for-profit entertainment sport) has come to rely so heavily on public investments, there is increasing interest in the means to manage sport in order to optimize its contribution to the local economy. Consequently, professional sport teams have increasingly found it useful to partner with their local convention-and-visitors bureau to package their games with other local attractions in order to entice tourists to come, stay, and spend in the local area. Many popular sports events—whether participation events (such as a marathon on a triathlon) or entertainment events (such as the Super Bowl or World Series)—do the same. Thus, effective management of sport increasingly requires the manager to understand the relationship between sport and tourism, and then to seek, use, and maintain effective partnerships with non-sport sectors of the economy, especially those having to do with tourism (hotels, restaurants, attractions, convention-and-visitors bureaus).

Participation-based sport programs less frequently partner with tourism organizations in order to enhance their economic impact. However, participation-based sport facilities and programs have been shown to enhance the desirability of communities with flow-on benefits for property values and stability of the local workforce (10). That is one reason communities often provide sport amenities (such as swimming pools, golf courses, tennis courts, and marinas), and typically offer sport programs, particularly through their parks-and-recreation programs. Consequently, a great deal of sport participation opportunities are provided directly or in partnership with local and county governments, with the result that there is a huge public sector demand for sport managers who understand the economic development value of appropriately designed sport participation opportunities.

The economic value of sport has created an entirely new sector of sport management—sports commissions. These are organizations that typically operate as private not-for-profit organizations at city or county level, although statewide sports commissions are beginning to emerge (in Florida and Delaware, for example). Nearly all large cities and counties in the United States have a sports commission. Although sports commissions vary in their design and responsibilities, they share the common objective of using sport to enhance the economy. They have been sufficiently successful at driving economic activity through sport that they are often supported by local businesses and/or through public subsidy. Sports commissions require employees who have a deep understanding of the ways sport can build the economy of the community in which it is offered, particularly by stimulating tourism.

Although, sports commissions typically seek to attract sports events to their community or region, and then to use those events to attract tourists, they may have other responsibilities. Some also work with local schools, universities, and/or parks-and-recreation to enhance sport programming and sport facilities. The extent of a sports commission's endeavors depends on its mandate, the interests of the partners who provide its funding, and the local vision for sport's place in economic development. See the next case study.

CASE STUDY: San Antonio Sports: Transforming a Community through Sport

San Antonio Sports, formed in 1984 as the San Antonio Sports Foundation, is a nonprofit sports commission created to bid on premier amateur athletic events. It has been very successful in attracting major events to San Antonio, beginning with the 1989 AAU Junior Olympics. Since that time, San Antonio Sports has hosted the 1993 U.S. Olympic Festival, six NCAA National Championships (three Men's Final Fours, two Women's Final Fours, and one Division I Women's Volleyball), the Rock 'n' Roll San Antonio Marathon and ½ Marathon, the TAAF Games of Texas, All Can Ski (the largest waterskiing clinic for people with physical disabilities in the United States), and the Big 12 Women's Soccer Championship. San Antonio has benefited from hosting these events, which have had an estimated economic impact of $446 million over the past two decades. The NCAA has designated San Antonio as a Championship City—a designation that recognizes its quality as a host city, as well as its ability to successfully host quality events in quality facilities.

Like the majority of sports commissions, San Antonio Sports has strong ties to the Chamber of Commerce, local government, and local business. Unlike most sports commissions, San Antonio Sports has a vision beyond economic impact, which includes a commitment to provide sports and fitness programs that inspire children and their families to live active, healthy lives and a responsibility to build and maintain facilities to support a sporting lifestyle. With a mission to "transform our community through the power of sport," San Antonio Sport actively pursues a joint vision—one that integrates economic and social development through events, health lifestyle, and tourism. This is reflected in its vision statement that reads: "To have healthy kids, places to play and events that impact."

San Antonio Sports has programs in 290 elementary schools and provides programs for the entire family, such as the Fit Family Challenge, a series of family-friendly activities across the community in which families participate and track their activities throughout a 12-week summer program. The Challenge includes activities such as the K Love Summer Fun Day that provides families with the chance to play soccer with the Scorpions (the local pro club), and participate in Zumba, nature hikes, a bicycle rodeo, and hamster ball races. School programs include the ING Kids Rock Marathon training program and Go!Kids Challenge. San Antonio Sports i Play afterschool program provides coaches, equipment, nutrition, and life lessons to inner-city children while introducing them fundamental sport skills. In this way, San Antonio Sports affects the lives of over 185,000 youth each year.

San Antonio Sports recognizes the interrelationship of elite and mass participation sport and the difficulties inherent in creating elites from a mass participation base. It is one of only seven cities selected by the United States Olympic Committee as a site for a Community Olympic Development Program. Through this program, San Antonio provides sports programs in fencing and diving to assist talented young people to become candidates for college scholarships, national, and Olympic teams. Core to this program are highly educated and experienced coaches, year-round training in sport-specific skills and conditioning, and a supportive environment. In many ways, this intermediary program bridges the link between the mass participation focus of San Antonio's participation-based events, and its elite sport focus represented by the major entertainment events hosted in the city.

The full range of sport opportunities that make up the offerings of San Antonio Sports build from three key requirements: funding, human resources, and community support. Not surprisingly, the three are highly interrelated. San Antonio Sports is a model organization in all three respects. The organization uses events such as the Annual San Antonio Sports Hall of Fame dinner (and silent auction) to raise funds to support its programs and services. This event, like all events run by San Antonio Sports, provides sponsorship opportunities for local businesses. Further funds are raised through sponsorship of the organization itself; through the sale of individual, business, and corporate memberships in the organization; and via donations. Membership provides individuals and businesses of all sizes with the chance to show their commitment to "implement innovative youth sports and fitness programs and attract major economic-generating sporting events to San Antonio."

The sheer number of events and programs supported by San Antonio Sports require significant community support. Support in the form of volunteer hours assists in two ways. First and most obvious, volunteers make most events feasible by providing inexpensive labor at the event, as well as before and after the event. Second, the skills, experience, and expertise of the volunteer force in San Antonio are continually being developed. This is a huge benefit for the community, which can then make good use of this expertise for local events and sport program implementation, but it also significantly strengthens the city's bid for major events. This is a win/win situation for the volunteers (and the community), who gain valuable skills, and the events that are able to take advantage of the constantly improving human resources in San Antonio.

Volunteers, members, and sponsoring organizations are the most obvious forms of community support enabling the success of San Antonio Sports. However, broader community support is invaluable to a successful event bid, as well as the success of local programming. The broader remit of San Antonio Sports assists to create a groundswell of community support. Sports commissions that focus only on high-profile entertainment sport events can be accused of catering to elites. These events are often priced out of the reach of many residents. Although San Antonio plays host to many such events, it also provides programs and events that are accessible and appealing to nearly all sectors of the city.

In summary, San Antonio Sports is a model sports commission. It has been successful in attracting events of all kinds to the city, with economic impact nearing half a billion dollars over the past 29 years. At the same time, the organization has had significant impact on the lives of its citizens, particularly its youth, through participation-based programming. It has been recognized for its excellence by the NCAA (i.e., Championship City status), and by the USOC (i.e., site for Community Olympic Development Program). Notably, San Antonio Sports has accomplished this through a blend of entertainment and participation sport programs and events.

Social Change

Social entrepreneurs and social change agents are increasingly turning to sport as a way to affect social change in individuals, communities, and society (6). Labeled "sport-for-development," organizations are seeking to harness the power of sport to make a positive impact in people's lives (see sidebar on the *First Tee* for an example). These organizations provide sport programs with one or more of the following objectives: (a) to provide sport to underserved or at-risk populations; (b) to substitute sport activities for antisocial behaviors such as substance abuse, violence, or destruction of property; and/or (c) to use sport as a hook to interest participants in a program that also provides social welfare services such as job training, reading, or other life skills (6, 9). The overarching objective of these programs is to enhance personal and/or community development. Sport is not the end goal; it is used as a tool to change social conditions for the better. Consequently, these programs do not look like traditional sport programs, nor can they be managed like traditional programs.

Consider the key management functions discussed in the first half of this chapter. The core management functions remain, yet new objectives alter the planning, organizing, and evaluation of staff, programs, and activities. The human resources needed to implement sport-for-development programs require a different skill set than their traditional sport counterparts. Coaches, for example, must provide sport training, but must also understand the overarching issues facing participants and support their overall development, not just their development as an athlete. That may require coaches to become mentors in life skills, to assist immigrants to adapt to their new country, or to enable players from groups that do not normally get along (e.g., from ethnic or religious groups that are in conflict) to develop productive social relationships. Coaches and administrators may also need to work in partnership with professionals from other fields in order to deliver on a sport program's social mission. In many programs, sport managers hire social workers, educators, or even substance abuse counselors as adjunct components of their program. Clearly, the shift in mission also creates a shift in training, supervision, and evaluation of staff. Yet these organizations are still part of the sport delivery system. Consequently, managers have an obligation to provide quality sport and to coordinate with traditional sport organizations within the overall sport system.

Marketing sport-for-development organizations is similar to marketing other sport organizations. Products and services are designed to meet the needs of participants. Promotions are created and implemented to increase awareness of programs and activities, develop interest, and move people to take action. The distribution system is developed to deliver programs that are convenient and enhance satisfaction. Pricing is developed

---

Sidebar Sport for Social Development: The *First Tee*

The *First Tee* is an example of a successful sport-for-development program with chapters across the globe. It is a private, not-for-profit organization that provides youth ages 5 to 18 with golf instruction combined with life skills by instilling the values inherent in the game of golf. The purpose of the program is to prepare young people for success in school, college, and life. It is a prime example of a sport development program that seeks to use the sport context to teach skills beyond the sport itself. Although the program is open to all, many chapters seek to provide the golf experience to children who would not normally have access to golf, for example, children from low-income families and/or minorities.

The curriculum focuses on five core life skills: (a) how to manage emotions, (b) how to set goals, (c) how to resolve conflicts, (d) how to introduce themselves, and (e) how to communicate with others. Each of these is incorporated into lessons delivered by mentors throughout the program. Further, participants are exposed to nine core values: honesty, integrity, sportsmanship, respect, confidence, responsibility, perseverance, courtesy, and judgment. These values are part of the game of golf and are, consequently, reinforced through participation in the game and interactions with mentors and other participants. The program has been successful, reporting the following impacts on participants' lives:

- Participants unanimously identified school as a setting in which they transferred life skills.
- 73% reported high confidence in their ability to do well academically.
- 82% felt confident in their social skills with peers.
- 57% credited the First Tee for their meeting-and-greeting skills.
- 52% credited the program for their ability to appreciate diversity.

The *First Tee* program has over 700 active programs building youth who are successful on the golf course and in life.

References

www.thefirsttee.org/club/scripts/section/section.asp?GRP=17346&NS=WWD
Weiss, M., First Tee impact report. Saint Augustine, FL: World Golf Foundation, 2010.

---

to facilitate revenue generation. However, the primary target market for these activities is not program participants. Rather, marketing efforts focus on revenue generation necessary to sustain the program's mission, including adjunct activities that support the mission. The marketing focus shifts to donors, sponsors, and granting organizations such as government and foundations. Similarly, marketing communications are necessary to recruit and retain volunteers to implement many of the program components. In short, marketing remains a way to generate revenue for the organization, but the targets of the marketing strategies and tactics add a focus on funding bodies and individual donors. As these sport organizations operate in the not-for-profit sector, managers typically devote a significant proportion of their time to fundraising.

ANCILLARY SPORT SERVICES

Organizations that use sport are varied in their mission and objectives, as well as the managerial focus required to grow and sustain their business. They are even more interdependent than traditional sport organizations, relying on participation sport organizations as well as high-profile events and media-friendly leagues and competitions. As the sport industry has grown to encompass participation sport, entertainment sport, economic development through sport, and sport for social change, a plethora of ancillary sport services has emerged to support and extend the business of sport.

Ancillary sport services offer a rich and diverse array of products and services to support existing sport offerings or extend those offerings for further profit. Some businesses have grown around the demand for sport participation, while others have grown as a function of the explosion of entertainment sport. Others highlight interrelationships between the two. Media coverage of sport has created demand for products and services among sport participants for clothing, equipment, sports drinks, and other goods that allow participants to imitate professional athletes. Entrepreneurs have capitalized on participants' and fans' aspirations by selling licensed products such as replica jerseys and key rings bearing a team or league logo, building facilities that re-create iconic ballparks, stadia, and arenas, and even providing adults with fantasy camp experiences that are a cross between a vacation and training camp. These latter businesses succeed by blurring the line between participation and entertainment sport. They provide experiences that allow average (or even well below average) participants to get a brief glimpse of what it is like to be a professional athlete playing with the best equipment, wearing a professional uniform, playing in facilities used by the pros, and even competing with or against a favorite professional athlete. Businesses offering ancillary services like these require managers and marketers who can identify new licensed product opportunities, and negotiate with manufacturers to provide them, or who can design new sport experiences that will appeal to the imagination of sport fans.

Similarly, businesses use sport and athletes in their advertising and marketing campaigns to take advantage of the positive feelings participants associate with sport, or the perceived expertise of professional and elite athletes. The use of sport celebrity endorsers is one of many opportunities often handled for athletes by a sports agent. Legal and financial services along with athlete representation by an agent are significant components of the ancillary services that have become integral to the entertainment sport system. Sports agents must be able to help athletes manage themselves as a commercial product. That requires agents to be adept not merely at negotiating contracts for athletes, but also at helping athletes keep their schedules and finances in order.

Sponsorship is a multibillion-dollar industry that, like advertising, seeks to capitalize upon positive associations with athletes, teams, events, and sport organizations. Sponsors may seek to associate with large, entertainment sport organizations and events that provide media coverage and exposure to a mass audience. Alternatively, sponsors may seek to associate themselves with local, amateur sport events, teams, and organizations. The choice is largely a function of the target market they are trying to reach and the objective of the sponsorship. Many professional athletes and teams are now able to offer sponsors both types of sponsorship—association with a large, mediated, entertainment sport *and* association with a community sport event or organization associated with the professional team's community relations department. In this way, the sponsor can meet multiple objectives through a single sponsorship. Many sport organizations, particularly large teams and events, have sponsorship specialists on their staff. Many non-sport businesses also employ sponsorship specialists to manage their sponsorship portfolios.

Sponsorship is only one of several ancillary businesses that links entertainment and participation sport. Training and educational services position themselves to help participants "make it to the next level" of their sport. The next level could be professional sport, collegiate sport, high school sport, or even a club travel team. Numerous sport services assist athletes with their physiological training, provide nutritional counseling, improve specific sport-related skills, provide parents of players with assistance creating highlight films and strategies to obtain college scholarships, work to obtain and manage media attention, and teach leadership skills. If there is a perception that improving a skill, knowledge, or ability will help an athlete who aspires to perform at a higher level, then a business has been (or will be) created to assist athletes to acquire the skill, knowledge, or ability. These businesses offer an array of career opportunities to sport managers who have the necessary vision and skills.

SUMMARY

It is common to think that sport management is a field focused on the management and marketing of entertainment sport. Entertainment sport is, like the tip of an iceberg, the most visible aspect of the sport industry. However, the vast majority of sport management jobs are not in entertainment sport contexts.

Sport managers work in numerous capacities across a wide array of organizations. These organizations operate in the government, private for-profit, and private not-for-profit sectors. Each requires skills in management, marketing, and finance. Yet each operates under a different context and with different contingencies. Consequently, the tasks within each functional area vary by organization type and location. An understanding of the ways in which these differences manifest, the ability to recognize customer needs, and a capacity to build partnerships with other elements of the system are vital for developing a career in sport management.

REFERENCES

1. "London 2012: Olympics success down to 70,000 volunteers." *The Independent.* (2012, 10 August). Retrieved June 5, 2013 from: www.independent.co.uk/sport/olympics/news/london-2012-olympics-success-down-to-70000-volunteers-8030867.html

2. Cialdini, R. B., R. J. Borden, A. Thorne, M. R. Walker, S. Freeman, and L. R. Sloan, "Basking in reflected glory: Three (football) field studies." *Journal of Personality and Social Psychology,* 34(3)(1976): 366–375.

3. ESPN. (2013). "The complex." Retrieved June 5, 2013 from http://espnwwos.disney.go.com/complex

4. Etoe, C. (2010, 6 February). *Attendance doubles as Mansfield fans pay what they want.* BBC. Retrieved June 5 from http://news.bbc.co.uk/sport2/hi/football/teams/m/mansfield_town/8502204.stm

5. Green, B.C., "Building sport programs to optimize athlete recruitment, retention, & transition: Toward a normative theory of sport development." *Journal of Sport Management* 19(2005): 233–253.

6. Green, B.C., "Sport as an agent for social and personal change." In *Management of sport development,* V. Girginov, ed. Oxford, UK: Elsevier, 2008, pp. 129–146.

7. Green, B.C., and L. Chalip, L. "Sport volunteers: A research agenda and applications." *Sport Marketing Quarterly* 7(2)(1998): 14–23.

8. Kelso, P., "London 2012 Olympics: Sport England claim participation surge despite missing targets." *The Telegraph* (2012, June 23). Retrieved June 5, 2013, from www.telegraph.co.uk/sport/olympics/news/9349173/London-2012-Olympics-Sport-England-claim-participation-surge-despite-missing-targets.html

9. Lyris, A., and J. Welty-Peachey, "Integrating sport-for-development theory and praxis." *Sport Management Review* 14(2010): 311–326.

10. Philips, P. L., *Developing with Recreational Amenities: Golf, Tennis, Skiing, Marinas.* Washington, DC: Urban Land Institute, 1986.

11. Shank, M., *Sports Marketing: A Strategic Perspective,* 3rd ed. Upper Saddle River, NJ: Prentice Hall, 2004.

12. SI.com. (2013). *Inside the NFL's money machine.* Retrieved June 5, 2013, from http://sportsillustrated.cnn.com/multimedia/photo_gallery/1103/nfl-inside-money-machine/content.1.html

13. Taylor, T., A. Doherty, and P. McGraw, *Managing People in Sport Organizations: A Strategic Human Resource Approach.* Oxford, UK: Butterworth-Heinemann, 2008.

14. Wakefield, K., *Team Sports Marketing.* Burlington, MA: Elsevier, 2007.

15. Wakefield, K. L., and H. J. Sloan, "The effects of team loyalty and selected stadium factors on spectator attendance." *Journal of Sport Management* 9(2)(1995): 153–172.

16. Wann, D.L., M. P. Schrader, and A. M. Wilson, "Sport fan motivation: Questionnaire validation, comparisons by sport, and relationship to athletic motivation." *Journal of Sport Behavior* 22(1) (1999): 114–139.

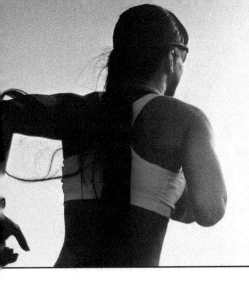

Chapter 21 ///

RECREATION AND LEISURE

OUTLINE

OBJECTIVES

1. Compare and contrast leisure and recreation.
2. Discuss the nine benefits of leisure and recreation.
3. List the three main services that leisure and recreation professionals provide.
4. Discuss the challenges that are facing the recreation and leisure field.
5. Discuss the eight different sponsoring agencies of the leisure service delivery system.

Defining *leisure* and *recreation* is often a difficult task. The Greek philosopher Aristotle considered leisure as occurring at various levels, defined as amusement, recreation, and contemplation. Viewed this way, recreation may be considered some form of activity that occurs during leisure, therefore becoming a subset of it. Abraham Maslow's hierarchy of human needs model claims that people have to take care of life's essentials before having access to leisure. Leisure, then, is simply time free from life's obligations (Figure 21.1).

There is a distinct difference between recreation and leisure. Recreation is more narrowly construed and is considered any discretionary activity that has socially redeeming qualities. This would imply, for example, that the phrase "recreational drug use" is not a correct usage of the term. Illicit drug use and abusing gambling and alcohol, for example, would not fall into the category of recreation. Therefore, for an activity to be considered recreation it must conform to certain moral and social norms.

A good starting point then for defining recreation is that it is voluntary participation in leisure activities that are meaningful and enjoyable for the person thus engaged. There are a wide variety of activities that can be defined as recreation and some that we might find hard to place in that category. Can you name a few?

Leisure is a broader term. To define leisure it is important to consider other aspects of life as those pieces of the 24-hour pie when leisure is not happening. There are constraints on leisure time with most agreeing that these limitations include at a minimum work time and family time. Constraints are things that restrict our ability to enter into leisure. Leisure is accomplished in unobligated time, therefore, leisure is that period of time when an individual has a choice in how to spend it.

Leisure does not include time spent doing activities of necessity (hygienic tasks, driving) or those activities centered on work or school. While we are doing such tasks we are not at leisure and are certainly not recreating. Leisure, then, is that time when we are not centered on things that are obligatory. In the modern age it seems obvious that leisure time has expanded because necessities such as gathering food have become easy. However, other factors, such as economic forces (requiring people to work two jobs) or a compulsive drive to multitask, can be seen as stealing leisure time, leading to the notion that what we perceive as freedom has been reduced.

This chapter provides an overview of the field of recreation and leisure and examines employment opportunities and professional issues and challenges. Recreation and leisure are often overlooked when studying kinesiology. This is unfortunate, because it can be said that we recreate best when it is expressed through our ability to move.

THE PROFESSION OF RECREATION AND LEISURE: AN OVERVIEW

The recreation professional often gets stereotyped as a party planner and an individual who is only in it to have fun. However, fun is an important part of recreation and leisure. While there are opportunities to have a good

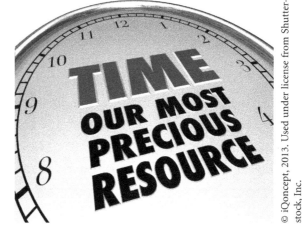

Figure 21.1. *Time is an important commodity. Recreation and leisure professionals are aware that consumers trust them with this valuable resource by providing experiences to fill their leisure hours.*

© iQoncept, 2013. Used under license from Shutterstock, Inc.

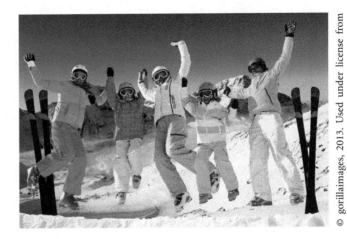

Figure 21.2. *Family vacations are recreational experiences that create lifelong memories.*

time while on the job, these fields require work and have their own distinct difficulties. Therefore, viewing fun as the only work requirement in recreation and leisure greatly underplays what these professionals provide to the community.

What Do Recreation and Leisure Professionals Do?

Think about the best memories of your life. Many of these memories come from experiences taking part in leisure and recreation. Whether it was traveling with family on a vacation or enjoying the company of friends at a park, the wide spectrum of experiences received is often the work of recreation professionals. These individuals are often not seen, but they are at work to create the memories most of us enjoy (Figure 21.2). Other benefits are also experienced from their work. This section presents three main services that recreation and leisure professionals plan and implement and the benefits provided by these services.

Programs

Programs are planned opportunities for leisure and recreation to occur. The activities offered to a community over a period of time may be viewed in different categories—arts and crafts, aquatics, athletics, social, outdoors/nature, fitness, educational, and self-help (Figure 21.3). The key to a good community recreation department is to offer a variety of programs to meet the interests and needs of the people.

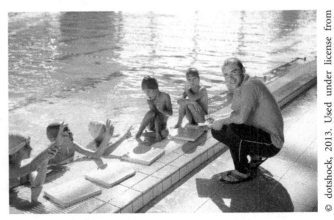

Figure 21.3. *Recreation programs, such as this youth aquatics program, have lasting impacts on the participants.*

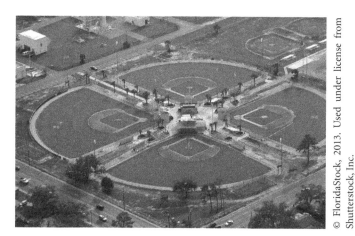

Figure 21.4. *Recreational professionals manage facilities and program activities that occur there. This facility could handle programs as well as special events to meet the needs of the consumer.*

Facilities

It is important to offer facilities where recreation can occur. Facilities refer to the locations and venues where people go to enjoy recreational experiences. They may include gymnasiums, pools, parks, amphitheaters, gardens, trails, arenas, and playgrounds just to name a few (Figure 21.4). Recreation professionals manage these facilities and the employees that work in them to make sure they provide a quality experience to participants.

Special Events

Special events are similar to programs, but usually more intensive. Whereas a program occurs over a longer period of time (six weeks), a special event occurs during a one day period or perhaps over several days.

Benefits of Recreation and Leisure

As mentioned previously just looking at recreation and leisure as fun greatly undersells the role they play. Nine benefits are discussed here.

Physical

Physical benefits refer to the changes in physical fitness that can occur because of participation in recreation programs and activities (Figure 21.6). Improvement can occur in the health-related components of fitness (cardiovascular endurance, muscular strength and endurance, flexibility, and body composition) and also in skills related fitness (speed, power, coordination, balance, reaction time, and agility).

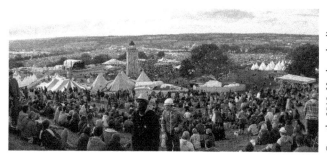

Figure 21.5. *Special events may take many different forms. This picture shows a music and performing arts festival.*

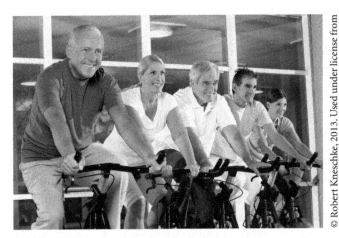

Figure 21.6. *People of all ages enjoy the fitness benefits of participating in exercise-based recreation programs.*

Social

The opportunity to meet new people and those from different backgrounds and ethnicities are social benefits recreation programs offer. Participation in recreational activities breaks down stereotypes by exposing people to others. Ask yourself how many friends you made playing sports or participating in a summer camp (Figure 21.7).

Educational

Recreation and leisure provide participants an opportunity to learn new skills and gain new knowledge. Whether it is developing leadership skills and sportsmanship through an athletic program or learning the different types of edible plants through a scouting program, recreation provides participants an additional way to learn rather than in the formal school setting. Learning through recreational experiences provides practical learning that is not based on grades and written tests.

Psychological

Participation in recreation can lead to psychological benefits (increased self-esteem, self-efficacy, and self-identity). Learning new skills assists in building feelings of worthiness and improving one's attitude toward self. Self-efficacy refers to a person's ability to work toward and achieve goals. Recreation programs are often challenging. When program goals are achieved self-efficacy is enhanced. Through the challenges and opportunities provided in recreation people get to know themselves better, which builds self-concept.

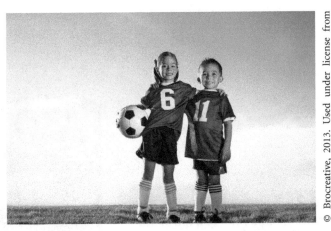

Figure 21.7. *Recreational sport programs offer children the opportunity to learn socialization skills.*

Emotional

Emotional benefits refer to those that reduce depression, assist with relaxation, and reduce stress. Participating in active forms of recreation can reduce levels of depression. Other forms of recreation such as reading a book, taking a walk in a park, or socializing with friends can be used as a means of relaxation and stress reduction.

Economic

Recreation can impact the finances of an individual, the community, and private businesses. An individual can be economically impacted by recreation employment in the field. Recreation employees many people in each community across the country and the world. The community is impacted by recreation through tax dollars generated. An additional trend that affects the local economy is sport tourism. Communities are capitalizing by offering tournaments and sporting events to draw a large number of participants and spectators to the area where they spend money on hotel rooms, meals, and other amenities. Private businesses such as commercial recreation providers offer recreation experiences for a profit. This profit supports not only the owner of the business, but the employees and the community through taxes. An area of particular interest is the high cost of health care. Recreation can be a proactive way to reduce these costs by offering incentives to business owners and individuals that encourage participation in exercise programs.

Spiritual

The spiritual benefits are the most abstract of the benefits of recreation. The spiritual benefits refer to the capacity for exhibiting moral values, compassion, and respect for others and for the environment. Spiritual recreation helps participants develop a sense of order and purpose in life as well as behaving responsibly. This development can occur through outdoor recreation experiences. Communing with nature is often viewed as a religious experience in which the participant learns about one's place and role in the world (Figure 21.8). Leisure and recreation often give individuals over to a better understanding of themselves and they are often better able to express themselves more fully (7).

Environmental

Programs in recreation and leisure help increase participants' understanding of stewardship and preservation, public involvement in environmental issues, and protection of ecosystems (Figure 21.9). For example, nonprofit organizations such as Ducks Unlimited work very hard to protect and conserve the natural habitats of ducks and other wildlife. The Sierra Club's purpose is to explore, enjoy, and protect the country's natural resources.

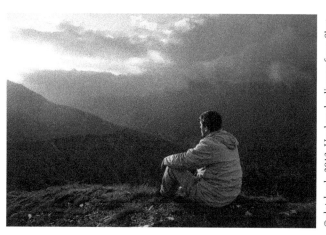

Figure 21.8. *Experiencing the beauty and wonder of nature can be a spiritual experience for people.*

© dotshock, 2013. Used under license from Shutterstock, Inc.

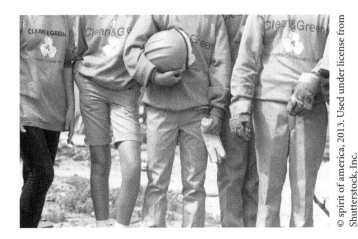

Figure 21.9. *People often come together for a cause like this Earth Day cleanup activity. Stewardship of the natural resources is an important benefit of recreation and leisure.*

Cultural

Through recreation programming it is possible to learn more about one's culture and the culture of others. Many communities have special events such as festivals that highlight diverse cultures within the community (Figure 21.10). For example, New Braunfels, Texas, offers WurstFest to highlight its German influences. Beaufort, South Carolina, offers the Gullah Festival to highlight Gullah culture. This provides an opportunity to teach locals and visitors about the local cultural, thus providing an identity to the local area.

LEISURE SERVICE DELIVERY SYSTEM

The leisure service delivery system is a network of community agencies and businesses providing their constituencies with leisure opportunities and experiences. These providers include the government, commercial enterprises, the military, universities, nonprofit agencies, therapeutic, corporations, and private entities. These are ways recreation and leisure programs are delivered to the public. One of the keys to developing a successful career in recreation and leisure is to find an agency with a philosophy that matches your value system.

Local, State, and Federal Government

Starting during the Great Depression, the government on all three levels took on more of a role in the provision of recreation. Recreation began to be seen as a service that needed to be provided by the government. The government on the local (city or county) level is the most likely of the three to offer direct services to the participant. The state and federal government main means to provide recreation is to offer the space for recreation to occur. State and federal governments manage lands and resources in the form of state and national parks and wildlife and national historic sites.

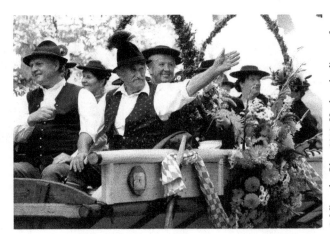

Figure 21.10. *German heritage is showcased in this Oktoberfest celebration.*

Opportunities in recreation abound in government agencies. Starting at the community level and advancing to the federal government, most recreation professionals can probably find a position within government. Examples of positions in the local government include programmers for sports, seniors, outdoors, youth, or fitness; facility managers; groundskeepers; and special events planners. State and federal government positions include park rangers, fish and game wardens, superintendents, and interpreters.

Fact about Government Recreation: The federal government manages approximately 636 million acres of land throughout the United States (3). These lands are managed by agencies such as the National Park Service, U.S. Forest Service, Bureau of Land Management, U.S. Fish and Wildlife, Bureau of Reclamation, Tennessee Valley Authority, and the U.S. Army Corps of Engineers. Each of these agencies has other purposes such as flood control, preservation, electricity production, logging, and mineral mining as their primary purposes. Recreation and leisure have evolved into a secondary purpose of these agencies.

Commercial Enterprises

Commercial enterprises refer to those providers of recreation that are offered for a profit. These businesses, unlike some providers of recreation, cannot rely on tax dollars to support them and also pay taxes based on the profits they make. A person interested in working in this realm of recreation is driven by the profit margin. The commercial recreation realm is the largest provider of recreation to the community. Examples of commercial recreation enterprises include bowling alleys, miniature golf courses, zip-lines, skating rinks, outdoor guides/outfitters, campgrounds, sporting good stores, professional sport teams, movie theaters, amusement parks, health clubs, and casinos (Figure 21.11).

Fact about Commercial Recreation: Commercial recreation has a large impact on the economy of the United States. One such example of this impact is outdoor recreation. The money spent by participants on equipment, experiences, vehicles, and travel add up quickly. According to the Outdoor Industry Association (2012), Americans spent $646 billion on outdoor recreation in 2010. Outdoor recreation also creates 6.1 million jobs and $80 billion in federal, state, and local tax revenue (6).

The Military

Each branch of the U.S. military offers recreation for their military personnel and families. It is commonly known as Morale, Welfare, and Recreation (MWR). Recreation is seen as being an important service in the military because it contributes to the readiness, productivity, morale, and quality of life for soldiers and their families. The MWR offers programs that include sports, aquatics, outdoor recreation, physical fitness, hobbies, arts and crafts, special events, and music. Military active service is not a requirement to work in military recreation.

Fact about Military Recreation: The military offers resorts called Armed Forces Recreation Centers (AFRC) in the United States and worldwide for servicemen and servicewomen to enjoy their vacation time. Shades of

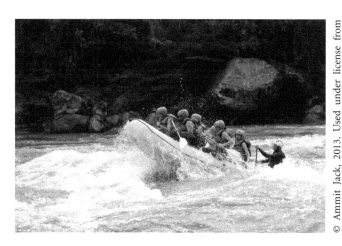

Figure 21.11. *Guiding tours, such as whitewater rapid excursions, for tourists and locals is one way that recreation professions make money using their skills and interests.*

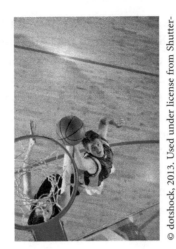

Figure 21.12.   *Intramural sports are often very popular on college campuses because they allow all students the opportunity to continue to play sports at a varying levels of competition.*

Green, the only one in the continental United States, provides military personnel a cost effective option for staying at the Disney World Resort in Florida. Another example is the Hale Koa Hotel in Hawaii. You can learn more about other AFRCs at www.armymwr.com/travel/recreationcenters.

Universities

Campus recreation is the provision of recreation for faculty, staff, and students at universities. Every university across the United States offers some form of recreation programming for its constituents. The purposes of campus recreation are to recruit and retain students, serve the personal needs of the constituents, and promote physical health. To accomplish these purposes campus recreation programming often falls into common categories such as intramural sports, sports clubs, fitness and wellness, facilities, outdoor recreation, and aquatics (Figure 21.12).

Fact about Campus Recreation: A recent study conducted by the National Intramural-Recreational Sports Association (NIRSA) showed that 174 colleges and universities across the United States planned for over $8 billion in recreation facility construction, expansion, or renovation through 2013 (5). The focus on growth and development of recreation facilities suggest that administrators of institutions of higher education see the significant role that campus recreation can play on their campuses.

Therapeutic

Recreation therapy is a means used by professionals that relies on activities and games to assist people with illnesses and disabilities gain new skills and restore skills that have been affected by an injury or illness (Figure 21.13). Professionals who work in this fieldwork in a variety of settings and with a wide variety of

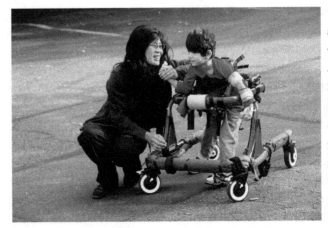

Figure 21.13.   *Therapeutic recreation enables people with disabilities opportunities to experience recreation. It also is used as a modality to improve the person's condition.*

illnesses and disabilities. The settings include hospitals, skilled nursing facilities, Special Olympics, local recreation departments, psychiatric facilities, and drug rehabilitation facilities. As these settings suggest, the illnesses and disabilities vary greatly. Some of the conditions that a person may work with in recreation therapy include developmental disorders, psychiatric conditions, addictions, physical disabilities, and amputations. Of the different providers in the leisure service delivery system, it is most beneficial for a professional working in therapeutic recreation to be certified.

Fact about Therapeutic Recreation: The Wounded Warrior Project (WWP) is a therapeutic recreation program serving veterans and service members who incurred physical or mental injury or illness because of their military service since September 11, 2001. Using recreation as a treatment modality the WWP assists participants to gain confidence and independence and adjust to life after injury. Activities such as adaptive sports and health and fitness training as well as a Soldiers Ride, which is a four-day cycling experience, are examples of some of the means used to reengage the wounded soldiers back to civilian life and maximize their independence (10).

Corporations

After World War II, companies and corporations began to look for ways to improve the often adversarial relationship between employers and employees. One of the ways that companies accomplished this was to offer recreation opportunities and experiences to their employees. Corporation- and company-sponsored recreation refers to recreation programs and services offered to employees and their families. Employers view recreation as offering several benefits such as promoting fitness and efficiency, decreasing health care costs, decreasing absenteeism and injuries, improving recruitment and retention of employees, improving the corporate image and community role to their companies and employee. Google and Nike have model programs and have built their companies' cultures on the concept of recreation.

Facts about Employee Recreation: Google offers its employees a wide variety of recreation programs and services, including massage, free beer and wine Fridays, free fitness classes and gyms, and organized intramural sports. Learn more about the benefits of working at Google by visiting www.cbsnews.com/8301-505266_162-57565097/inside-google-workplaces-from-perks-to-nap-pods.

Private

Private recreation is recreation services and experiences offered to members of an organization. While on the surface private membership recreation is similar to commercial recreation because an individual pays to belong to the organization and receives the benefits of membership. The major difference between the two is that anyone can go to a commercial recreation enterprise, while only members of the private organization can use their facilities and services. It is not unusual for members of a private membership organization to provide leadership in making administrative decisions. Many of these private recreation agencies are focused on a major recreation interest such as boating, sailing, hunting, tennis, golf, or skiing that is shared among the members. All of these agencies have a sense of exclusiveness in that there is an element of status in being a member of the agency.

Additional types of private-membership organizations have developed to serve individuals. Residence-connected clubs, vacation homes, and retirement communities are types of private organizations that have evolved in the past 50 years. Residence-connected clubs are tied to the growth of subdivisions in housing development. To gain an edge in selling houses, developers realized they needed to add amenities such as clubhouses, swimming pools, playgrounds, tennis courts, and golf courses to the subdivisions. Leaders and facility managers are hired by the subdivisions to manage and maintain the amenities. Vacation homes and time shares are other examples of private-membership agencies. Recreation services, amenities, and facilities are offered to members who own the homes. Retirement or age-segregated communities offer their members (residence) may different opportunities for recreation. These leisure villages include Sun City, Arizona, which was one of the first. This house development offers its residents seven community centers, seven swimming pools at each community center, 11 golf courses, two libraries, two bowling alleys, two lakes, and more than 350 social and civic clubs (4). Other developers have taken on a similar model.

Fact about Private Recreation: A trend that occurred in the United States was for country clubs and other private clubs to hand over their leadership to for-profit management companies. One such management company is ClubCorp, which owns 150 golf and country clubs, sports clubs, and alumni clubs in 23 states, the District of Columbia, and two foreign countries. These clubs have 350,000 members and employs 14,000 workers (1).

Nonprofit Agencies

A nonprofit recreation organization differs from other forms of recreation in that it has a public service orientation or mission. These agencies are focused on improving the lives of others and have a commitment to altruistic values. Altruism refers to putting aside one's personal needs and interests to serve others. Since these agencies have a public service focus and altruistic values, they are tax exempt. The agencies are further governed by a voluntary board which does not receive a financial gain from this service.

Nonprofit providers of recreation are very diverse and serve a variety of groups and missions. Some agencies have youth at their focus: Boy and Girl Scouts of America, Boys and Girls Clubs of America, Camp Fire USA, Big Brother Big Sisters, and 4-H Clubs (Figure 21.14). Other agencies are focused on promoting religious beliefs and instilling morals and values of religion into their participants: Young Men's Christian Association (YMCA), Catholic Youth Organization (CYO), Salvation Army, Jewish Community Centers (JCC). Many individual churches also use recreation as a means to reach people and teach these values as well as build fellowship among members. Agencies such Little League, Youth Basketball of America, United States Tennis Association, Young American Bowling Alliance, and Pop Warner Football are all nonprofit agencies that exist to promote youth sports and games. Additional nonprofit agencies are focused on conservation of natural resources and outdoor recreation: The Sierra Club, Ducks Unlimited, Wildlife Federation, and Outward Bound International.

Facts about Nonprofit Recreation: The term *nonprofit* often confuses people. Most students are at first not interested in working in the nonprofit sector because they think they cannot make money. In fact, people working in entry-level positions in this realm usually make a salary that is comparable to school teachers in the area (11). The nonprofit title refers to the agency as a whole. These organizations can be profitable. The issue is that the profits have to be put back into the organization, which usually means that the revenue generating programs pay for (or subsidize) the programs that are not making money or actually losing money. YMCAs commonly make money through their gym memberships and youth sport programs, but they use these profits to cover the losses incurred by afterschool programs, summer day camps, and community outreach.

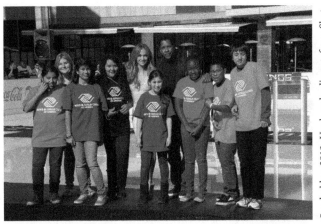

Figure 21.14.   *The Boys and Girls Clubs of America work with at-risk youth to help them achieve their fullest potential. Some celebrities lend their names and talents to help support these nonprofit organizations.*

© s_bukley, 2013. Used under license from Shutterstock, Inc.

PROFESSIONAL ISSUES IN RECREATION AND LEISURE

Funding

When the economy falters, many forms of recreation are hindered by lack of funding or revenue. For example, government-sponsored recreation feels the effects of a bad economy through a reduction in the tax base that supports the programs. People put off vacations and trips and other activities that rely on disposable income, so commercial recreation agencies feel the effects of the bad economy. Corporations are affected by a bad economy through reduction in sales and profits, so they cut their employee recreation programs.

Hours

Hours of work are mentioned here as a warning to people thinking about going into the field of recreation. The hours do not fit the traditional idea of an 8-hour workday. Recreation and leisure professionals must be willing to work when others want to take part in these activities. This means weekends and nights. It may also include holidays like Independence Day, Labor Day, and Memorial Day. While the job is very fulfilling and enjoyable, a young professional has to be prepared to work when others are playing.

Obesity Epidemic

A major issue confronting Americans is obesity. It is estimated that almost 68.8% of the American population is overweight and of those 35.7% are obese (2). One of the major causes of obesity is lack of physical activity. Recreation and leisure professionals have a role to play in the health care system rather than only its traditional participation as a social service agency.

Changes in Demographics

The United States has been going through a major demographic shift that will impact the recreation and leisure industry. The average age of citizens in the United States is increasing. It is projected that by 2025 there will be twice as many Americans 65 and above as there will be teenagers (4). Another change occurring is the increase in racial and ethnic diversity in the United States. In the past, the largest percentage of immigrants to the United States came from European countries. Now the largest percentage is from Mexico (8). Hispanics are expected to make up 30% of the total U.S. population by 2050 (4). A final demographic change that will impact the delivery of recreation and leisure services is the change in the American family. The traditional nuclear family of a father, a mother, and one or more children is reported to be just one-fifth (20%) of the total American households according to the 2010 U.S. Census (9). This becomes a particular area of importance because single-parent households are often challenged when recreation and leisure services are wanted or needed.

Influence of Technology

A final issue that will impact the delivery of recreation in the future will be technology. Information is literally at one's fingertips. Americans spend more time communicating and using media devices than any other activity (4). Communication has become easy and immediate. Participants can post comments on social media about programs, events, and experiences before they are even over. Word of mouth has taken on a whole new role in which telling one or two friends is now magnified to thousands.

Technology is also affecting how people participate in recreation. Improvements in equipment and resources have helped people enjoy forms of recreation that were not possible in the past. Changes in golf clubs such as larger head sizes and synthetic shafts have increased the size of the "sweet spot" of the club and increased the accuracy and distance the average player can hit the ball. Global Positioning Systems (GPS) have created activities such as geocaching and made knowledge of one's exact position in hiking more achievable.

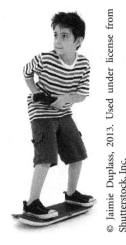

© Jaimie Duplass, 2013. Used under license from Shutterstock, Inc.

Figure 21.15.   *Exergaming uses physical skills and conditioning to promote success in the video games. In this example, the child is balancing and adjusting his weight on a skateboard to control the skateboard in the video game.*

Synthetic materials used for outdoor gear and clothing have made outdoor activities dryer, warmer (or cooler), and more enjoyable for individuals. The rapid growth and improvement of home gaming systems such as Xbox and Wii have impacted the way people enjoy their leisure time.

Exergaming, which is a combination of exercise and virtual gaming, is an example of how technology is impacting the recreation industry. In these types of activities, the participant has to move to actually play the video game (Figure 21.15). For example, to participant in a NASCAR racing game, the participants have to pedal stationary bikes to control the speed of their cars. Coastal Carolina University and the University of South Florida are two examples of universities that have exergaming rooms in their fitness centers.

SUMMARY

This chapter provided a brief overview of the field of recreation and leisure. The field of recreation and leisure serves a broad and diverse spectrum of constituencies and to do that a diverse array of programs, events, and facilities have to be offered. The nine benefits these programs, events, and facilities offer people were discussed. In addition, the chapter covered the eight providers of the leisure service delivery system. Based upon these eight providers the readers became aware of areas not only of service but employment if they decide to enter this profession. Finally, issues facing the profession were discussed to increase the awareness of readers to these challenges.

REFERENCES

1. ClubCorp. (2013). *About ClubCorp: Company profile*. Retrieved May 1, 2013, from www.clubcorp.com/About-ClubCorp/Company-Profile

2. Flegal, K. M., M. D. Carroll, B. K. Kit, and C. L. Ogden, "Prevalence of obesity and trends in the distribution of body mass index among U.S. adults, 1999-2010." *Journal of the American Medical Association* 307(5) (2012), 491–497.

3. Lipton, E., and C. Krauss. (2012, August 23). Giving reins to states over drilling. *New York Times*. Retrieved April 29, 2013, from www.nytimes.com/2012/08/24/us/romney-would-give-reins-to-states-on-drilling-on-federal-lands.html?_r=0

4. McLean, D. D. and A. R. Hurd, *Kraus' Recreation and Leisure in Modern Society*, 9th ed. Sudbury, MA: Jones & Bartlett.

5. National Intramural-Recreational Sports Association (2011). *NIRSA 2011 Outstanding Sports Facilities Awards*. Retrieved May 1, 2013, from www.nirsa.org/AM/Documents/about/awards/osf/OSF2011-WinnersBrochure_Final.pdf

6. Outdoor Industry Association, *The Outdoor Recreation Economy*. Boulder, CO: Outdoor Industry Association, 2012.

7. Pieper, J., *Leisure: The Basics of Culture*. San Francisco: Ignatius Press, 2009.

8. U.S. Department of Homeland Security, *Yearbook of Immigration Statistics: 2011*. Washington, DC: U.S. Department of Homeland Security, Office of Immigration Statistics, 2012.

9. Tavernise, S. (2011, May 26). "Married couples are no longer a majority, census finds." *New York Times*. Retrieved May 1, 2013, from www.nytimes.com/2011/05/26/us/26marry.html?_r=0

10. Wounded Warrior Program. Retrieved May 1, 2013 from www.woundedwarriorproject.org

11. Zimmerman, J. M., "Recreation in non-profit organizations." In *A Career with Meaning: Recreation, Parks, Sport Management, Hospitality and Tourism*, C.A. Stevens, J. F. Murphy, L. R. Allen, & E. Sheffield. Urbana, IL: Sagamore Publishing, 2010.

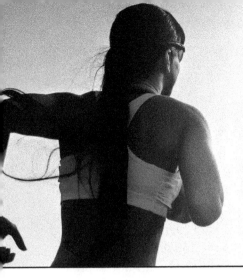

Chapter 22

HEALTH-FITNESS

OUTLINE

OBJECTIVES

1. Identify the diseases that plagued the United States in the early 20th and 21st centuries.
2. Describe the link between lifestyle and the chronic diseases.
3. Describe the components of organic-related physical fitness.
4. Identify key roles of the health-fitness specialist.
5. Understand the importance of Health Risk Assessments.
6. Understand the importance of communication with and screening of clients.
7. Understand the three primary functions of an exercise prescription.
8. Discuss the importance of credentials (i.e., certifications, licensure programs) in the health-fitness profession.

Health is defined as physical, mental, and social well-being, and not merely the absence of disease. Fitness is the capacity to perform a physical challenge with enough energy reserve for leisure-time activities and to meet emergency demands without becoming overly fatigued. The intersection between the definitions of health and fitness centers on the concept of well-being. The individual who is physically fit is ill less often and the older person who is fit is more apt to be independent than their unfit counterpart. For example, obese employees have higher rates of depression, absenteeism, low productivity, and medical claims. The health care cost of obesity is thought to be about $5,000 more per year than that incurred by individuals of normal weight. Being physically fit drives down the cost of personal health care, a benefit that could be seen on a national scale if a large cross section of the population would exercise regularly. And that is the crux of the matter—how to get people to become more physically active? This chapter explores the health-fitness profession, whose main goal is to help individuals achieve a better life through the benefits physical fitness brings.

HEALTH GOALS FOR THE NATION

The three leading causes of death in 1900 were pneumonia, tuberculosis, and diarrhea/enteritis. Together with diphtheria these three diseases caused one-third of all deaths (Figure 22.1). By the end of the 20th century, however, chronic lifestyle diseases (CLD), most notably heart disease and cancers, accounted for 55% of all deaths. Currently, that percentage hovers around the 50% mark. By the end of the 20th century deaths from infectious diseases (particularly pneumonia, influenza, and human HIV) dropped to nearly 5% of the total (Figure 22.2) and have remained at about that level.

Life expectancy increased steadily throughout the 20th century because people no longer died of infectious diseases at a young age. But with longer life came a greater incidence of CLD and the need for better medical and surgical interventions. Primary through tertiary medical care, aided by a massive effort at public risk factor education in the last half of the 20th century, produced a steady decline in CLD from the peak incidence years of the late 1960s. Nevertheless, in the second decade of the 21st century CLD is still the leading cause of death.

Epidemiological research in the 1990s established physical inactivity as a primary risk factor for CLD alongside smoking, hypertension, and high blood cholesterol. Notwithstanding this advance in knowledge, over the last 20 years there has been a trend toward declining levels of physical activity across the population. During this time period, obesity reached epidemic proportions, accompanied by a sharp rise in metabolic syndrome and diabetes.

Clearly, people are living longer, yet just as clearly they are not necessarily living as well as they could. Is the solution more medical intervention or better preventive methods? The answer is both. Medical science has done a remarkable job in extending life by ameliorating the effects of both infectious and chronic diseases, but people can do much for themselves by changing destructive lifestyle habits and modifying the risk factors associated with chronic disease.

Exercise Is Medicine

The key to approaching the problem of low physical activity rates is to establish better methods of risk factor modification and an important way to approach that is for primary-care physicians to play a key role. With that in mind, the American College of Sports Medicine and the American Medical Association in 2007 initiated a worldwide effort called, *Exercise Is Medicine.* The initiative calls for physical activity and exercise to be included as necessary parts of standard medical care. It urges members of the health care team (especially physicians) to review patients' physical activity levels at every visit, including exercise clearance and prescription or referral to a qualified health-fitness professional. Patients are encouraged to begin a conversation with their physician about physical activity and to learn how to best continue or improve upon their exercise regimens.

Exercise Is Medicine focuses on the physiological and medical benefits of physical activity and how these benefits contribute to longevity and quality of life. Accordingly, health-fitness professionals can have a direct impact on the effort to get people to include physical activity as a part of their everyday life experience. The

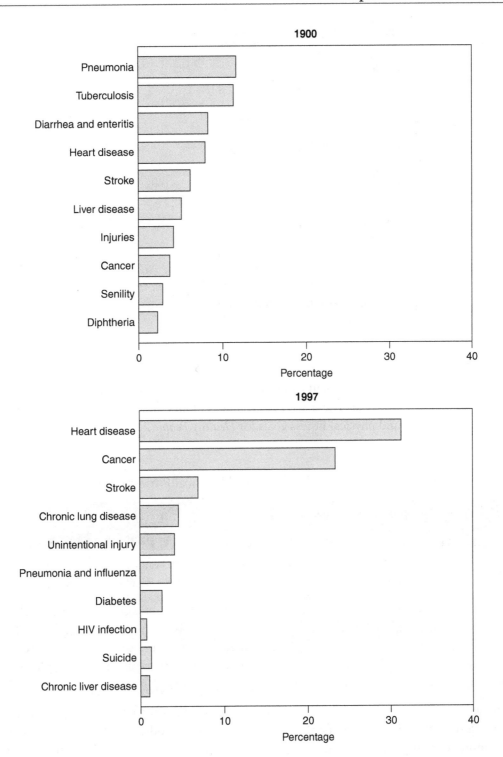

Figure 22.1. *The 10 leading causes of death as a percentage of all deaths—United States, 1900 and 1997.*

overarching goal of the health-fitness specialist, therefore, is to impart to clients an appreciation for the value of physical activity and turn that appreciation into regular participation. The task is enormous. To affect rising health care costs and stop and reverse the triplet epidemics of obesity, diabetes, and metabolic syndrome, a larger portion of the population will have to be reached with risk factor modification, especially increased levels of physical activity. That goal, thus far, has not been accomplished, but the effort continues.

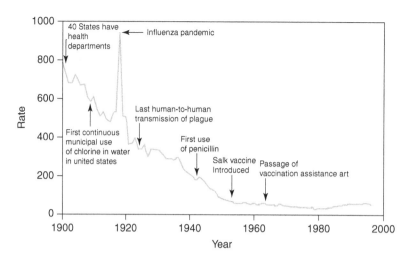

Figure 22.2. *Death rate per 100,000 population per year for infectious diseases—United States, 1900–1996.*

Healthy People 2020

Each decade since 1980 the U.S. Department of Health and Human Services established a set of "Objectives for the Nation" called *Healthy People*. These are policy goals to guide the American public to better health. Some of the physical activity and physical fitness goals for *Healthy People 2020* are presented in Table 22.1 (3).

Table 22.1. *Healthy People 2020* Physical Activity and Physical Fitness Objectives

Select Objectives for Adults	Baseline from *Healthy People 2010* / 2020 Target
PA-1. Reduce the proportion of adults who engage in no leisure-time physical activity.	36.2% of adults engaged in no leisure-time physical activity in 2008 / 32.6% (10% improvement)
PA-2.1 Increase the proportion of adults who engage in aerobic physical activity of at least moderate intensity for at least 150 minutes/week, or 75 minutes/week of vigorous intensity, or an equivalent combination.	43.5% of adults engaged in aerobic physical activity of at least moderate intensity for at least 150 minutes/week, or 75 minutes/week of vigorous intensity, or an equivalent combination in 2008 / 47.9% (10% improvement)
PA-2.2 Increase the proportion of adults who engage in aerobic physical activity of at least moderate intensity for more than 300 minutes/week, or more than 150 minutes/week of vigorous intensity, or an equivalent combination	28.4% of adults engaged in aerobic physical activity of at least moderate intensity for more than 300 minutes/week, or more than 150 minutes/week of vigorous intensity, or an equivalent combination in 2008 / 31.3% (10% improvement)
PA-2.3 Increase the proportion of adults who perform muscle-strengthening activities on two or more days of the week	21.9% of adults performed muscle-strengthening activities on 2 or more days of the week in 2008 / 24.1% (10% improvement)
PA-2.4 Increase the proportion of adults who meet the objectives for aerobic physical activity and for muscle-strengthening activity.	18.2% of adults met the objectives for aerobic physical activity and for muscle-strengthening activity in 2008 / 20.1% (10% improvement)

The health-fitness specialist is uniquely qualified to help achieve the objectives. Accordingly, the job of the health-fitness specialist is to:

1. Perform pre-exercise health risk assessments.
2. Conduct physical fitness assessments.
3. Develop exercise prescriptions based on the results.
4. Apply behavioral and motivational strategies to apparently healthy individuals in support of clients adopting and maintaining healthy lifestyle behaviors.

These job tasks are typically carried out in commercial, community, studio, corporate, university, and hospital settings. Through the remainder of this chapter these tasks will be covered, but first the concept of physical fitness is presented more fully.

PHYSICAL FITNESS DEFINED

The health-fitness specialist's main content expertise is in the area of physical fitness—how to measure it, how to prescribe exercise and physical activity to achieve it, and how to develop strategies to help people maintain it. At the beginning of the chapter a definition of physical fitness was presented for the purpose of an initial comparison to concepts of health and well-being. However, physical fitness can also be defined as a set of characteristics people have or accomplish that give them the ability to perform physical activity. This definition is taken from *Physical Activity and Health: A Report of the Surgeon General* (4). Important to the definition is the fact that these characteristics exist in two categories and several components within each of the categories (Table 22.2).

This chapter focuses solely on organic-related physical fitness because health-fitness professionals rarely assess skill-related fitness, which is more often measured in school-aged children and athletes. Assessing skill-related physical fitness is largely of interest to strength and conditioning coaches or physical education teachers.

An important job task of the health-fitness specialist is assessing the components of organic physical fitness and with this information writing individualized exercise prescriptions. Organic physical fitness pertains to the integrity of bodily systems at rest and during the application of exercise stress. Organic fitness is closely tied to health outcomes, and, as such, is inseparable and functionally equivalent to the concept of medical fitness.

Skill-related physical fitness, however, pertains to how well the body moves and is especially tied to sport performance. It is possible, for example, to be a high-level athlete while being modestly endowed with one or more of the components of organic fitness. The opposite is also true: A person with a superb level of organic fitness may only be an average athlete.

Notice that Category 1, Organic Fitness, lists in parentheses five additional qualities: body composition, muscular strength, muscular endurance, cardiorespiratory endurance, and flexibility. These are the traditional components of health-related fitness, a term synonymous with organic fitness. The components of organic

Table 22.2. The Categories and Components of Physical Fitness

Category 1: Organic-Related Physical Fitness	Category 2: Skill-Related Physical Fitness
Metabolic integrity (body composition)	Agility
Neuromuscular integrity (muscle strength & endurance)	Balance
Cardiorespiratory integrity (aerobic fitness)	Coordination
Joint integrity (flexibility)	Power
Bone integrity	Reaction time
	Speed

fitness are re-conceptualized here due to the increasing prevalence today of obesity (greater than one-third of adults and nearly 17% of youth), metabolic syndrome (currently 25% of the U.S. population), diabetes (over 8% of the U.S. population), and osteoporosis (2% of men 50 years and over and 10% of women 50 years and over). These numbers point to the general lack of metabolic health across the population. Therefore, the concept of health-related fitness has been necessarily expanded to account for the aging population and for the level of disease-producing physical inactivity that exists today.

Metabolic Integrity

Metabolic health is a state in which the chemical processes in cells are sufficient to provide at least two things: resistance to sickness and disease and enough vigor to function optimally and remain independent throughout life. As mentioned previously, the epidemics of obesity, diabetes, and metabolic syndrome are a triple threat to the health of people today. Yet, these conditions may be ameliorated or at least substantially improved by regular physical activity and exercise.

Body Composition

Increasing body fat is associated with rising rates of diabetes and metabolic syndrome. Obesity rates are of epidemic proportions in the United States and other developed nations. For adults, overweight and obesity ranges may be determined by using weight and height to calculate body mass index (BMI) by dividing body weight (pounds) by height (inches squared). The unit derived is $lb \cdot in^{-2}$.

For most people BMI correlates with the amount of body fat carried. For example, an adult who has a BMI between 25 and 29.9 is considered overweight, and one with a BMI of 30 or higher is considered obese. Fifteen percent body fat is considered average for young healthy males (25% for young healthy females). Twelve percent body fat is ideal for young healthy males (18% fat for young healthy females). A normal body weight is usually defined as a BMI between 18.5 and 24.9.

Although BMI fails to account for the relationship between lean body mass and fat mass, an increased risk of cardiovascular disease is associated with a BMI greater than or equal to 30. Approximately 65% of Americans are today classified as overweight and 34% of these are classified as obese. In 1960, only 13.4 % of the population met the criteria for obesity. Tables 22.3 and 22.4 present BMI data across a wide range of heights and weights. For assessing someone's likelihood of developing overweight or obesity-related diseases, the National Heart, Lung, and Blood Institute guidelines recommend observing two other predictors: the individual's waist circumference (because abdominal fat is a predictor of risk for obesity-related diseases) and other risk factors the individual has for diseases and conditions associated with obesity (diabetes, metabolic syndrome, high blood pressure, or physical inactivity).

Metabolic Syndrome

Metabolic syndrome is a complex disorder defined by a cluster of interconnected factors that directly increase the risk of atherosclerotic diseases and type 2 diabetes. Its main components are: elevated triglycerides and apolipoprotein B, low levels of high-density lipoproteins, elevated arterial blood pressure, irregular glucose homeostasis, insulin resistance, and abdominal obesity. An evolving aspect of metabolic syndrome is its increasing prevalence in both childhood and young adulthood.

Preventing metabolic syndrome entails (a) exercising on most days of the week for 30 to 60 minutes; (b) eating a healthy diet with plenty of fruits and vegetables, lean protein, low-fat dairy, limited grain products (including whole wheat) and saturated fats, and limiting trans fats, cholesterol, high glycemic index foods, and salt; (c) losing weight if overweight, and (d) quitting smoking.

A 2005 study showed how well lifestyle changes prevent metabolic syndrome (2). The study involved more than 3,200 people who already had impaired glucose tolerance, a pre-diabetic state. One group exercised 2.5 hours a week and ate a low-calorie, low-fat diet. After three years, people in the lifestyle group were 41%

Table 22.3.   Body Mass Indexes, 19-35

BMI	19	20	21	22	23	24	25	26	27	28	29	30	31	32	33	34	35
Height (inches)	Body Weight (pounds)																
58	91	96	100	105	110	115	119	124	129	134	138	143	148	153	158	162	167
59	94	99	104	109	114	119	124	128	133	138	143	148	153	158	163	168	173
60	97	102	107	112	118	123	128	133	138	143	148	153	158	163	168	174	179
61	100	106	111	116	122	127	132	137	143	148	153	158	164	169	174	180	185
62	104	109	115	120	126	131	136	142	147	153	158	164	169	175	180	186	191
63	107	113	118	124	130	135	141	146	152	158	163	169	175	180	186	191	197
64	110	116	122	128	134	140	145	151	157	163	169	174	180	186	192	197	204
65	114	120	126	132	138	144	150	156	162	168	174	180	186	192	198	204	210
66	118	124	130	136	142	148	155	161	167	173	179	186	192	198	204	210	216
67	121	127	134	140	146	153	159	166	172	178	185	191	198	204	211	217	223
68	125	131	138	144	151	158	164	171	177	184	190	197	203	210	216	223	230
69	128	135	142	149	155	162	169	176	182	189	196	203	209	216	223	230	236
70	132	139	146	153	160	167	174	181	188	195	202	209	216	222	229	236	243
71	136	143	150	157	165	172	179	186	193	200	208	215	222	229	236	243	250
72	140	147	154	162	169	177	184	191	199	206	213	221	228	235	242	250	258
73	144	151	159	166	174	182	189	197	204	212	219	227	235	242	250	257	265
74	148	155	163	171	179	186	194	202	210	218	225	233	241	249	256	264	272
75	152	160	168	176	184	192	200	208	216	224	232	240	248	256	264	272	279
76	156	164	172	180	189	197	205	213	221	230	238	246	254	263	271	279	287

less likely to have metabolic syndrome than those in the non-treatment group. Lifestyle changes were twice as effective as using medicine common in the treatment of diabetes.

The prevalence of metabolic syndrome increases with each succeeding age group for both sexes. Twenty percent of males and 16% of females under 40 years of age meet the criteria for metabolic syndrome, compared to 41% of males and 37% of females 40 to 59 years of age, and 52% of males and 54% of females 60 years of age. Males and females 40 to 59 years of age were about three times as likely as the youngest age group to meet the criteria for metabolic syndrome. Males 60 years of age and over were more than four times as likely as the youngest age group to meet the criteria.

Diabetes

Diabetes is a disease in which the body has a shortage of insulin, a decreased ability to use insulin, or both. Insulin is a hormone that allows glucose to enter cells and be converted to energy. When diabetes is not controlled, glucose and fats remain in the blood and, over time, damage vital organs and other tissues.

Table 22.4. Body Mass Indexes, 36-54

BMI	36	37	38	39	40	41	42	43	44	45	46	47	48	49	50	51	52	53	54
Height (inches)	Body Weight (pounds)																		
58	172	177	181	186	191	196	201	205	210	215	220	224	229	234	239	244	248	253	258
59	178	183	188	193	198	203	208	212	217	222	227	232	237	242	247	252	257	262	267
60	184	189	194	199	204	209	215	220	225	230	235	240	245	250	255	261	266	271	276
61	190	195	201	206	211	217	222	227	232	238	243	248	254	259	264	269	275	280	285
62	196	202	207	213	218	224	229	235	240	246	251	256	262	267	273	278	284	289	295
63	203	208	214	220	225	231	237	242	248	254	259	265	270	278	282	287	293	299	304
64	209	215	221	227	232	238	244	250	256	262	267	273	279	285	291	296	302	308	314
65	216	222	228	234	240	246	252	258	264	270	276	282	288	294	300	306	312	318	324
66	223	229	235	241	247	253	260	266	272	278	284	291	297	303	309	315	322	328	334
67	230	236	242	249	255	261	268	274	280	287	293	299	306	312	319	325	331	338	344
68	236	243	249	256	262	269	276	282	289	295	302	308	315	322	328	335	341	348	354
69	243	250	257	263	270	277	284	291	297	304	311	318	324	331	338	345	351	358	365
70	250	257	264	271	278	285	292	299	306	313	320	327	334	341	348	355	362	369	376
71	257	265	272	279	286	293	301	308	315	322	329	338	343	351	358	365	372	379	386
72	265	272	279	287	294	302	309	316	324	331	338	346	353	361	368	375	383	390	397
73	272	280	288	295	302	310	318	325	333	340	348	355	363	371	378	386	393	401	408
74	280	287	295	303	311	319	326	334	342	350	358	365	373	381	389	396	404	412	420
75	287	295	303	311	319	327	335	343	351	359	367	375	383	391	399	407	415	423	431
76	295	304	312	320	328	336	344	353	361	369	377	385	394	402	410	418	426	435	443

Type 1 diabetes is usually first diagnosed in children and young adults, but may occur at any age. Type 1 diabetes is an autoimmune disease that may be caused by genetic, environmental, or other factors. It accounts for about 5% of diabetes cases. There is no known way to prevent it, and its treatment requires the administration of insulin.

Type 2 diabetes accounts for 90 to 95% of all diabetes cases and is usually associated with older age, obesity, and physical inactivity, or a family history of its occurrence. Physical activity offers specific benefits for type 2 diabetics since exercise has been shown to dramatically improve glucose metabolism via skeletal muscle mediated translocation of glucose transporter type 4 (Figure 22.3). This is one reason (among several) type 2 diabetics are heavily encouraged to engage in physical activity.

Diabetes rates vary by race and ethnicity. Native American, Alaska Native, African American, Hispanic/Latino, and Asian/Pacific Islander adults are about twice as likely as Caucasian adults to have type 2 diabetes. It can be prevented and controlled through healthy food choices, physical activity, and weight loss. Insulin or oral medication also may be necessary.

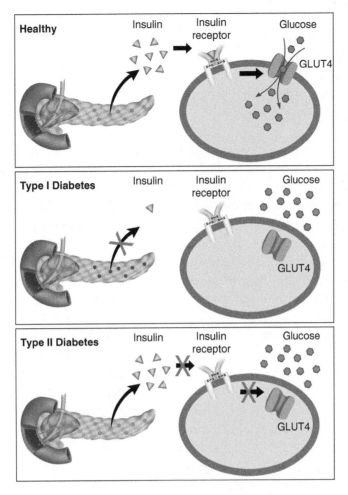

Figure 22.3. *Insulin action and diabetes type 1 and type 2.*

Metabolic syndrome and diabetes are endemic today just as obesity rates and levels of physical inactivity have steadily risen. The associations are obvious. People who exercise and eat responsibly are more likely to be at a normal weight and have a higher level of metabolic integrity.

Neuromuscular Integrity

Neuromuscular integrity refers collectively to the viability of the nervous system and the motors (muscles) that cause movement. Traditionally, the components of health-related physical fitness targeted the strength and endurance of the muscular system. This new conceptualization goes beyond that because of the prevalence of neuromuscular diseases in the general population.

- Spinal Muscular Atrophy: 1 per 6,000–10,000 people
- Muscular Dystrophy (Duchenne and Becker type): 1 per 3,500–5,000 male newborns
- Parkinson's Disease: 7–10 million people worldwide
- Paralysis: 9 per 1000 (paralysis of extremities complete/partial)
- Amyotrophic Lateral Sclerosis: 6–8 per 100,000
- Myasthenia Gravis: 14–20 per 100,000
- Fibromyalgia: 10 million people in the United States (3–6% of the world population)
- Guillain–Barre Syndrome: 1 in 100,000

- Primary Lateral Sclerosie: rare
- Progressive Supranuclear Palsy: rare
- Alternating Hemiplegia: rare
- Friedreich Ataxia: rare
- Congenital Myotonic Dystrophy: 5 per 100,000
- Paramyotonia Congenita: 1 per 100,000

Muscle strength refers to the capacity of a muscle or muscle group to exert maximal force against resistance through a full range of motion. Muscular endurance is the ability to perform many repetitions with a sub-maximum resistance over a given period of time. Resistance exercise enhances muscle strength and endurance in several ways. The first and simplest to understand is that resistance exercise causes an increase in muscle mass. The larger the cross sectional area of a muscle, the greater potential force development during contraction.

The second way to understand how muscle strength and endurance improves with resistance exercise is to consider the basic organizational unit of skeletal muscle. The motor unit is defined as an alpha motor neuron and all the muscle fibers it innervates. Muscles create more force when more motor units are recruited during contractions. Muscle force also depends on the rate at which motor units discharge action potentials. Physical activity requires the activation of multiple muscle groups using numerous motor units. The sedentary individual activates motor units at different times, which causes inefficient movement. Strength training aids the synchronization of motor unit recruitment so that, after training, activation of these motor units happens simultaneously for optimal strength production and performance.

Human muscle contains fast-twitch and slow-twitch muscle fibers. Slow-twitch fibers perform low-intensity contractions, which are found during endurance forms of exercise. Fast-twitch fibers, however, support power-based activities, such as sprinting or lifting heavy weights. Greater activation of fast-twitch fibers increases speed and strength during physical activity. Resistance training results in a greater activation of these fibers. These basic neuromuscular adaptations can occur within weeks of a new resistance-training program.

The increase in muscle strength and endurance has profound health benefits. Resistance training enhances the functional capacity of the neuromuscular system, improves the risk profile for cardiovascular disease, and increases quality of life. These factors are well-known predictors of higher risk of mortality. The benefits of resistance training are evident across sex, age, various weight individuals, and people with or without disability. In addition to decreasing body fat and reducing the risk of obesity, strength training stimulates a variety of positive adaptations including increased blood glucose utilization, reduced resting blood pressure, improved blood lipid profiles, enhanced vascular condition, increased gastrointestinal transit speed, increased bone mineral density, and improved body composition. It also has been shown to improve function in post-coronary patients and chronic obstructive pulmonary disease patients. It also reduces discomfort in people with low back pain and arthritis. Strength training has been shown to be effective for decreasing depression and for reducing the risk of metabolic syndrome and cardiovascular disease.

Cardiorespiratory Integrity

Aerobic endurance is dependent on the ability of large muscle groups to perform dynamic exercise for extended periods of time. These activities require the pulmonary and cardiovascular systems to provide sufficient oxygen, remove waste products, and deliver nutrients necessary to sustain rhythmic activity. To improve aerobic capacity, the working muscles must become more efficient in utilizing oxygen, the heart must contract with greater force, and the lungs must transport air more efficiently within the pulmonary system. Training interventions improves aerobic capacity by enhancing the efficiency of the heart, lungs, vasculature, and muscles. Aerobic training also enhances the thermoregulatory response to endurance exercise and heat stress.

Cardiorespiratory endurance is measured by determining the maximal amount of oxygen the body can consume per minute (VO_2 max). Oxygen consumed by the body is used in aerobic energy production. When an individual desires information as to how best to improve his or her health status, a health-fitness professional usually assesses aerobic exercise capacity first. An ideal $\dot{V}O_2$ max for young healthy adults is from 42 ml/kg/min to 47 ml/kg/min for males and females (females generally have lower values then males). There is a gradual decline in $\dot{V}O_2$ max with age. However, this decline is attenuated when vigorous exercise training continues throughout the lifespan.

Joint Integrity

Flexibility is defined as the ability to move a joint through a complete range of motion (ROM). Resistance training and various stretching activities can influence flexibility. Ball-and-socket joints (hip and shoulder) can execute movements about all anatomical planes and have the greatest ROM. Ellipsoidal joints (such as the wrist) are those that can execute movements in both sagittal and frontal planes and have less flexibility compared to ball-and-socket joints. Hinge joints have the least flexibility compared to the aforementioned and are primarily responsible for executing movements about the sagittal plane.

Flexibility is also limited by the muscles, with muscle temperature being the major influence. Unless flexibility is a limiting factor in performance, static stretching activities should only be performed *after* a muscle has already been warmed. Static stretching prior to activities such as 1RM testing and sprinting may decrease muscular force output and lead to a decrease in performance. The chosen method of warm-up before such events should be dynamic stretching, which has not been shown to be detrimental to performance.

Resistance training is one of the best ways to maintain joint integrity and stability, and, together with stretching interventions, can be performed to improve flexibility. However, resistance training activities should be performed through a full range of motion; failure to do so can lead to a decrease in flexibility. Individuals should train both agonist and antagonist muscles. Among athletes and resistance trained individuals, two high-risk areas for injury include the shoulder and knee. Both of these areas can be protected by maintaining optimal strength ratios between agonist and antagonist musculature.

Stretching sessions performed at least twice a week can significantly improve flexibility. For optimal flexibility, static stretches should be held for 15 to 30 seconds, and performed after exercise while the muscles are still warm, which allows for optimal muscle and tendon elasticity. This method may also be beneficial in terms of reducing muscle soreness. Individuals who have experienced an increase in muscular flexibility often report a reduction of low-back pain, reduction of muscular injury, and improved posture. They are also less likely to develop sclerosis.

Bone Integrity

Often seen with increasing age is an increase in the prevalence of osteoporosis, a condition described by weak and fragile bones that can result in fractures from minor shear forces, falling, or even other minor occurrences. Osteoporosis is defined as having a bone mineral density that is 2.5 standard deviations below the normal range for healthy adult values (Figure 22.4). Osteopenia is defined as having a bone mineral density between 1 and 2.5 standard deviations less than the normal range for healthy adults. Both men and women are at an elevated risk for low bone mass and osteoporosis beyond the age of 50. This is largely due to a progressive decrease in the production of the sex hormones known to have bone strengthening properties. Older women, however, are at a greater risk than their male counterparts due to the role of estrogen in the inhibition of osteoclastic activity. A loss of estrogen coupled with inactivity contributes to a significant reduction of bone mineral density. These risks can be significantly decreased if individuals maintained a physically active lifestyle. This principle goes hand-in-hand with the need to maintain joint integrity, since physical activity can strengthen musculature about joints as well as provide for favorable bone adaptations that lead to an increase in dynamic stability. These characteristics are much needed, especially among osteoporotic individuals. Taken together, these are the reasons why individuals (especially older individuals) should maintain a physically active lifestyle. Some specific risk factors for osteoporosis include genetic predisposition, gender, age, physical inactivity, hormonal factors that affect bone metabolism, smoking, alcohol consumption, and low dietary calcium and vitamin D intake.

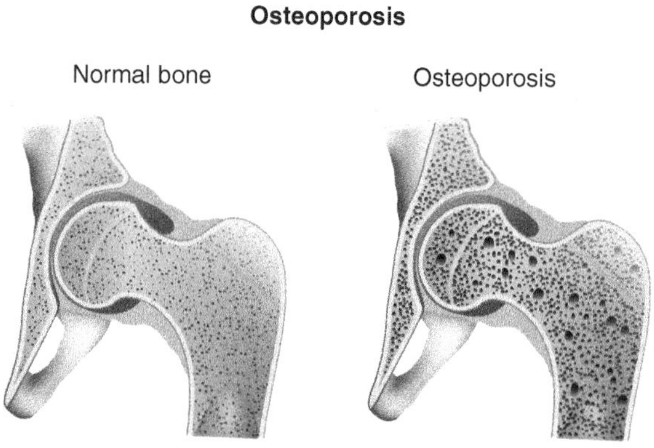

Osteoporosis

Normal bone   Osteoporosis

Figure 22.4. *Healthy bone and bone with osteoporosis.*

Resistance training produces both axial tension and axial compressive forces upon bones that can induce beneficial adaptations. This principle is well explained by Wolff's law, which states that bone tissue adapts in response to the stresses placed upon it. Although heavy resistance training is the preferred method of stimulating osteoblastic activity, all types of physical activity including both endurance and resistance exercise are beneficial for osteoporotic individuals. Greater loads result in greater bone stress, which is optimal for stimulating tissue growth. However, it is not advisable for an individual with osteoporosis to begin a physical activity program with heavy resistance exercise (>70% 1RM). It is important to consider proper progression of exercise since even moderate aerobic activity such as walking has been shown to improve bone mineral density. Exercise programs should include a combination of both endurance and resistance training to seek optimal benefits.

Working as a Health-Fitness Specialist

Employment in the health-fitness industry offers a promising career path and a sense of fulfillment by contributing to and changing the lives of others. The role of the health-fitness specialist has evolved from simply a basic knowledge of program design and motivation to a more comprehensive approach including health screening, fitness assessments, behavioral modification and coaching strategies, and the integration of specific recuperation strategies for clients. As discussed in the Careers section, there are many specialty areas in the health-fitness setting with responsibilities ranging from greeting clients to employee training and staff supervision. In this section, we will address the following question: What is the health-fitness professional's role with the client?

Communication, Screening, Assessment, and Referrals

A health-fitness specialist's ability to communicate both verbal and nonverbally is essential to create rapport with client. Rapport will allow the health-fitness professional to connect, gain trust, and understand how to motivate the client to achieve his or her fitness goals.

Another important facet performed by health-fitness specialists is screening, assessing risk, and distinguishing between healthy clients and those needing additional medical clearance by a health care provider such as a clinical exercise physiologist, physician, or physical therapist. Combined with effective communication skills, tools such as the health history form and the Physical Activity Readiness Questionnaire (PAR-Q) provide the health-fitness specialist with valuable insight into the client's past and current state of health. These tools provide the following:

• Determination of the number of risk factors and the client's signs and symptoms to assess whether the client is classified as low, moderate, or high risk for a chronic disease
• Determine whether a medical clearance or referral is in order

- Understand level of social influence both positive and/or negative from family, friends, and coworkers/colleagues
- Determine potential negative behavioral triggers that may impose challenges during the exercise regimen.

Finally, assessments are tests and measurements used by health-fitness specialists to evaluate a client's current physical and functional state. The assessments commonly used in the health-fitness industry are discussed in the upcoming sections.

Pre-Exercise Health-Risk Assessments

Resting heart rate (HR) and blood pressure (BP) are simple and effective indicators of cardiovascular status. Subjects should be in a rested state, which can best be attained when individuals are calm and in a stable environment for at least 10 minutes prior to assessment. The resting state assures that plasma concentrations of catecholamines are stable, which assures stable BP and HR measures.

The clinical norm for resting HR is between 60–100 beats per minute, although it is not uncommon for the resting HR of a highly trained individual to be lower than 60 beats per minute. This is a condition called bradycardia. BP values for normal, prehypertension, and hypertension are shown in Table 22.5.

Working as a health-fitness specialist involves encountering individuals who meet the criteria for hypertension and/or type 2 diabetes, since these are very common health issues. Clinical settings can utilize blood tests to analyze lipid profiles, during which an assessment of high density lipoprotein (HDL), low density lipoprotein (LDL), and triglycerides might be made. Total cholesterol should be less than 200 mg/dl; values between 200 and 239 mg/dl are identified as being borderline high, while 240 mg/dl or greater is identified as high cholesterol. Optimal values for HDL and LDL cholesterol are above 40 and below 100, respectively. A good HDL/LDL ratio is important to reduce the likelihood of developing hyperlipidemia and atherosclerosis, as well as other potential health issues. Fasting glucose should also be assessed. The normal range for fasting glucose levels is between 60–90 mg/100 ml, whereas pre-diabetics have a fasting glucose between 100–125 mg/100 ml and type 2 diabetics have a value of 126 mg/ml or greater. An oral glucose tolerance test may be considered to assess glucose metabolism.

Physical Fitness Assessments

Physical fitness assessments are necessary to ascertain baseline fitness levels for the purpose of prescribing exercise. Muscular strength assessments are often quantified as low- or high-velocity strength. Low-velocity muscle strength assessments involve activities that require a significant amount of force output and are performed at low speeds using the one repetition maximum (1RM) test. Traditional 1RM tests utilize free weights and dynamic contractions as seen, for example, during traditional free-weight barbell lifts. However, force transducers allow for the assessment of maximal voluntary isometric contraction and isokinetic machines allow for maximal force output tests performed at fixed speeds. 1RM tests are performed following a dynamic warm-up protocol. The goal of the test is to reach 1RM within three to five sets while utilizing 1–5 minute rest periods between sets.

Table 22.5.   Normative Blood Pressure Values

	Systolic	Diastolic
Optimal (Normal)	< 120	< 80
Pre-hypertensive	120–139	80–89
Hypertension 1	140–159	90–99
Hypertension 2 (Severe)	160+	100+

High-velocity muscular strength is considered anaerobic power. Since power is the product of force and velocity, muscular power is defined and assessed by an individual's ability to exert high force while contracting at high speeds. 1RM tests that incorporate more explosive movements are preferred for high-speed strength assessments. Examples of these types of exercises include the power clean, snatch, or push jerk. The vertical jump can also be used to calculate anaerobic power. Maximal exertion attempts of these exercises generally take only a few seconds to complete.

Longer duration anaerobic power tests can also be used. The most common test for maximal anaerobic power is the Wingate test. This is a 30-second test performed on a cycle ergometer following a warm-up protocol. During this test, resistance on the pedals is predetermined as proportional to the individual's body weight. Power is calculated during each 5-second interval during this test and quantified as work divided by time. Peak power is obtained during the first 5 seconds of the test, while other variables such as fatigue index and mean power are also assessed.

Muscular endurance is defined as the ability of a muscle or group of muscles to sustain repeated contractions at a submaximal load and can be assessed in a relative or absolute sense. Relative tests prescribe loads relative to a certain percentage of 1RM or relative to body weight and are preferred when comparing individuals, since body weight can have an effect on lifting performance. Examples of tests that can be performed include YMCA bench press, leg press, pullups, parallel bar dips, pushups, or situps. A metronome may be used to standardize lifting speed, which can also have an effect on performance. Some tests may be administered with the purpose of recording the maximum number of repetitions performed in a given time frame.

Aerobic capacity is assessed during a $\dot{V}O_2$ max test. Since direct measurement of $\dot{V}O_2$ max is expensive, indirect methods to estimate $\dot{V}O_2$ max are usually preferable in most health-fitness settings. Aerobic capacity can be estimated via many different submaximal tests such as the 1.5-mile run, 12-minute run, Rockport 1 mile walk test, or by using ergometer protocols.

Flexibility assessment involves the use of electric goniometers to quantify joint angle. Less expensive devices, such as a sit-and-reach box or just a simple meter stick can be used. The most common flexibility assessment is the sit-and-reach test, which measures flexibility of the lumbar and hip extensors. During any flexibility assessment, a warm-up procedure should be performed that involves static stretching prior to the test to ensure reliability.

Body composition is not only a marker of health, but also an indicator of athletic performance. Excessive body fat increases an individual's risk for developing type 2 diabetes and cardiovascular disease and also inhibits athletic performance. Body composition is often estimated via BMI and girth circumference measurements. Although BMI correlates with the amount of body fat, it is not a direct measurement. Rather, it provides a superficial assessment of body size as a whole. Athletes, for example, may have a BMI identifying them as overweight even though they may not have excess body fat. This may contribute to situations where athletes with minimal body fat are falsely classified as obese since these methods do not measure the composition of the body. Other methods of estimating body fat and body fat distribution include measurements of skinfold thickness, waist circumference, and calculation of waist-to-hip circumference ratios.

Body composition can also be determined using bioelectrical impedance analysis (BIA), dual x-ray absorptiometry (DEXA), and hydrostatic weighing. DEXA provides accurate body composition assessments and is also used for bone mineral density analysis as well. While DEXA may be the gold standard for body composition assessment, skinfolds are the most commonly performed method. The principal assumption with the skinfold method is that total body fat is proportional to the measured subcutaneous fat. Other techniques are ultrasound, computer tomography, and magnetic resonance imaging (MRI).

Exercise Prescription

An exercise prescription is a plan for physical activity formulated to achieve specific beneficial outcomes while minimizing accompanying risks. Exercise prescriptions have at least three primary functions: (a) to increase physical fitness, (b) to improve health by reducing risk factors for chronic disease, and (c) to ensure safety during exercise.

A properly conceived exercise prescription is an important tool to manage apparently healthy individuals. Inappropriate exercise for a given individual and a lack of sound counseling about exercise can lead to dangerous situations in which the health and sometimes the life of the person can be compromised. While these three common purposes of the exercise prescription should be considered in every activity plan, each should be weighted differently with regards to the particular needs of the individual client.

The idea of individualization is paramount in developing the exercise prescription. While exercise prescriptions have a sound physiological foundation, personal health behavior often dictates how successful the exercise prescription will be in bringing about its intended goal. Health-fitness specialists should be aware of the psychosocial aspects of behavioral change that is a necessary part of the successful exercise prescription.

Individualized exercise prescriptions are necessary for at least three reasons: (a) physiological and perceptual responses to acute exercise vary among individuals and within an individual across the lifespan or when performing different types of exercise, (b) the magnitude and rate of development of chronic adaptations to exercise training vary, and (c) exercise programs considerably different in structure and makeup may still achieve desired outcomes in individual clients, necessitating the need to consider individual interests, abilities, and limitations when writing the prescription.

The components of the exercise prescription are (a) mode, (b) intensity, (c) duration, (d) frequency, and (e) progression. Each individual will respond differently, which is to say that each dose-response relationship will be different. *Dose* refers to the components of the prescription and *response* is how well the individual tolerates the dose. These five components are the parameters around which the exercise prescription is built and individualized for different clients. For both healthy and chronically ill (considered in Chapter 16) people, the exercise prescription in influenced by a variety of factors, including needs, goals, physical and health status, available time to exercise, personal preferences, and practical considerations such as cost, equipment, and facility availability. In all cases, the parameters of the exercise prescription are the same whether dealing with a young athlete, a middle-aged apparently healthy man, or an aged patient who has just had heart surgery.

How the exercise stressor is applied to clients and the rate of physiological adaptation they attain must be followed closely and, as much as possible, be based on objective test data. The overriding concern is for safety, but beyond that, the well-formulated exercise prescription must provide a therapeutic benefit while minimizing risks. It is important to understand, however, that physical fitness is multifaceted, and a complete exercise prescription covers neuromusculoskeletal as well as cardiopulmonary aspects. The major factors essential to the attainment and maintenance of optimal functional capacity through exercise training include more than improved cardiorespiratory endurance. Body composition, muscular strength and endurance, and joint flexibility are also essential components to be considered in developing the exercise prescription. Developing each physical fitness component requires specific exercise training techniques, necessitating the need to adhere to the principle of "specificity of training."

Heart rate is a simple assessment and can be used in aerobic conditioning programs to prescribe training intensities based on a predetermined target heart rate. The Karvonen method is the most common method to determine target heart rate training zones. The steps for determining target heart rate (THR) based on the Karvonen method are as follows:

$$\text{Age predicted maximum heart rate (MHR)} = (220 - \text{age})$$
$$\text{Heart rate reserve (HRR)} = \text{MHR} - \text{resting heart rate (RHR)}$$
$$\text{Target heart rate (THR)} = [\text{HRR} \times \text{desired intensity (\%)}] + \text{RHR}$$

Consider the following case study. A 25-year-old moderately trained male weighs 200 lbs, has a resting heart rate of 80 beats per minute, scores relatively high on the 1RM anaerobic power assessments but relatively low on muscular endurance assessments, and reports that he wants to increase lean tissue and improve his body composition. To write a complete exercise prescription, two separate areas need to be addressed: endurance training and resistance training. While it is possible to prescribe a resistance training protocol that is accommodated for the purpose of increasing caloric expenditure, the majority of the caloric expenditure resulting in weight loss will come from the endurance training aspect of the exercise prescription. Especially consider that this individual wants to increase muscle mass, therefore proper guidelines for hypertrophy training should be followed.

A resistance training protocol designed to maximize caloric expenditure—reduced resistive load and reduced rest between sets—will likely prove to be counter-productive since a heavy enough load needs to be implemented to achieve the desired muscular adaptations. In addition, caloric expenditure is known to be higher in endurance training versus resistance training. Also note that if improved body composition is a goal, a program that focuses *solely* on resistance training is not optimal. A common misconception is that significant hypertrophy contributes to an increase in basal metabolic rate, which can in turn lead to improvements in body composition. The amount of lean tissue required to stimulate this type of adaptation is tremendous. Therefore, if weight loss is a goal a separate portion of the exercise program must emphasize caloric expenditure.

To first address the goal of hypertrophy, an adequate resistance training regimen will consist of a training frequency at least three to four times per week. The general recommendations for hypertrophy are sets of eight to 12 repetitions with loads between 65 to 85%1RM. A training split must be considered to avoid localized overtraining. This means that even if the individual's goal is to increase bench press strength, it is not advised to perform bench presses on every training day. At least 48 hours of recovery is required between training sessions to avoid overtraining of muscle groups utilized. An example of a training split that allows the appropriate frequency is as follows:

Day 1 : Chest, deltoids, abdominals
Day 2: Back, trapezius, calves
Day 3: Quadriceps, hamstrings
Day 4: Biceps, triceps, abdominals
Day 5: Rest

Training volume for hypertrophy programs is quite high. Therefore, training for each muscle group will consist of at least three exercises per group (consisting of three to six sets for each exercise), while maintaining the target load range of 65 to 85% 1RM and short-to-moderate rest between each set (10 seconds–120 seconds). The reason for this wide range in rest time is that although the general training regimen will utilize between 30 and 90 seconds rest, certain principles of "shock" training may often be used to introduce variation into the training regimen when necessary. Some methods may include supersets (sets performed back-to-back of opposing muscle groups), pyramid sets (load of ascending/descending weight), and giant sets (two or more exercises performed back-to-back). In addition, the two-for-two rule should be followed as a guideline regarding the timing of load increase. This means that if the individual can perform two repetitions beyond assignment for two consecutive workouts, then it is time to increase the load assignment.

With regards to the caloric expenditure aspect of training, both endurance (steady state aerobic) and high-intensity interval training (HIIT) should be performed when appropriate. Endurance or aerobic training has been shown to be beneficial for improving body composition by increasing caloric expenditure and increasing excesses post-exercise oxygen consumption (EPOC). Recently, HIIT has been receiving a significant amount of attention for the ability of this approach in providing additional cardiovascular benefits beyond traditional steady state training. Interval training might be more effective at improving $\dot{V}O_2$ max, lactate threshold, EPOC, and caloric expenditure. This type of training involves short bursts of extremely high (maximal or near maximal) intensity, followed by active recovery periods.

Many different variations have been introduced regarding this style of training. Some approaches include the performance of three intensities (low, moderate, and high). Depending on the training status of the individual and his or her ability to tolerate lactate and fatigue, steady-state exercise is likely to be performed more frequently than HIIT due to the fatigue and exhaustion that occurs during the latter. However, both should be incorporated into a training program to maximize caloric expenditure and cardiovascular adaptations. Before moving forward with the endurance training prescription, it is first necessary to differentiate between the "fat-burning zone" (FBZ) and "aerobic-training zones" (ATZ) frequently discussed in relation to endurance training, as these are two common areas of misconception.

The term *fat burning zone* is misleading, since it seems as though this is the optimal intensity to perform exercise if the goal is fat loss or improvements in body composition. The fat-burning zone is generally performed at lower intensities (60–75% max heart rate), whereas the aerobic training zone is performed at higher intensities (75–80% max heart rate). The metabolic response to exercise at lower intensities is such that energy is derived primarily from lipids. However, as exercise intensity increases, the relative energy from lipid stores decreases as energy from carbohydrate stores increases. The notion behind the fat-burning zone is that exercise performed in this intensity range will result in the most amount of fat loss, since this intensity produces the greatest amount of energy derived from lipids. However, it should be noted that even though there is a higher percentage of energy coming from lipids, this *lower* level of intensity requires a significantly *longer* duration of training, since the ratio of calories expended per time is much lower with this approach. That being said, HIIT produces the highest ratio of calories expended per time and thus does not need to be performed for the same duration. The key point being that the fat-burning zone does derive more relative energy from lipid stores. However, exercise at this intensity requires a significant duration of each training session to achieve weight-loss goals.

To complete the training for the case study mentioned above, both traditional steady-state exercise will be performed in combination with interval training for the purpose of maximizing cardiovascular adaptations and caloric expenditure. The goal of the intervention should be to increase training frequency over time. However, at the beginning of the program, this individual is training four times per week and thus endurance training will be four times per week as well. Two to three of these sessions will consist of steady-state exercise performed at 70–85% target heart rate that should be determined based on the Karvonen method as follows:

$$APHRM = 220-25 = 195; HRR = 195-80 = 115$$
$$\text{Target heart rate (THR)} = [HRR \times \text{desired intensity (\%)}] + RHR$$
$$THR_{minimum} = (115 \times .7) + 80 = \textbf{160.5 (161) bpm}$$
$$THR_{minimum} = (115 \times .85) + 80 = \textbf{177.8 (178) bpm}$$

Therefore, the target heart rate range will be between 161 and 178 bpm for 40 minutes for these training sessions. For the remaining one to two sessions, a high-intensity protocol will be followed that incorporates a 1:2 work rest ratio performed repeatedly for 20 minutes. This means that the individual will perform extremely high intensity (sprint) for 30 seconds, followed by 1 minute of active recovery. These times can be adjusted based on the tolerance of the individual, as a longer recovery time might be required at first. Over the duration of the training program, the overall goal will be to increase training frequency and accommodate the program accordingly to avoid overtraining.

Behavioral and Motivational Strategies

In order to find the proper motivational strategies, it is important to consider potential barriers keeping individuals from maintaining a healthy lifestyle. Individuals are influenced by both external and internal factors. Often, a reciprocal relationship exists between these factors such that external factors tend to influence internal and vice versa. One of the largest internal factors that should be an area of focus is the development of self-efficacy. Self-efficacy is defined as an individual's perceived ability to perform a specific behavior. There is a direct relationship between self-efficacy and positive health behaviors. Individuals who have well-established self-efficacy also tend to have a well-established internal locus of health. Individuals are said to have a high internal locus of health when they attribute the majority of their health status to their own behavior. Both self-efficacy and locus of control can be assessed via surveys. If individuals have a low internal locus of health (high external) that means that they tend to attribute most of their health status to external factors as opposed to internal (i.e., their own behavior). It is essential for individuals to be aware that their own actions and health behaviors make a large contribution to their health status. Individuals who have a low internal locus of control tend to attribute their health status to external factors such as their doctor or just by luck or chance.

Another major internal issue that can serve as a limiting factor or a barrier in relation to a healthy lifestyle could simply be a lack of perceived benefit in the activity, or just the lack of knowledge regarding how to perform physical activity to benefit health. It is possible that individuals are not performing physical activities due to a lack of perceived benefit in the activity. If a lack of perceived benefit is the issue, knowledge-based interventions can be beneficial. These are prime examples of microlevel issues that tend to affect an individual's health status. Interventions should seek to assess and develop self-efficacy and internal locus of health.

In order to achieve the aforementioned, it may be imperative to consider the macro or external factors that affect health behaviors. One of the best ways to promote positive health behaviors is to create conducive environments that support the target behavior. Individuals are influenced by their environment; this means that it can be very difficult to quit smoking if everyone in the environment is smoking. The same goes for exercise and healthy eating habits. Simply stated, the attitudes of individuals in the environment can affect health behaviors. Another external factor that may be present is a lack of accessibility to fitness facilities. Consider, though, that it may not be necessary to access a fitness facility to perform physical activities. Observational learning could be utilized in this regard. The presence of a role model may be beneficial to provide behavioral acquisition and provide knowledge and reinforcement when necessary.

When considering behavioral motivational strategies, it is also important to think about what should *not* be done in attempt to induce motivation. It often may be tempting to make threatening statements such as "if you don't stop smoking, you'll die" or "if you don't lose weight, you will develop diabetes." These types of threatening statements should be avoided when attempting to induce behavioral modification. As mentioned earlier, motivation is a product of self-efficacy. However, a series of factors act as barriers that are keeping individuals from positive health behaviors. All possible barriers should be considered and addressed as appropriate in attempt to create conducive environments for change, and seek to develop self-efficacy.

Health-Fitness Jobs

Aerobic Fitness Instructor

Instructors may lead individuals or groups exercise sessions. Classes may include, but are not limited to, spin, zumba, boot camp, core training, step and body combat. Aerobic instructors must gauge the level of intensity to suit the clientele.

Employee Fitness Director

An employee fitness director is usually responsible for overseeing staff members such as personal trainers, fitness instructors, nutritionists, and a sales team. This position entails proper education and certification and relevant work experience.

Fitness Attendant

Fitness instructors embrace a wide range of roles including designing exercise programming, client instruction, spotting, to fixing and cleaning equipment. The primary role is to be out in the fitness area greeting members and maintaining a health-positive relationship with the cliental.

Fitness Coach

Fitness coaches assess, evaluate, educate, and motivate clients wishing to improve their fitness levels. Coaches may train individuals or lead groups of people (i.e., boot camps) through a series of exercises that enhance aerobic fitness, muscular strength and endurance, and flexibility.

Fitness Consultant

Fitness consultants may perform many of the duties relegated to a personal trainer or fitness coach; primarily, their duties revolve around familiarity with exercise science and exercise technique. The consultant must have the capacity to distill knowledge for others. Teaching requires much greater mastery than simply instructing or modeling exercises for clients.

Fitness Director

A director of fitness position is multifaceted role including, but not limited to, supervision, enforcement of policies, staff training, assessment of clients, and basic fitness skills. Additionally, many directors of fitness serve as ambassadors for the program and do public speaking to promote their programs. The staff reporting to the director includes exercise technicians, exercise instructors, personal trainers, nutritionists, fitness assistants, and volunteers. This position entails proper education and certification and relevant work experience.

Fitness and Wellness Program Coordinator

A coordinator assists the director with the day-to-day supervision and administration of the fitness center. Duties include supervising and coordinating group exercise classes, youth fitness programs, health promotion activities, and wellness/fitness lectures and screenings. Supervision may also include exercise instructors, personal trainers, etc.

Fitness Manager

Fitness managers are generally in charge of membership sales and managing equipment and instructors. Educating and training staff may be common duties depending on the size of the facility/center/organization. The manager also ensures that employees have the proper certification and training for their positions. Typically, a bachelor's and/or a master's degree with relevant experience are required for this position.

Group Exercise Instructors

Group instructors lead, instruct, and motivate individuals and/or groups in exercise activities, including aerobic fitness, muscular strength and endurance, and flexibility.

Personal Trainer

A personal trainer's primary responsibility is to assist individuals to create and execute customized workout plans to reach optimal health and fitness.

Personal Sports Trainer

Personal sports trainers' primary responsibility is to assist their clients in reaching their athletic goals. For these individuals, health and fitness benefits are desirable, but the primary goals are to motivate, design, and train individuals to reach their athletic goals.

Yoga Instructor

Yoga instructors help guide clients (individual or group) in yoga through a variety of body postures in yoga exercise and breathing exercises. Primarily, providing hands-on instruction to make sure clients are performing movements properly and applying the breathing techniques.

Yoga Coordinator

The yoga coordinator's primary role is to hire, train, and oversee yoga instructors. The coordinator may maintain a class if he or she enjoys teaching or the situation demands it.

Careers in Health-Fitness and Wellness

The U.S. Department of Labor estimates that employment in the health-fitness industry will increase faster than all occupations between 2008 and 2018 (see Table 22.6), with a projected growth of 29% during this period (1). As the American population accepts that individual responsibility is the key to well-being, health-fitness programs will continue to increase. Growth in the health-fitness industry has been classified by the U.S. Department of Labor into three distinct categories: personal trainer, group exercise instructor, and fitness director. Each of these roles has evolved into specialty areas over time, thus spawning different educational demands. See the sidebar on health-fitness jobs.

Table 22.6. Overview of the Health-Fitness Industry

45.3 million	U.S. health-fitness and wellness club members
29,750	U.S. health-fitness and wellness centers
$19.5 billion	U.S. health-fitness and wellness center revenues for 2009
261,000	U.S. health-fitness professionals
337,900	U.S. projected health-fitness professionals in 2018

As reported from the International Health, Racquet & Sportsclub Association (IHRSA) Industry Statistics 2010 Global Report: Available at www.ihrsa.org/media-center/2010/6/7/ihrsa-releases-the-2010-global-report-the-state-of-the-healt.html

Commonly Asked Questions

Question: How do you obtain the appropriate certification in order to be qualified to work in the health-fitness industry?
Answer: Contact the National Commission for Certifying Agencies (NCCA) for a listing of accredited certified programs. (See the next section for a complete listing of agencies)

Question: Do you need a degree in order to be a certified trainer?
Answer: While a degree in kinesiology is advantageous, most agencies only require a high school education to sit for the examination. Additional study material is generally offered to individuals preparing for certification at an additional cost.

Question: What are my occupational opportunities in the fitness industry?
Answer: This varies depending on current market demands and your level of expertise, but generally it can range from personal and group fitness trainer to fitness director. (see *Careers in Health-Fitness and Wellness*)

Question: What can I expect to earn as a health-fitness professional?
Answer: The median pay for health-fitness trainers and instructors was approximately $31,090 per year and $14.95 per hour. Health-fitness managers and directors earned approximately $80,000 per year.

Recommended Certifications for Individuals Desiring Employment in the Health-Fitness Profession

*Academy of Applied Personal Training Education (www.aapte.org)

- Certified Personal Fitness Trainer

*Aerobics and Fitness Association of America (www.afaa.com)

- Personal Trainer Certification
- Group Exercise Certification
- Step Certification

*American College of Sports Medicine (www.certification.acsm.org/get-certified)

- ACSM Certified Personal Trainer
- ACSM Certified Health-Fitness Specialist
- ACSM Certified Group Exercise Instructor

*American Council on Exercise (www.acefitness.org)

- Advanced Health and Fitness Specialist
- Group Fitness Instructor
- Personal Trainer

*American Fitness Professionals & Associates (www.afpafitness.com)

- Personal Trainer Certification
- Advanced Personal Trainer Certification
- Master Personal Trainer Certification
- Children's Fitness Specialist Certification
- Sports Conditioning Specialist Certification
- Strength Trainer Specialist Certification
- Functional Training Specialist Certification
- Group Fitness Instructor Certification
- Yoga Fitness Instructor

The Cooper Institute (www.cooperinst.org)

- Personal Trainer Certification

International Fitness Professionals Association (www.ifpa-fitness.com)

- Certified Personal Fitness Trainer

*National Academy of Sports Medicine (www.nasm.org)

- Certified Personal Trainer

*National Council for Certified Personal Trainers (www.nccpt.com/User/Index.aspx)

- National Certified Personal Trainer

*National Council on Strength and Fitness (www.ncsf.org)

- National Certified Personal Trainer

---

*National Exercise and Sports Trainers Association (www.nestacertified.com)

- Certified Personal Fitness Trainer

*National Exercise Trainers Association (www.netafit.org)

- Certified Personal Trainer
- Certified Group Exercise Instructor

*National Federation of Professional Trainers (www.nfpt.com)

- Certified Personal Fitness Trainer

*National Strength and Conditioning Association (www.nsca-lift.org/Home)

- Certified Personal Trainer
- Certified Strength and Conditioning Specialist

*Indicates the agency is accredited by the National Commission for Certifying Agencies as of May 2013.

The knowledge required to be an effective health-fitness professional is extensive, thus a bachelor's degree in kinesiology is a base requirement. The following box lists some typical questions students ask, and the next box lists the current certifications available.

SUMMARY

This chapter provides an overview of the health-fitness profession's role in advocating active lifestyles, gives a brief look at the job activities of the health-fitness specialist, and surveys the various occupational opportunities available in the field. The chapter identified the various diseases that plagued the United States into the 20th century and those lifestyle diseases that active today that helped birth the health-fitness profession. To educate individuals regarding the nature of what produces bad health, the U.S, Department of Health and Human Services established a set of "Objectives for the Nation" called *Health People*. The health-fitness specialist intersects with *Healthy People* by helping clients achieve their personal fitness goals.

REFERENCES

1. Bureau of Labor Statistics, U.S. Department of Labor, *Occupational Outlook Handbook, 2010–2011* edition [Internet]. Available from: www.bls.gov/oco/ocos296.htm

2. Orchard, T. J., M. Temprosa, R. Goldberg, S. Haffner, R. Ratner, S. Marcovina, and S. Fowler, "The effect of metformin and intensive lifestyle intervention on the metabolic syndrome: the diabetes prevention program randomized trial." *Annals of Internal Medicine* 142(2005): 611–619.

3. U.S. Department of Health and Human Services, *Healthy People 2020: The Road Ahead*, Revised 2009, www.healthypeople.gov/HP2020.

4. U.S. Department of Health and Human Services, *Physical Activity and Health: A Report of the Surgeon General.* Atlanta, GA: U.S. Department of Health and Human Services, Centers for Disease Control and Prevention, National Center for Chronic Disease Prevention and Health Promotion, 1996.

Chapter 23 ///

STRENGTH AND CONDITIONING COACHING

OUTLINE

OBJECTIVES

1. Describe the current professional standing of strength and conditioning.
2. Discuss the roles and responsibilities of a strength and conditioning coach.
3. Learn the path to becoming a strength and conditioning coach.
4. Discuss the state of strength and conditioning certifications and licensure.
5. Learn the importance of a scientific approach to strength and conditioning coaching.
6. Discuss issues in sport science education.
7. Discuss current issues in strength and conditioning coaching.
8. Discuss formulating the training prescription utilizing periodization concepts.
9. Present the process of athlete monitoring.

BRIEF OVERVIEW OF THE PROFESSION

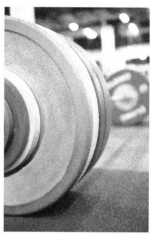

© Nico Traut, 2013. Used under license from Shutterstock, Inc.

Strength and conditioning (SC) coaching can be broadly defined as individuals charged with the responsibility of physically and mentally preparing athletes for competition. They are an integral part of the sport performance enhancement group working alongside sport medicine, sport coaches, and sport scientists in an effort to maximize the adaptation process. This chapter presents the scope and aim of SC coaching. It focuses on the coach's responsibility, the plan's execution, and some practical situations often facing SC coaches.

Paid positions in SC include working with athletes ranging from youth (primarily in the private sector), to college (the largest group of employed SC coaches in the United States), to professional, and military personnel (currently the fastest growing area of SC). Salaries in SC span a wide range. For example, many NCAA assistant SC coaches or head SC coaches at smaller colleges/universities earn from $30,000–$50,000. Head SC coaches at large universities or those working with professional teams can earn well over $100,000. In general, SC is a male-dominated profession. 62.9% of Division 1 Football Bowl Division (FBS) schools have at least one female SC coach compared to 29.3% of FCS schools.

Strength and conditioning coaching can be a very stressful position because it is a high-energy job typically requiring a high volume of work hours (50+), often including weekends, dealing with departmental politics, and just like other jobs in sport, the importance of winning is paramount. Top-level athletics is big business, as evidenced by the number of cable channels exclusive to sports and even the popularity of local broadcasts (21).

Goals and Challenges

SC coaching requires diligence and a detail-oriented mindset. One could argue that being passionate about SC is perhaps the first requirement to being a good SC coach. An excellent example of this is the individual's willingness to train like the athletes being coached. Undergoing rigorous training alongside his or her athletes enables the coach to better understand what the athletes are experiencing, which allows for better direction.

An example of being detailed is keeping records. Extensive recordkeeping is required in the job because of the number of athletes typically trained, usually 100 or more at any given time, as well as the high prevalence of lawsuits in sport due to injury or poor performance. Being able to justify decisions, training loads, and relative intensities can help protect SC and sport-specific coaches. Additionally, SC coaches must be well versed in the various rules and regulations of their employer (team or school) *and* the sports league (NCAA, NFL).

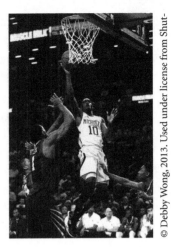

© Debby Wong, 2013. Used under license from Shutterstock, Inc.

Perhaps the most difficult thing a SC coach does is produce a scientifically supported annual training plan. An individual coach can be inspiring and enthusiastic, but if the plan lacks the necessary scientific underpinning, its execution may fail to induce the necessary adaptations for improving performance.

Training for sport is a complex, multifaceted, and integrative process in which an athlete is prepared physically, technically, tactically, and psychologically to perform at the highest level possible (22). This makes SC coaching a complicated endeavor with many considerations coexisting within an intricate and often perplexing process. Taking the scientific approach is imperative if the process is to have the desired effect.

Historical Perspective

SC coaching came into existence in the United States in the late 1970s thanks to the efforts of several groundbreaking coaches such as Alvin Roy and Boyd Epley (16). However, physical training for enhanced performance is not a new concept. For example, strength training of soldiers for the purpose of preparing for warfare was routine during the Chou dynasty (1122–249 B.C.). Gladiators underwent strength training and conditioning practices to better prepare them for battle/competition (17).

Coaches Highlight

Strength and Conditioning Spotlight: Mike Favre, M.Ed., RSCC*D, CSCS, SCCC Director of Strength and Conditioning for Olympic Sports at the University of Michigan

Coach Favre, The recipient of the 2011 NSCA College SC Coach of the Year, is currently the Director of Olympic Sports at the University of Michigan. Coach Favre has led an impressive and successful career in SC that includes five-plus years as an SC coach at the U.S. Olympic Committee Sports Performance Center in Colorado Springs, CO, and two and a half years as the Lead SC Coach for The Scottish Institute of Sport. Coach Favre has consistently utilized a scientific approach, staying on top of the scientific literature as well as being involved in the process. He has contributed several scientific papers to peer-reviewed journals and presents at national and international sport science and coach education meetings (NSCA Coaches Conference, UKSCA International Conference). When explaining his rationale for utilizing a scientific approach to training and demanding it of his staff, Coach Favre explains, "I have always been very interested in why something does what it does. The end result wasn't good enough, I needed to know the 'how' and 'why.' In addition, I wanted to be able to support my decisions when asked by others as to the 'how' and 'why.' I don't want to be considered an irrational person who does things based on 'emotion' or 'feeling,' but rather rational, objective science."

The National Strength Coaches Association, later renamed the National Strength and Conditioning Association (NSCA), was formed in 1978. Prior to this, if a school had a weight room, it was likely to be managed by a sport coach, an athletic trainer, or a volunteer. This was problematic in that persons from these fields lacked the required knowledge to be successful SC coaches.

Over the last few decades the number of SC coaches has steadily grown. In the early 1980s these coaches were primarily employed by large Division I universities. Presently, all BCS schools employ a SC coach, and they can also be found at Division II, Division III, and NAIA schools. All of the major professional sports teams (NFL, NBA, NHL, MLB) employ SC coaches. College coaches may have somewhat greater autonomy and freedom to make training decisions for their athletes compared to professional SC coaches. However, college SC coaches certainly have their own hurdles/issues, such as dealing with NCAA rules (accountable hours), having to work around the academic calendar (most athletes are gone for summer and winter break), working around the sport coaches' practice schedules, and an inability to override the sport coach regarding certain training decisions.

PREPARATION AND PLANNING FOR THE PROSPECTIVE STRENGTH AND CONDITIONING COACH

Realizing a passion for physical training is a crucial first step to becoming a SC coach. Based on job postings where the required and preferred qualifications are introduced, an applicant must possess a bachelor's degree in exercise science or a related field and possess a certification, typically the NSCA CSCS. Preferred qualifications typically involve a master's degree in exercise science or related field and from two to five years of experience working with athletes.

Planning a Path

Beginning the journey to becoming a SC coach typically involves pursuing a bachelor's degree in exercise science. While there are literally hundreds of exercise science programs, most do not emphasize sport and/or strength and conditioning. Consequently, during the four years of undergraduate work, it is recommended that students read SC and sport science literature outside the classroom.

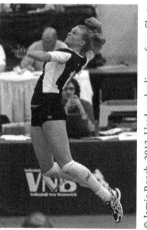

© Jamie Roach, 2013. Used under license from Shutterstock, Inc.

It is also important to get field experience. For example, volunteering at the student's college or university as an unpaid intern is critical. It is also worthwhile to train as an athlete trains in order to look the part. It is true that ex-collegiate athletes may have an advantage in acquiring SC coaching positions because of their prior experience in competitive athletics. Many SC coaches once competed at the collegiate level. However, athletic experience at the scholastic level is necessary in the absence of collegiate experience.

During the last year of undergraduate work the prospective SC coach may be advised to do two things: prepare for the NSCA CSCS exam and submit applications to schools for graduate assistant (GA) positions. The NSCA CSCS requires a bachelor's degree, but the exam can be taken within the last semester of enrollment and, if passed, awarded immediately after graduation. Graduate assistant opportunities can be found on the NCAA marketplace website (ncaamarketplace.ncaa.com). For a prospective SC coach, a prior GA position can strengthen the resume in that it improves academic qualifications while also counting as two years of experience in training collegiate athletes.

Due to the number of those applying for GA spots, it has become fairly common for those recently graduated to pursue either an unpaid or slightly paid (usually a small stipend) position for a semester (sometimes a year) before pursuing their master's degree. These internships can also strengthen the resume and are available at various places (professional teams, private sector) in addition to the NCAA. Paid or stipend internships at places such as the U.S. Olympic Training Center or Athletes Performance Institute can often be as competitive as applying for GA SC positions. These internships cost employers less money (and in many cases no money) and usually last only a semester. There are also more internships available at any given time, and they are posted much more frequently.

With this basic guideline or path to becoming a SC coach, the rest of this chapter covers nuances, issues, and important information about SC as well as conceptual ideas once an individual enters the SC coaching profession.

CERTIFICATIONS, LICENSURE, AND EDUCATION

SC coaches bear a tremendous responsibility for their athletes, who often place much of their development in the hands of these coaches (22). Dedicated, determined athletes will often place as much or more importance on their sport as anything else in their life, so much so they will even identify themselves by their particular sport (I am a baseball player). These athletes expect, and demand at times, that their SC coach help them realize their goals (make an Olympic team or achieve professional status). Thus, qualified SC coaches should be knowledgeable, have a background in sport science, and remain up to date. These coaches must ensure evidence-based training practices. Therefore, education and certification are often the primary indicators of a SC coach's knowledge base.

SC lacks an agreed-upon body of knowledge and the necessary certification standards required to be considered to a true profession. This lack of a body of knowledge is not due to a lack of existing scientific information, but to a lack of agreement within the SC community. This can be traced to the lack of serious coach education and sport science in the U.S. collegiate system (21). The literature indicates that SC coaches often put little priority on peer-reviewed literature and commonly implement training practices they underwent themselves as athletes or that they "borrowed" from the most recent successful team (5).

The National Strength and Conditioning Association (NSCA) and the Collegiate Strength and Conditioning Association (CSCCa) offer the two better-known certifications for SC coaches in the United States, but there is no official governing body for SC coaches in the United States. Both the NSCA and CSCCa represent strong interest groups and, as professional organizations, operate to provide guidelines and networking opportunities for SC coaches. The need for licensure for coaching has been proposed, specifically for NCAA SC coaches, noting the many serious injuries athletes have endured. In some documented cases athletes have died due to poor decisions by the sport-specific and/or the SC coach (4).

The NSCA offers two levels of certification available to SC coaches: the CSCS and the Registered Strength and Conditioning Coach (RSCC). The certification offered by the CSCCa currently is not an accredited certification. The CSCS has been accredited by the National Commission for Certifying Agencies (NCCA) for nearly 20 years. The CSCCa also offers an advanced certification "Master" SC coach, which is available to those coaches who have been active continuously in a full-time job for 12 years or more. Table 23.1 presents a comparison of the NSCA and CSCCa's certifications while Table 23.2 presents a comparison between the two organizations.

A primary difference in the two certifications and organizations at present appears to be a focus on the educational background necessary to become certified and the use of evidence-based protocols and programming. Based on the data obtained from the NSCA, the scientific knowledge required to pass the CSCS exam may have created a barrier leading to resistance of CSCCa members to the NSCA certification process. Upon further investigation of CSCS records, it appears that 20% of the CSCCa Master Strength Coaches who attempted the CSCS exam failed. This was particularly evident in the scientific portion of the test. This is not to denigrate the CSCCa certification process. It appears to be developing into an excellent certification. It is still evolving; however, the findings suggest that these coaches who had been in the SC coaching field for more than 12 years did not have the minimum level of sport science and sport medicine background to pass the CSCS exam, but

Table 23.1. Comparison between Various NSCA and CSCCa Certifications

	NSCA		CSCCa	
	RSCC	CSCS	SCCC	MSCC
Bachelors required	x	x	x	X
Internship required			x	X
CEUs required	x	x	x	X
Annual renewal course required	x			
Accredited with NCCA		x		
Textbook available	x	x		
Scientific journal available to members	x	x		
Evidence based practitioners journal available to members	x	x		
Certification available to college or pro SC Coaches	x	x	x	X
Available to physicians		x		
Available to physical therapists		x		
Available to athletic trainers		x		
Available to nutritionists		x		
Available to personal trainers		x		

*This table compares the NSCA's RSCC distinction and CSCS certification as compared to the Collegiate Strength and Conditioning Coaches Association Strength and Conditioning Coach Certified and Master Strength and Conditioning Coach certifications.

yet were in charge of training athletes at their schools. This finding suggests that (a) there is a lack of scientific rigor associated with the certification process of the CSCCa and (b) individuals receiving their qualifications through the CSCCa may lack the knowledge to understand basic principles of sport science and conditioning. This could reduce student-athletes' development and place them at greater risk for injury or death by being trained by unqualified coaches.

Currently, in the United States it may be argued that the NSCA, as an interest group organization, provides a greater level of the scientific foundation for the application of SC compared to the CSCCa. However, this is not to indicate that the NSCA certifications are of a sufficiently high standard. It could also be argued that the NSCA certifications are not of sufficient quality. The written exam may not be scientifically rigorous enough, and the education requirements to sit for the exam are minimal (any undergraduate degree will suffice; history is as good as exercise science). The NSCA certainly falls short on the practical side as well: No internship or evidence-based "hands-on" experience is required.

NSCA and CSCCa certifications have strengths and weaknesses. In studying certifications from around the world, it becomes apparent that the United Kingdom (UKSCA) and Australian Strength and Conditioning Associations (ASCA) provide far more comprehensive certifications than either U.S.–based group. The

Table 23.2.   NSCA's CSCS vs. CSCCa Organizations

NSCA vs CSCCa	NSCA	CSCCa
Recertification Fee	$50	$45
CEU Requirements (3 year)	60 contact hours	45 contact hours[*]
Accepted CEUs	Identical	Identical
Clinics & Workshops	4 national conferences, 9 regional conferences and 50 state clinics	National conference, USAW clinics
Accreditation	NCCA	None[**]
Online Courses	>75 quizzes, online modules	13 available
Certifications	Certified Strength & Conditioning Specialist (CSCS) & NSCA—CPT	Strength & Conditioning Coach Certified Master Strength & Conditioning Coach

*CEU calculation value is virtually identical to NSCA; for example, attendance at an event is worth 0.75 where the NSCA is worth 1.0 (contact hours).

**Based on current NCCA requirements: assuming that CSCCa eventually has its certification accredited, it may have to discontinue some of its membership requirements and all of its CEUs cannot all come from its own organization.

Accredited Strength and Conditioning Coach (ASCC) offered by the UKSCA is particularly sound. To become certified and to become eligible to vote in UKSCA elections, you must be an active SC coach and pass the following tests:

1. Present an annual plan for the athlete(s) *that you have been working with* and be able to defend this before a group of expert coaches and sport scientists. This annual plan would include all of the competition, training, and nutrition, for the athlete(s) in question for the coming year or competitive year. Also required is a paper detailing the same subject area.
2. A written test dealing with basic science (physiology, biomechanics, psychology) as well as the scientific foundations of training.
3. A practical test of ability to actually teach (not simply demonstrate) a snatch or a clean, and a squat.
4. A practical/applied test of the ability to construct a non-weight-room conditioning session for a sport drawn out of a hat. This session requires the implementation of plyometric, agility and other such drills.

At present:

- The NCAA has no real educational standards for coaches, particularly for SC coaches.
- Athletic departments have no real standards for coaches, including the SC coach, nor do athletic departments strongly promote coaching education.
- Most academic programs are based on participation not performance and are generally devoid of classes dealing with the training process, use of monitoring programs, appropriate SC practices, or how to interface with sport science and sport medicine.
- Sport science programs are in the minority among exercise science academic programs in the United States.

Application of Strength and Conditioning Education: A Common Issue

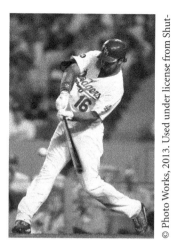

© Photo Works, 2013. Used under license from Shutterstock, Inc.

When comparing the fields of Sport Medicine and SC, a few interesting contrasts are apparent. Due to the professional nature of sport medicine (medical doctors and NATA-certified staff), the sport medicine staff is able to overrule sport-specific coaches on training/practice procedures. This, however, is not the case for the SC coach. If poor coaching/training decisions are being made by the sport coach, the SC coach, who should be more educated in psychological and physiological responses to training, cannot override the sport coach's decision. Many coaches do not have a degree in physical education, exercise physiology, sport science, or anything related, believing that on-the-job experience is of prime importance. While experience is essential, it cannot take the place of a sound science background.

The current environment in sport is that the head coach has the final word on everything (except allowing participation with severe injury or illness). In contrast, the SC coach is looked upon as a service provider rather than a professional. For example, if the head coach (or an assistant) makes poor decisions with the athletes' training program that will likely increase the potential for injury or overtraining, the SC coach is usually powerless to alter the course of events. An interesting dilemma occurs when the SC coach realizes deficiencies in the program or potential injurious practices. By allowing poor training practices to proceed, the SC coach is essentially sanctioning the activity. However, if the SC coach speaks up, he or she is rarely acknowledged or taken seriously by the coaching staff or the Athletic Department, and the SC coach often gets blamed for the poor outcome. Job and livelihood could be at stake. Speaking up can be perilous. A major effort of SC advocates should be to change this situation.

Non-Evidence-Based Coaching

Sport coaches are certainly not alone in making poor, non-evidence-based training decisions. SC coaches all too often commit these errors as well. There is no doubt that mental toughness is an important attribute in sport. A popular idea in both the sport coaching and SC coaching arena is that increasing mental toughness will enhance sport performance during critical points in competition. Thus, the coach's idea of increasing mental toughness is usually to make athletes extremely fatigued and having to "push through it." This line of reasoning is flawed. Mental toughness has been shown to be specific to the task. For example, if one increases mental toughness to run long distances, this is unlikely to make this person mentally tough in unrelated situations, such as staying off a breaking ball, an important skill in baseball. Furthermore, this approach can greatly interfere with planned training. Simply applying a training stimulus for the sake of creating fatigue is to misunderstand the importance of the training process. Poor fatigue management can disrupt the positive adaptive stimulus of an otherwise well-planned training process. The addition of extra work, or very fatiguing work, at the wrong time during training limits positive adaptation (22). Furthermore, SC coaches are limited in the amount of time spent with athletes, especially in the collegiate setting, and having to deal with the issue of conflicting adaptations further reduces the effectiveness of both the coach and the prescribed training stimuli (2). As one noted sport scientist explains, "It doesn't take a genius to make an athlete tired" (3). This is not implying that training may not incorporate important psychological characteristics. It should. Simply put, the focus of the overload (training stimuli) principle should be focused and specific to the sport.

Another example of non-evidence-based coaching practices can be found when training fads enter the SC realm. This is problematic for several reasons. Most fads are intended for the general population and are meant to enhance health or looks, not as a developmental process for athletes. Examples of these types of fads are crossfit, unstable surface training, and P90X. These programs generally lack any scientific backing and are not supported in peer-reviewed literature.

While some may claim that a new training paradigm produces greater results, and over time this will be demonstrated in the scientific literature, one must ask if this "new" mode of training adheres to evidence-based training principles and processes (overload, specificity, variation, fatigue management). If this is not the case, the SC coach should proceed with caution. Those who claim they do not have time to wait for the science are ignoring the mountain of research that currently exists.

© Aspen Photo, 2013. Used under license from Shutterstock, Inc.

SPORT SCIENCE: THE FOUNDATION OF STRENGTH AND CONDITIONING KNOWLEDGE

The science underpinning the training process allows SC coaches to justify their training prescription. It also allows them to analyze and critique other SC coaches' training prescriptions. Most importantly, however, it enables the SC coach to evaluate his or her own training processes, which eventually results in more optimal training. Sport science can help guide the decision-making process, allowing the SC coach to provide evidence-based training prescription for athletes.

An understanding of basic and applied sport science allows for training mechanisms and theories to be established, increasing the knowledge base from which the training process is built upon (2, 22). Due to the multifaceted nature of the training process, SC coaches should have a firm grasp of the various scientific disciplines involved. These include anatomy, physiology, biomechanics, and bioenergetics. An understanding of basic training principles and more advanced training theory is also required.

Numerous sport scientists have contributed, those working in the East (Nadori, Matveyev, Verkhashonsky, Bompa) and those in the west (Stone, Garhammer, Sands), to further sport science research (6). Countries such as Hungary (1940s–1950s), the old Soviet Union (1960s–1970s), East Germany (1970s–1980s), and Australia (1990s– 2000s) are examples of countries that have invested a tremendous amount into sport science and subsequently found success on the world stage. Perhaps German super-heavyweight lifter Matthias Steiner summed up the role of sport science best shortly after winning the gold medal in Beijing (2008). When asked the reason behind his victorious performance, he said, "German sport science is the best" (19).

Medvedyev, a well-known Russian sport scientist, explains that, "At the present time, considerable scientific methodological material has accumulated . . . . this constantly raises the knowledge requirements of the coach, with respect to planning rationally, the athletes training." He continues, "A definite contradiction arises when instructions are designed by highly qualified specialists, but their implementations, to put it mildly, are carried out by lesser qualified coaches." (10)

A thought-provoking paper titled, "The Downfall of Sport Science," argued that essentially all coaches in the United States who received a degree focused on coaching received a degree concentrating on participation and not performance (21). The paper also explained how there are few or no true sport science positions in the United States. At the 2009 NSCA national conference, the keynote speaker presented the idea that perhaps those most similar to sport scientists in the United States are highly educated SC coaches that utilize a scientific approach (20). Unlike exercise science faculty members who focus on sport, SC coaches can dictate and influence the overall training prescription, implement athlete monitoring programs, and help drive the sport performance team.

Sport Science: Guiding the Formulation of the Periodized Training Plan

Planning and organizing the training program is arguably the most important thing an SC coach does. It is important to understand that periodization and the process of planning the athlete's training cycle are not exactly the same thing.

Periodization is an organized approach to training that involves progressive cycling of various aspects of a training program during a specific period in order to achieve specific fitness parameters and meet specific timelines. Planning deals with exercise selection, set and repetition manipulation that allows the protocol to meet the periodization requirements.

Periodization deals with appropriate, logical application and timing of fitness phases, timelines, and is an inclusive theoretical paradigm that SC coaches and sport scientists use to direct training adaptations. Thus, periodization can be viewed as a conceptual roadmap to optimize performance. Planning, however, deals with the detailed manipulation of training variables such as exercise selection, sets, and reps that make periodization work. Periodization is the tool with which the SC coach manipulates and structures all of the training variables, systematically allowing the athlete to optimize performance at the appropriate time as well as inducing long-term adaptations.

Planning is probably the most important thing coaches do when constructing their training programs (2). They should be constructed methodically and based upon scientific evidence. Implementing a training plan that is unstructured, random, and aimless does a disservice to the athletes involved. Coaches should plan their training programs three to five annual plans ahead of time (1). In many settings this is unreasonable due to too many future unknowns (i.e., next year's team roster). However, the idea that long-term planning is important certainly holds true. Annual plans should include not just sets, reps, and percentages of weight room, but the overall training plan such as conditioning, practice, and travel, among other variables. Furthermore, annual plans should be viewed as modifiable to allow for unforeseen scheduling adjustments and coaching decisions. In short, the use of periodization allows the SC coach to plan and structure the training process logically and with purpose.

Brief History of Periodization

Periodization in some form has been around since the ancient Olympic Games (776 B.C. to 339 A.D.) (6). The term *periodization* comes from the word *period*, or segment of time (6). Originally, periodization was used to describe the photo periods of the sun because coaches and scientists noted that their athletes performed better in the summer months when the days were longer and warmer and fresher produce was available (6). During the 1920s and 1930s the term *periodization* became more applied to training methodology and as a means of dividing training phases into smaller, more manageable divisions of time (6, 22).

Several sport scientists and coaches from various countries, notably northern and eastern Europe, have made contributions toward the concept of periodization. The old Soviet Union and allied countries made effective use of the concepts of periodization. At the end of World War II the Soviet Union made a commitment to athletics, funding a statewide sports program with the intention of demonstrating the superiority of its political system (6). Russian sport scientist and pedagogist Lenoid Matveyev published a model of an annual training plan in 1965 (9). This model was developed through the monitoring and recording of how the Russian athletes trained and prepared for the 1952 Olympic Games in Helsinki, Finland (6). Matveyev analyzed the training programs implemented by the Russian Olympic coaches and divided the annual plan into phases, subphases, and training cycles (6). Matveyev then compared the training approaches of the more successful athletes to the approaches of the athletes of lesser success.

Matveyev based his periodization model on these data proposing relatively gradual, wavelike increases in volume and intensity over each phase (22). He used the term *periodization* based on the historical significance of measuring time and noted that the human body experiences natural monthly biocycles (typically four). Consequently 4 ± 2 weeks is often considered one block of training because it conforms to Matveyev's idea of biocycles lasting approximately 4 wks (6). It could be argued that Matveyev's periodization studies are more relevant and applicable to today's athletics than more contemporary studies due to the extensive length (multiple years), type of subjects (athletes including elite athletes), and sample size.

Modern Periodization Models

Matveyev's basic periodization models are considered by many to be the traditional or classic model of periodization. However, it should be noted that Matveyev's models were not created with the intent of being universally applied. Matveyev's periodization model originally culminated with only one competition phase because the athletes he was observing had few competitions and even fewer major competitions (one or two major contests in a calendar year).

Sport is quite different now than it was 50 years ago with the number of competitions being much greater. Undertraining and overcompeting can result in decreased training time along with increased competition stress (travel stress, interrupted/decreased training, physiological and psychological fatigue) (7). Additionally, it is difficult to develop different physical and physiological characteristics or motor abilities (speed and long-term endurance) simultaneously. Matveyev noted these problems in his original work (9).

Several sport scientists have recently proposed periodization models that modify the traditional approach in a manner fitting modern competition schedules (2, 7, 13, 22,). Phase potentiation or block periodization enables coaches to plan around modern competitive schedules by training specific fitness components in sequential blocks (2, 7, 13, 22). This helps obviate negative interactions of "mixed training" and allows for multiple peak performances during a season (2, 7, 13, 22). This process utilizes specific phases and subphases that make up the annual plan in which a specific fitness characteristic is emphasized during each subphase while other fitness characteristics are de-emphasized (2).

Implementing Periodization

Although periodization has grown in popularity in the United States, many coaches still struggle with understanding and mastering the concept (22). Modern concepts of periodization appear to have originated in Eastern Europe, thus many of the original terms do not translate well into English (13). Also, this confusion may exist due to the differences in educational backgrounds between most American sport coaches and sport scientists. Periodization theory contains primarily scientific terminology, resulting in a more complicated language that may distance coaches from attempting to completely grasp certain advances.

SC coaches attempt to optimally manipulate training variables (volume, intensity, exercise selection) to enhance adaptation and avoid overtraining. Just like coaches prepare to defeat an opposing team by tactically outsmarting the opponent, the coach can use periodization and planning to implement "planned unpredictability," which is designed to outsmart "the body's adaptive mechanism" (13). *Planned unpredictability* is a term used to mean that sudden and large alterations in training variables can "shock" the physiological mechanisms into creating positive adaptations leading to improved performance. As stated by Plisk, "This is no easy task considering that this adversary (adaptation) is very smart, having the collective wisdom of millions of years of evolution" (13).

Training is the process of imposing physical stress resulting in enhanced fitness capabilities (17). Training adaptations or "effects" can differ based on their physiological mechanisms, timing, and duration (8). These adaptations (Table 23.3) are classified as acute, immediate, cumulative, delayed, and residual (8).

Periodization seeks to take advantage of these effects by emphasizing fitness phases in a logical order. Typically, an annual training plan is broken down into three main phases: preparatory, competition, and transition (2). The preparatory and competition phases can be divided into general and specific, while the transition phase simply consists of a rest and restitution period following the end of the competition phase (2). The focus of the general subphase is to develop a base (e.g., alterations in body composition and increased work capacity), which increases the ability to meet the physiological and psychological demands of the sport by emphasizing less specific exercises along with typically higher volume loads and less technical work (2). The specific/special subphase employs more sport-specific technical work along with typically higher training intensities and

Table 23.3. Generalized Training Effects

Types	Definition	Duration of Event
Acute Effects	Alterations in physiology during exercise	Seconds, minutes
Immediate Effect	Alterations in physiology resulting from a single workout and/or a single day of training	Hours
Cumulative Effect	Alterations in physiology and level of motor/technical abilities resulting from a series of workouts	Days, months, year
Delayed Effect	Alterations in physiology and level of motor/technical abilities attained over a given time interval after a specific training program	Days, Weeks
Residual Effect	Retention of physiological adaptations and motor abilities after cessation of training	Days, Weeks

Modified from Issurin (8)

somewhat lower volume loads (2). During the competition phase, training intensity may be further increased, volume is lowered, and emphasis on technical aspects intensified (2, 22).

Periodization also deals with time lines or time phases. Traditionally, macrocycles, mesocycles, and microcycles are subunits of the annual plan, each having a designated time length and each devoted to specific tasks that direct the objectives of the training plan. The duration of each phase or subunit depends on the time allowed by the competition schedule and the training status of the athlete. An athlete's training status as well as his or her inherent athletic ability significantly affects the adaptation process and consequently the optimal training dose.

A potential problem with the traditional approach is that within many phases the volume of training variables is raised or lowered simultaneously, thus long periods of low volume (as in long competitive seasons) can reduce fitness to the point at which performance deteriorates (7). Sequenced/block approaches to periodization in which each phase is highly specialized through the use of logically sequenced concentrated loads help to obviate this problem (7). A concentrated load is a period of training that emphasizes one specific aspect of fitness (or performance). A concentrated load typically fits into 4 ± 2 week blocks (22). However, the length of the block may vary according to the competitive time frame.

Sequenced periodization models rely on mesocycles, blocks, and concentrated loads to direct the macrocycle or annual plan. These blocks allow for the training and manipulating of specific training variables (volume, intensity, exercise selection). Blocks or concentrated loads are the structural building blocks that serve as the vehicle driving the macrocycle. Four-week blocks appear to be the optimal window for integrating various stimuli (13). Training decay has been cited as the rationale for one-month training cycles (23, 24). After four weeks a change in the focus of the training stimulus is necessary to avoid a plateau in performance and to continue physiological adaptations. Furthermore, four-week blocks allow for delayed training responses to summate cumulative training effects (2, 22). Classifying mesocycles by their objectives and foci allows for purposeful sequencing of the training plan (2, 22).

Appropriate sequencing of training blocks within a mesocycle is crucial because one block potentiates the next due to the aftereffects of one training stimulus altering and influencing future training stimuli (2, 12, 22). This is a basic tenet of periodization. What a SC coach implements during one phase or block affects the adaptive responses and physiological expressions of the athlete down the road (22). For an intermediate or advanced athlete systematically converging, the cumulative effects over the long term is referred to as long-term phase potentiation and is due to the nature of residual or delayed training effects (22).

An intermediate periodization strategy related to the manipulation of microcycles or intra-mesocycle variation termed summated microcycles is proposed (22). Summated microcycles are a type of block and are based on the summation phenomena of training effects and the involution of training effects (22). Summated microcycles are characterized by a series of three- to four-week blocks with an extensive to intensive workload progression followed by a short restoration period.

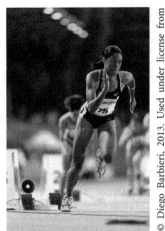

© Diego Barbieri, 2013. Used under license from Shutterstock, Inc.

This concept allows corresponding stimuli to be introduced and reintroduced in a cyclical manner while minimizing the decay of these stimuli (22). Summated microcycles are unique compared to other periodization models in that a whole block of training (four-week mesocycle) targets a very specific training factor such as strength endurance, maximum strength, or speed strength (22).

Two variations of this concept are illustrated, a model for increased strength and a model for increased power (22). The strength-summated microcycle or block follows a loading progression of increasing intensity, which can increase the volume (work) followed by an unloading week (for example, 3:1:3 weeks of increases followed by a decreased loading week). The highest workloads occur during week 3. Consequently, cumulative fatigue is highest during week 3 and necessitates an unload week during week 4.

The power-summated microcycle implements the largest training volumes during week 1 (usually with an emphasis in strength) in the form of planned overreaching. The subsequent three weeks follow a decrease in training volume with an unload week during week 4. In this model decreases in power production can occur during week 1 as a result of fatigue. However, during the following weeks, power increases back to baseline or further and during the unload week (week 4) there is the possibility of markedly enhanced power performance.

SPORT-PERFORMANCE ENHANCEMENT GROUPS

Sport is unique because, unlike many other facets of life, it represents a pursuit of excellence and rewards the best performer as champion. Consequently, sport is the quest to become a champion and requires a commitment not only by the athlete, but by the entire sport enhancement team (coaches, sport scientists, athletic trainers, sport physicians, sport psychologists, among others). It is truly a unique undertaking.

In addition to developing and executing the training prescription, SC coaches should also monitor how their athletes are responding to the training program. If a SC coach does not record daily training volume loads and intensities, and periodically measure training effects via performance testing, valid conclusions about the effectiveness of a particular training prescription become impossible. Essentially, if the coach doesn't know what the athletes did and doesn't know what the individual results were at a particularly moment in the training process, then he or she is not only unable to ascertain the effectiveness of a particular training program, but it becomes difficult to claim that the program itself worked or didn't work.

Since fatigue and responses to various training stimuli are cumulative, the SC coach is not only monitoring how the athlete is responding to the SC program, but all of the training the athlete encounters. This can allow for training integration among SC coaches, sport coaches, sport scientists, and sport medicine staff. For example, during data returns from performance testing, the various parts of the sport performance team can discuss the data as a group and better determine the efficacy of the training program for individual athletes. An integrated plan allows for better fatigue management (sport practice and weight training) and optimized training practices (athletic trainer and SC coach planning injured athletes' training/rehab prescription).

Athlete Monitoring

"In theory there is no difference between theory and practice. In practice there is."—Yogi Berra

The objective of monitoring is to describe the athlete psychologically and physiologically at a specific moment (a biological snapshot). This allows the sport performance team to assess the effects of the training program (and other stressors) on that athlete since the last monitoring session. One of the primary reasons athletes may not respond as expected to a training program is poor fatigue management. If an athlete is not monitored closely, there is a chance that an acute period of accumulated fatigue may eventually evolve into long-term overtraining (18).

Ideally, there is very close interplay between the planning process and its subsequent execution (11). This interaction should result in an interrupted loop of: (a) planning, (b) executing, (c) measuring the training effects, and (d) revisiting the training plan to verify whether the predetermined training stimuli should be adjusted for upcoming mesocycles. Olbrecht refers to this as "training steering" and suggests that each feedback loop provides insight into an athlete's individual training responses, thus creating a greater training efficiency and a greater "return" from the training program (11).

SC coaches especially (through the sports performance enhancement group) can institute a monitoring system to provide feedback in order to make proper training adjustments (10). Periodic monitoring of the training process of an athlete is crucial in understanding how an athlete is responding to the training program and whether alterations or changes need to be made to the training plan (15). It is important to quantify both positive and negative effects of training. For example, it is important for the coach to understand the degree to which group and individual athletes' enhancement occurs and if the appropriate adaptations are occurring in concert with the design of the training program. Athlete monitoring includes training diaries to

---

Strength and Conditioning Spotlight: Tom Myslinski, MS, CSCS, RSCC Strength and Conditioning Coordinator Jacksonville Jaguars

Tom Myslinksi currently serves as the Head SC coach for the Jacksonville Jaguars. Before he began his coaching career, Myslinski spent nine seasons in the NFL as an interior lineman. Prior to working with the Jaguars, coach Myslinski served as the Head SC coach for the Cleveland Browns, the University of Memphis (football), and the University of North Carolina (football). In addition to his role as head SC coach Myslinski serves on the Jaguars Coaching Performance Committee and the Jaguars Human Performance Center Committee. Coach Myslinksi is incredibly diligent and committed to the monitoring process of his athletes. Coach Myslinksi explains, "My goal is to provide an all-encompassing athletic management data information system that will support and enhance the organization and programming of all physiological aspects of the professional football player."

Data returns from athlete monitoring sessions should be swift and rapid. If a SC coach sits on the data, by the time the coaching and sport medicine team receives the information the athletes will be in a different physiological state. Data return sessions should also include daily data collection in the form of volume loads and other more often measured variables (hydration status). Perhaps the most comprehensive approach to returning data to coaches is to give them a written paper while also providing an oral presentation. Data returns should be meaningful and as inclusive as possible. The SC coach should be mindful of the level of the language used in the paper and during the presentation in an effort to make it as easily consumable as possible.

record training volume, training intensity, exercises, tracking outside-daily stressors (for example, the Rusko heart rate test, body mass, and hours of sleep), and periodic field or laboratory tests to measure performance and performance variables. Given that training is a long-term process, the data should be handled as longitudinal data.

While we can predict the general direction of the adaptation process, we are much less effective at accurately predicting the magnitude of adaptation and specific performance outcomes (14). The quantification of training is a necessary step in understanding training outcomes. Quantification allows relationships to be established between the training program and physiological and performance variables as well as relationships between the training volume and the athlete's preparedness. Graphing these variables for extended periods enables the coach to ascertain if the athlete is going in the right direction.

Physiological and performance alterations as a result of the training program typically involve a lag time. However, the length of this delay is often impossible to predict, but may be longer in better trained athletes (15). Constantly monitoring and measuring performance variables enables the coach to receive cyclical feedback to make sure the changes the athlete experiences match the SC coach's expectations.

Since an athlete's preparedness fluctuates frequently, it is important to constantly monitor physiological and performance changes. If a coach only makes measurements at the beginning and end of a season or macrocycle, and the information obtained by those measurements shows a decrease in performance, no improvement, or much less improvement than expected, it is too late to make changes. A subpar performance at a major competition is not a good time for coaches to find out that their athlete was not adequately prepared. Athlete testing should be implemented regardless of the immediacy of a real competition (20).

SUMMARY

Being a SC coach is a major responsibility. Getting athletes as close to their genetic ceiling as possible, along with managing fatigue and optimizing performance at critical time periods, is no easy feat. It requires an education and understanding of sport science and an unwavering commitment to his or her athletes and the training process. An athlete monitoring program allows the SC coach to follow the adaptive process of his or her athletes as well as promoting integration among the sport performance enhancement group. Going forward, the landscape of education and certification and licensure will most likely be changing in that certain organizations will require a specific certification and, perhaps, eventually a uniformed licensure will be created similar to that received by athletic trainers. In short, being a SC coach can be a challenging and demanding profession. However, helping an athlete succeed can be more than enough reward as this is at the heart of what drives an SC coach.

REFERENCES

1. Banister, E. W., and H. A. Wenger, "Monitoring training." In *Physiological Testing of the Elite Athlete*, J. D. MacDougall, H. A. Wenger, & H. J. Green, eds. Ithaca, NY: Mouvement Publications, 1982, pp. 163–170.

2. Bompa, T. O., and G. G. Haff, *Periodization: Theory and Methodology of Training*, 5th ed.. Champaign, IL: Human Kinetics, 2009.

3. Brewer, C., "Some thoughts on athlete development." Presentation at the *Third Annual Coaches and Sport Science College*, Johnson City, Tennessee, 2007.

4. Casa, D. J., S. A. Anderson, L. Baker, L., et al., "The Inter-Association Task Force for Preventing Sudden Death in Collegiate Conditioning Sessions: Best practices recommendations." *Journal of Athletic Training* 47(4)(2012):477–480.

5. Durrel, D. L., T. J. Pujol, and J. T. Barnes, "A survey of scientific data and training methods utilized by collegiate strength and conditioning coaches." *Journal of Strength and Conditioning Research* 17(2003): 368–373.

6. Haff, G. G., "Roundtable discussion: Periodization of Training—Part 1." *Strength and Conditioning Journal* 26(2004): 50–69.

7. Issurin, V. B., "Block periodization versus traditional training theory: A review." *The Journal of Sports Medicine and Physical Fitness* 48(2008): 65–75.

8. Issurin, V. B., "Generalized training effects induced by athletic preparation: A review." *Journal of Sports Medicine and Physical Fitness* 49(2009): 4; ProQuest, p. 333.

9. Matveyev, L. P., *Periodization of Sports Training.* Moscow, Russia: Fizkultura I Sport, 1965.

10. Medvedyev, A. S., *A System of Multi-Year Training in Weightlifting.* Moscow, Russia: Fizkultura I Sport, 1986.

11. Olbrecht, J., *The Science of Winning.* England: Swimshop, 2000.

12. Plisk, S., "Periodization: Fancy name for a basic concept." *Olympic Coach* 16(2004): 14-1

13. Plisk, S., and M. H. Stone, "Periodization strategies." *Strength and Conditioning Journal* 25(19)(2003): 37.

14. Sands, W. A., and J. R. McNeal, "Predicting athlete preparation and performance: A theoretical perspective." *Journal of Sport Behavior* 23(3)(2000): 289–310.

15. Sands, W. A., and M. H. Stone, "Are you progressing and how would you know?" *Olympic Coach* 17(2005): 4–10.

16. Shurley, J. P., and J. S. Todd, "'The strength of Nebraska': Boyd Epley, Husker power, and the formation of the strength coaching profession." *Journal of Strength and Conditioning Research* 26(2012): 3177–3188.

17. Siff, M. C., *Supertraining.* Denver, CO: Supertraining Institute, 2003.

18. Smith, D. J., "A framework for understanding the training process leading to elite performance." *Sports Medicine* 33(15)(2003): 1103–1126.

19. Steiner, M., Television interview. Sky TV, 2008.

20. Stone, M. H., "What is sport science?" Presentation at the National Strength and Conditioning Conference, Las Vegas, Nevada, 2009.

21. Stone, M. H., W. A. Sands, and M. E. Stone, "The downfall of sports science in the United States." *Strength and Conditioning Journal* 26(2004): 72–75.

22. Stone, M. H., M. E. Stone, and W. A. Sands, *Principles and Practice of Resistance Training.* Champaign, IL: Human Kinetics, 2007.

23. Viru, A., *Adaptation in Sports Training.* Boca Raton, FL: CRC Press, 1995.

24. Zatsiorsky, V. M., *Science & Practice of Strength Training.* Champaign, IL: Human Kinetics, 1995.

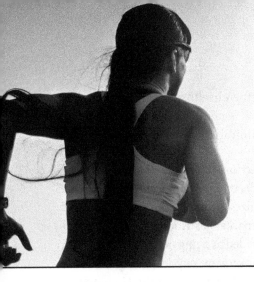

Chapter 24

FUTURE KINESIOLOGY

OUTLINE

Objectives

New Frontiers

Paradigm Shifts

Future Perspective

Summary

References

OBJECTIVES

1. Explain the paradigm shift associated with the development of exercise science as an academic discipline.
2. Describe two important distinctions between a profession and a discipline.
3. Explain how modern technology may continue to impact exercise science into the 21st century.

The future of kinesiology is to lower chronic disease prevalence, lengthen healthspan and average lifespan, and improve the quality of well-being/mental health. *Frank W. Booth, PhD, Department of Physiology, School of Medicine, University of Missouri* (personal communication, May 2013)

Who could have thought in the 1960s, when the challenge to physical education was made, that its offspring, kinesiology, would one day relegate the mother discipline to the narrow status of a pedagogical field of study, a mere teaching profession? That is not pejorative in any sense; it simply recognizes the enormous stature to which the transdisciplinary field of kinesiology has risen. Kinesiology has made remarkable strides in terms of its relevancy to higher education. A scant generation ago physical education was derided as being non-academic, a field not worthy of graduate education. Today, this bleak picture of the study of movement, physical activity, exercise, and sport is completely reversed. For example, by 2018 the number of physical therapists in the United States is projected to grow by 30%. But according to the American Kinesiology Association, the number of students majoring in kinesiology—a field in which many physical therapists hold a degree—grew 50% from 2003 to 2008.

Kinesiology has undoubtedly been the fastest-growing major at many universities due in no small part to its social significance, its importance in impacting general health (especially in relation to the triple epidemics of obesity, metabolic syndrome, and diabetes), and the growing societal prominence of sports. For example, one has only to input the term *exercise* in the search engine provided at the website of the *National Institutes of Health* to glean the importance placed on exercise science research by the federal government. In March 2016 a search was completed using the Research Portfolio Online Reporting Tools (RePORT) to access the database of the National Institutes of Health (NIH). Using the term "exercise" showed 1,896 active projects worth $826,227,804 in funding and 177 sub-research awards worth $44,642,228 in 2015–16. There were 807 active clinical trial studies related to "exercise." The Expenditures and Results Tool (RePORTER) database is a repository of NIH-funded research projects and access publications and patents resulting from that funding. This represents a massive amount of funding, indicating the need to continue to study the effects of exercise on health. But what of kinesiology's future? Will the discipline continue to progress as it has over the last several decades?

NEW FRONTIERS

The answer to the previous question should be a resounding yes if current health trends are of predictive value. For example, the *World Health Organization*, in discussing the root causes of obesity, cited the "decrease in physical activity due to the increasingly sedentary nature of many forms of work, changing modes of transportation, and increasing urbanization." Research on obesity, metabolic syndrome, and diabetes are at a fever pitch, with exercise-science-related studies at an all-time high on these problems and others. But is future kinesiology solely in the hands of researchers and the federal dollars that support them?

The maturation of any discipline certainly follows a path in the production of relevant science. If scientific productivity is the chief indicator of continued development and growing strength, then the future of kinesiology is bright indeed. Consider a review of the research conducted in exercise science over the first decade of the 21st century and where it is likely to go over the next decade or two (1). These researchers conducted a Pub Med search in 2010 using the word "exercise." Some of the results were as follows:

- Over the decade there were approximately 82,826 peer-reviewed articles published
- About 3,836 papers were linked to genetics, 45 to proteomics, 155 to genomics, 22 to epigenetics, 326 to signaling pathways.

When the word *obesity* was added to the search, there were 7,357 articles retrieved. In succession, each of the following terms produced a significant number of exercise science related papers:

diabetes 6,312, longevity 254, muscle 18,562, bone 4,038, metabolism 24,033, nervous system 4,505, hormones 6,954, brain function 2,644, circulation 3,426, immune system 1,281, respiratory 5,734, and hematology 126.

If nothing else, these data show the wide range of exercise-science research currently being conducted. Baldwin and Haddad mention several noteworthy achievements by exercise researchers in the last decade (1).

- Exercise genomics should enhance understanding of exercise responses and help the prescription of individualized exercise regimens for treating susceptible patients.
- Introduction of exercise "pills," (*exercise mimetics*)—pharmacological agents (orally active compounds that mimic the effects of exercise training) that activate certain pathways linked to, for example, enhancing running capacity and/or muscle growth.
- Exercise regulates muscle mitochondria—one researcher states, "As strategic regulators of life and death, mitochondria are deeply involved in human disease, but the depth and breadth of mitochondria-based diseases is only now starting to be recognized" (8). *Mitochondrial medicine*, connecting mitochondrial function and adaptation to health, disease and aging, should become even more clinically relevant.
- Muscles regulate other organ systems be releasing *myokines*, factors synthesized in skeletal muscle in response to physical activity.
- Exercise as *super-protector* (exercise-induced longevity)—physical exercise is more protective than might be predicted on the basis of exercise-induced changes in risk factors—exercise becomes an important contributor to longevity.
- The link between exercising muscle and brain plasticity for quality of life improvement for the aging population.

Exercise science seems ready to make an even greater contribution, perhaps one day soon earning for a currently working exercise scientist the Nobel Prize in Physiology or Medicine. See the sidebar on a serious exercise science breakthrough that nevertheless has a humorous ring to it (6). Probably the most important research direction exercise science will embark on is to determine the medical value of exercise and physical activity in preventing, treating, and managing individuals with chronic disease. As more data substantiate the important roles of exercise and physical activity on health, kinesiology will continue to gain acceptance in health care. In addition, as the evidence concerning the scientific basis of movement continues to grow, society will begin to expect these professionals to be more knowledgeable, certified, and academically prepared. The following were quotes given in May 2013 for inclusion in this chapter. These should help kinesiology students think about future directions.

- From Steven N. Blair, P.E.D., Department of Exercise Science, University of South Carolina (personal communication, May 2013). It is very exciting to see how the field of kinesiology has emerged from the old discipline of physical education over the past 50 years. The focus has broadened considerably, and now includes important research in many areas. I hope to see continued growth in many areas, but here are three near the top of my list.
  1. Continued expansion of physical activity as a major public health issue. The U.S. *National Physical Activity Plan* has been in place for a few years, and we are making progress, but much remains to be done. This will require innovative programs and projects in many sectors, such as community planning, clinical medicine, education, public health, worksites, and other areas. Let us continue to emphasize physical activity across society.
  2. The *Exercise Is Medicine* initiative was established by the American College of Sports Medicine and the American Medical Association, and now has many other partners. The program has been rolled out around the world in many countries, and will continue to emphasize the importance of implementing exercise advice into clinical medicine.
  3. I hope that we will continue to see creative uses of modern technology and social media to promote physical activity. This is an exciting new area of research and practice, and it offers great potential for addressing the major public health problem of inactivity.
- From Scotty K. Powers, PhD, Department of Applied Physiology and Kinesiology, University of Florida (personal communication, May 2013). It is very exciting to witness the growth in both volume and quality of research in kinesiology departments during the past three decades. Indeed, scientists based in kinesiology

The Lazy Gene

Studies show 97% of American adults get less than 30 minutes of exercise a day, which is the minimum recommended amount based on federal guidelines. New research from the University of Missouri suggests certain genetic traits may predispose people to being more or less motivated to exercise and remain active. Frank Booth, a professor in the MU College of Veterinary Medicine, along with his post-doctoral fellow Michael Roberts, were able to selectively breed rats that exhibited traits of either extreme activity or extreme laziness. They say these rats indicate that genetics could play a role in exercise motivation, even in humans.

"We have shown that it is possible to be genetically predisposed to being lazy," Booth said. "This could be an important step in identifying additional causes for obesity in humans, especially considering dramatic increases in childhood obesity in the United States. It would be very useful to know if a person is genetically predisposed to having a lack of motivation to exercise, because that could potentially make them more likely to grow obese."

In their study published in the *American Journal of Physiology: Regulatory, Integrative and Comparative Physiology* on April 3, 2013, Roberts and Booth put rats in cages with running wheels and measured how much each rat willingly ran on their wheels during a six-day period. They then bred the top 26 runners with each other and bred the 26 rats that ran the least with each other. They repeated this process through 10 generations and found that the line of running rats chose to run 10 times more than the line of "lazy" rats.

Once the researchers created their "super runner" and "couch potato" rats, they studied the levels of mitochondria in muscle cells, compared body composition and conducted thorough genetic evaluations through RNA deep sequencing of each rat.

"While we found minor differences in the body composition and levels of mitochondria in muscle cells of the rats, the most important thing we identified were the genetic differences between the two lines of rats," Roberts said. "Out of more than 17,000 different genes in one part of the brain, we identified 36 genes that may play a role in predisposition to physical activity motivation."

Now that the researchers have identified these specific genes, they plan on continuing their research to explore the effects each gene has on motivation to exercise.

This article, first appearing as *Couch Potatoes May Be Genetically Predisposed to Being Lazy, MU Study Finds: Genetics Could Be a Reason Some People are Motivated to Exercise More Than Others* (April 08, 2013), has been reprinted with permission from Nathan Hurst, Convergence Media Manager of the University of Missouri News Bureau.

departments are now actively involved in high quality research aimed at understanding the mechanisms of why regular exercise promotes a reduced risk of disease. This work will lead to future advances in both preventative medicine and the treatment of existing diseases in a wide variety of patient populations.

PARADIGM SHIFTS

In the 21st century, those professions and disciplines centered on human movement as their knowledge base will play a very important role in the lives of us all. But the skills required for the various jobs people do, like the world we live in, has largely changed. Globalization has produced a different marketplace, making it far more competitive. Thomas Friedman, in *The World Is Flat*, suggests that we should develop a new kind of education to make individuals more competitive (3). Now as never before, people need to network and make connections. They should learn to communicate increasingly through social media, which link individuals who are ever receding behind their computers and personal communications devices. These are the new learning tools and people need to embrace the new pedagogy they inspire, a new way to learn.

At no point in history is critical thinking needed more than now, but what people need to become are *critical learners*. Critical learners are those who have a passion and need for continual learning almost to the point of continually remaking themselves in a world that changes almost with every news cycle. Critical learners recognize that "24/7" defines the pace at which the world operates. They embrace this pace, think analytically about and process the information they receive, and then learn what is needed to stay ahead. As information continues to bombard us at breakneck speeds, critical learners receive and process it, then as Daniel Pink says, in *A Whole New Mind*, they reconceptualize (5). Critical learners then use creativity and empathic skills to see and respond to the "big picture" conceptualizations. These are the aptitudes for new mind thinkers in a flat world.

What does all this have to do with the world of kinesiology? Precisely everything! High-functioning kinesiologists at all levels need to embrace future thinking and learning and remain open to new ideas that challenge accepted fact. They think and learn through critical lenses. They ask the why question as a matter of course, but in turn do not wait for someone else to answer it before seeking answers for themselves. They embrace new paradigms.

We undertake our daily lives in a set pattern, an established way of perceiving the world. A set pattern such as this is the definition of a paradigm. Paradigms are powerful in that they often preclude the possibility that any other worldview is conceivable. However, paradigms can and often do change. After years of small often unnoticed adjustments, the once well-established daily patterns undergo complete modification, usually as a result of farsighted thinking by individuals, which then becomes established in the larger culture. The resulting new pattern is often much different from the original.

In *The Structure of Scientific Revolutions*, Thomas Kuhn called these changes *paradigm shifts* (4). Published in 1962, his book has subsequently become one of the most cited academic texts of all time. Kuhn advanced a version of how science develops over time that was dramatically different from the accepted version—steady, cumulative "progress" to Kuhn's discontinuities or sets of alternating "normal" and "revolutionary" phases in which communities of specialists in particular fields are plunged into periods of turmoil, uncertainty, and angst. These revolutionary phases correspond to great conceptual breakthroughs and lay the basis for a succeeding phase of "business as usual." In 1962 almost everything about Kuhn's book was controversial because of the challenge it posed to entrenched philosophical assumptions about how science should work. It is ironic that in coining the term *paradigm shift*, he succeeded in setting one in motion.

Think of a paradigm shift as a change from one way of thinking to another. It is a revolution, a transformation, a metamorphosis, and a massive shift of thought driven by agents of change. There have been examples of paradigm shifts throughout history:

- Agriculture changed primitive society from the prevalent hunter-gatherer stage.
- Scientific theory moved from the Ptolemaic system (the earth at the center of the universe) to the Copernican system (the sun at the center of the universe).
- Our worldview was altered when Newtonian physics gave way to relativity and quantum physics.

These transformations were gradual as new paradigms replaced old beliefs. Other key paradigm shifts are readily recognizable. The making of books using of the printing press and use of vernacular language had a direct effect on the scientific revolution. Johann Gutenberg's invention of movable type in the 15th century made books readily available, smaller and easier to handle, and less expensive to purchase. Masses of people acquired direct access to scriptures, resulting in relief from church domination. On a more popular level was the switch that occurred in the 1970s from the popularity of the mechanical watch made by the Swiss to the electronic watch made by the Japanese and Americans, which subsequently captured the world's watch market. When the electronic watch was first proposed, the idea was met with disdain by those who held 70% of the world market share of watches. Over time this new way to make watches caught the public's imagination, and the paradigm shift was under way. A much more recent example and more relevant to people today is the advent of personal computers. The introduction of the personal computer and the Internet has impacted business environments, shifting from primarily a mechanistic, manufacturing, industrial base to an organic, service-based, and information-centered society.

FUTURE PERSPECTIVE

The emergence of the disciplines of kinesiology when physical education was challenged 50 years ago is another example of a paradigm shift. The focus surrounding the study of physical education changed as a result of a desire to bring academic respectability to the study of human movement, but what of the future?

We have already seen what research might bring in the second decade of the 21st century. Predicting the future of human enterprise with any degree of success is at best tenuous, but at the same time future possibilities or trends frequently materialize in small or altered forms. Knowing our past does not always help in understanding what the future might bring, but by knowing history we may gain an appreciation for where we might go. An important activity in any disciplinary field of study is to attempt to understand future courses and directions. This has been largely neglected in kinesiology. In their chapter on future directions in exercise science published in 1997, Swanson and Massengale (7) explain that . . .

> The process of creating alternative futures, studying them, and then selectively choosing the most appropriate future is not currently being done in the field of exercise and sport science. The leadership of the field needs to focus attention upon the creation of alternative futures, the selection of one, and then take the necessary steps to make that future come true.
>
> A complicating factor is that the future will not be like the past, regardless of accurate trend extrapolation; it will be far more complex. New data that are yet to be established may not be like current data. Frames of reference will probably change. Demographics will change, as will science and technology. Social norms, cultural norms, and political institutions will vary independently of one another, as well as independently of science and technology.

In has been almost 20 years since these words were first published, and they are likely still true today. Leaders in the field of kinesiology can forecast many possible alternatives for future outcomes. The question is which alternative will be the correct one, or will there be more than one correct alternative, or will new unforeseen alternatives be created. Reviewing the historical development of kinesiology reveals two consistent points: (a) the direction and growth of kinesiology must continue to be assessed, and it must be determined whether the present curricula will continue to meet the needs of students in the future as they seem to be doing today: and (b) possibly the most important consideration is the continued development of science-based curricula so there is continued training of undergraduate and graduate students in the scientific disciplines of human movement.

The journey that began in the 20th century will lead inextricably to exciting new avenues of growth in the 21st century. How will kinesiology continue to develop? What will be the relationship between the various disciplines and professions of kinesiology with their respective parent disciplines? Will our understanding of human movement continue as rapidly as the pace of technological advancement possibly leading to, as some call for, more transdisciplinary research?

As we begin to think *prospectively* about possible or even probable futures, it is important to note that this is the type of intellectual activity that makes up a field of study known as *Futures Studies* (2). What is clear at the outset is that for any future to be bright it takes hardworking people with a vision to make it happen.

> The purposes of futures studies are to discover or invent, examine and evaluate, and propose possible, probable, and preferable futures (2).

Recent demographic projections of the U.S. population show that by the middle of the 21st century approximately 70 million Americans will be over the age of 65, with the number over the age of 85 increasing to nearly

The Kinecian: A Paradigm Shift for Kinesiology

Policymakers need to be encouraged further to emphasize physical activity and exercise for the maintenance of good health. As Steve Blair indicated in the quote cited earlier in the chapter, the last decade saw the beginnings of a massive effort toward bringing exercise recommendations to the average person via the *Exercise Is Medicine* initiative that began in 2007. Medical care must continue to integrate physical activity into the health care picture because the most cost-effective strategy for improving public health is to get sedentary individuals to become active. In this way, kinesiology professionals might take on a much more prominent role in society beyond merely the effort seen in research.

Market forces driving health care policy are likely to become increasingly more intense, leading to more reliance on the disciplines and professions that embrace movement as an everyday paradigm. As the population ages, exercise and physical activity will play a larger role in both medical and movement dysfunction diagnoses and treatment. It is not hard to envision, then, that over the next several decades the economic burden of the graying population could drive health care cost to heights that eclipse those seen today. How the national economies of Western nations are to be sustained in the face of this kind of economic strain is difficult to tell. Yet, the evidence that physical activity prevents potential medical problems from reaching an overt clinical state is powerful.

The fact that the health care delivery mechanism is ill equipped to adequately prescribe and implement physical activity interventions may prompt state legislators, lobbied by activists from professional organizations such as physical therapy, occupational therapy, and exercise science/kinesiology, to find a way to take the ideals of *Exercise Is Medicine* to a much higher level.

Conceptually, this could involve the creation of a new lobby, a professional group combining many currently independent professional organizations centered on movement dysfunction into a single, more powerful body that in time may equal the lobbying capability of the American Medical Association. Table 24.1 shows the way this *movement profession* may be juxtaposed with that of the medical profession by the year 2050. The evolution of the movement profession to a status equal to that of the medical profession would come with notable changes in status. The earning power of members of this professional group could more than double once its practitioners move from mere allied health status to something akin to direct access for the new type of care provided. These professionals would practice in private offices, clinics, and medical centers. Like the medical professional, several lines of specialties can become available including those left over from the restructuring of academic programs in occupational therapy, physical therapy, and kinesiology. Therefore, the professional landscape for the movement profession could be analogous to the medical profession, with the majority of *Kinecians* (movement doctors) in general practice and many in specialized fields, often in close alliance with *Physicians* and others in the medical field.

12 million. Due to medical advances that are evident in our day and that are sure to progress with technological advancement, this group will have a greater chance to be healthier than any people of similar age in previous generations. But at what cost to the health care industry? What is inevitable as any population ages is that health care costs rise. It has been projected that the "graying" generation will bring with it severe economic burdens if increasing costs are sustained into the future. Barring some great advance in genetic engineering that ameliorates aging and its attendant diseases, the evidence points to lifestyle interventions as being the best method for optimizing health and reducing health care costs. Based on this, the next sidebar presents one possible outcome of the current crisis in health care funding. While the vision presented in this sidebar may or may not come to pass, clearly there is value in this type of intellectual endeavor in order to take more definitive steps into the future and avoid stumbling about.

Table 24.1. Comparing Professions*

Medical Profession		Movement Profession
Physiological/Biochemical Sciences	Knowledge Base	Kinesiological Sciences
Medical Doctor (MD)	Degree	Movement Doctor (MvD)
Prescription of Medicine Medical Diagnoses Medical and Surgical Treatment	Scope of Practice	Prescription of Movement Therapy Movement Dysfunction Diagnoses Movement Dysfunction Treatment
American Medical Association	Regulating Organization	American Movement Association
Physician	Practitioner	Kinecian

*This is an exercise in *future thinking*.

SUMMARY

The disciplines of kinesiology have produced a substantial amount of research in recent years, making great strides in increasing our understanding of the benefits of exercise at the molecular level and higher. What is needed is a new paradigm shift that propels kinesiology, the study of movement, to a new and better status that equals this most fundamental of all human attributes, the ability to move.

REFERENCES

1. Baldwin, K. M., and F. Haddad, "Research in the exercise sciences; where we are and where do we go from here: part II? *Exerc Sport Sci Rev.* 38(2)(2010): 42–50.

2. Bell, W., "The purposes of futures studies." *The Futurist* (1997, Nov–Dec): 42–45.

3. Friedman, T. L., *The World Is Flat: A Brief history of the Twenty-First Century*. New York: Picador, 2007.

4. Kuhn, T. S., *The Structure of Scientific Revolutions*. Chicago: University of Chicago Press, 1962.

5. Pink, D. H., *A Whole New Mind: Moving from the Information Age to the Conceptual Age*. New York: Penguin Group (Riverhead), 2005.

6. Roberts, D. C., J. D. Brown, J. M. Company, L. P. Oberle, A. J. Heese, R. G. Toedebusch, K. D. Wells, C. L. Cruthirds, J. A. Knouse, J. Ferreira, T. E. Childs, M. Brown, and F. W. Booth, "Phenotypic and molecular differences between rats selectively-bred to voluntarily run high versus low nightly distances." *Am J Physiol Regul Integr Comp Physiol; published ahead of print April 3, 2013, doi:10.1152/ajpregu.00581.2012.*

7. Swanson, R. A., and J. D. Massengale, "Current and future directions in exercise and sport science." In *The History of Exercise and Sport Science*, J. D. Massengale & R. A. Swanson, eds. Champaign, IL: Human Kinetics, 1997.

8. Wallace, D. C., "A mitochondrial paradigm of metabolic and degenerative diseases, aging, and cancer: A dawn for evolutionary medicine." *Annu Rev Genet.* 39(2005): 359–407.

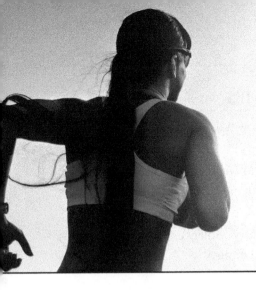

GLOSSARY

CHAPTER 1: INTRODUCTION TO KINESIOLOGY

Disciplinarity—phases of human activity to seek, develop, and produce knowledge manifesting in four forms—singular, multiple, inter-relational, and boundary-breaking pursuits.

Exercise—any movement with the purposeful intent of producing bodily fitness.

Exercise Science—any aspect of science applied to the phenomenon of exercise.

Generalist—an academician capable of teaching in a number of the disciplines of kinesiology.

Kinesiology—the academic field that specifically pursues the study of movement, physical activity, exercise and sport.

Specialist—an academician who teaches in a specific discipline of kinesiology.

CHAPTER 2: EXERCISE, SPORT AND PHYSICAL CULTURE

Culture—the patterns of life which individuals create in a society through interacting with each other and consisting of behaviors, feelings, beliefs, norms, objects, values and other shared characteristics of a group of people.

Cultural Studies—cultural, interpretive, philosophical, anthropological, sociological and semiotic study of exercise and culture. The field of cultural studies is comprised of many "parent" disciplines, among them literary criticism, sociology, economics, political science, history, psychology, anthropology, English, and pedagogy. Some major categories of work in cultural studies include gender and sexuality, nationhood and national identity, identity politics, colonialism, aesthetics, popular culture, narrative and rhetoric, and transnational economies.

Hegemony—power or dominance of an idea, ideal, or value over other ideas, ideals or values. Usually the power is hidden, subtle and assumed to be the natural and received way things are done.

Postmodernism—a broad, vague label for a time period, literary form, or artistic style. The label is used to refer to changed contemporary society.

Subculture—a subunit of a culture which has values different from the larger culture and may be represented by concepts such as age, gender, religion, race, ethnicity, social class, physical ability, and sexual orientation for example.

CHAPTER 3: DISABILITY: EXPLORING HEALTH DISPARITIES

Americans with Disabilities Act (ADA)—federal law, passed in 1990, to allow full and equal access to services and facilities by persons with disabilities.

Disability—the consequence of an impairment that may be physical, cognitive, mental, sensory, emotional, developmental, or some combination of these that result in restrictions on an individual's ability to participate in what is considered "normal" in their everyday society.

Health Disparities—preventable differences in the burden of disease, injury, violence, or opportunities to achieve optimal health that are experienced by socially disadvantaged populations.

CHAPTER 4: PROFESSIONAL CONCERNS

Certification—The process by which an individual, institution, or educational program is evaluated and recognized as meeting certain predetermined standards through successful completion of a validated, reliable examination.

Encroachment—the act of working outside the established role of an occupation.

Licensure—Granting of permission by a competent authority (usually a government agency) to an organization or individual to engage in a practice or activity that would otherwise be illegal.

Profession—an occupation requiring detailed knowledge in a course of study, accompanied by advanced education and training involving intellectual skills.

Professional organization—association of individuals formed for the purpose of self-regulating and advancing common goals and interests.

Registration—Recording of professional qualification information relevant to government licensing regulations.

Role Delineation—a study of the specific responsibilities of an occupation based on the knowledge, skills, and abilities expected of that professional.

CHAPTER 5: SPORT PHILOSOPHY

Deductive Reasoning—the logical process in which a conclusion is based on the concordance of multiple premises that are generally assumed to be true. Sometimes referred to as top-down logic.

Ethics—moral philosophy, the branch of philosophy that involves systematizing, defending, and recommending concepts of right and wrong conduct.

Inductive Reasoning—the logical process in which multiple premises, all believed true or found true most of the time, are combined to obtain a specific conclusion. Often used in applications that involve prediction, forecasting, or behavior. Sometimes referred to as bottom-up logic.

Philosophy—specifically, the love of wisdom, of more broadly, the study of the fundamental nature of knowledge, reality, and existence.

CHAPTER 6: SPORT HISTORY

Historiography—the methodological process of producing historical accounts of the past through analyzing not only facts, but the assumptions and values of society and its people.

History—the study that gives meaning and life to what people of the world have done, said and thought in the past.

History of Sport—The accumulative body of knowledge that recounts past practices and purposes of sport, games, athletics, leisure pursuits, and exercise through the ages.

Primary Sources—works written at or near the time something occurred and usually by a party who was present to observe the occurrence.

Qualitative Research—examines meanings, concepts, characteristics, definitions, symbols, and descriptions of things. Conclusions from this research are most often drawn from analysis of descriptive data rather than from mathematical treatment of data.

Quantitative Research—refers to counts and measures of things; a collection of data that can be tested through statistical means in order to draw conclusions.

Secondary Sources—works based on primary sources; books, journal articles, newspaper accounts, and other material written about a subject in later years and by a person who was not an eye witness to the occurrence.

Sport History—a scholarly field concerned with the historical study of sport. Studies in sport history encompass the practices and meanings of exercise, recreational pastimes, play, games, and athletics from the past.

CHAPTER 7: SPORT SOCIOLOGY

Conflict Theory—a theory which contends that sport is an opiate of society deadening our awareness to social concerns.

Critical Theory—focuses on concepts of power in social life and are about action and political involvement.

Patriarchy—political and social control of women by men in which the subordination of women is implicit.

Sociology—the study of human behavior and social interactions as they occur in social and cultural settings.

Sport sociology—a subdiscipline of exercise science focusing on sport as a part of social and cultural life.

Values—socially determined and shared ideas regarding what is good, right, and desirable.

CHAPTER 8: EXERCISE PHYSIOLOGY

Adenosine Triphosphate (ATP)—energy "currency" of the cell, responsible for delivering free energy to accomplish cellular activity.

Aerobic—with oxygen, especially referring to a class of exercise using aerobic metabolic processes.

Anabolism—bodily chemical reactions resulting in the buildup of large molecules from smaller molecules.

Anaerobic—without oxygen, especially referring to a class of exercise using anaerobic metabolic processes.

Beta Oxidation—metabolic pathway that catalyzes fatty acids.

Bioenergetic—energy processes in living organisms.

Cardiac Output—volume of blood pumped by the heart per minute.

Catabolism—chemical reactions resulting in the breakdown of large molecules to smaller molecules.

Cellular Respiration—series of metabolic processes involved in the aerobic production of ATP.

Chronic—continuing over a long period of time or recurring frequently.

Core Temperature—deep internal temperature of the body (normal is 37°C, but may easily exceed 40°C during heavy aerobic exercise).

Electron Transport Chain—final metabolic pathway that oxidatively phosphorylates ADP to form ATP, with water produced as a by-product.

Endurance Exercise—exercise that can be performed with a steady-state oxygen consumption for long periods of time.

Exercise Physiology—the study of how body structures and functions are altered when we are exposed to acute and chronic exercise.

External Respiration—exchange of gases between the atmosphere and the lungs, and the lungs and the blood.

Free Energy—form of energy that is "free" to do various kinds of cellular operations, i.e., powers muscle contraction.

Glycolysis—process whereby glucose is broken down to pyruvic acid or lactic acid.

Heart Rate—frequency of cardiac contractions in beats per minute.

Homeostasis—tendency of various control systems in the body to regulate physiological processes within narrow limits (i.e., blood glucose levels, blood pH, and body temperature are all tightly controlled by homeostatic mechanisms).

Homeothermic—same body temperature (mammals - including humans - maintain body temperatures within narrow limits regardless of the external environmental conditions).

Krebs Cycle—cyclic reactions in the mitochondria that metabolize pyruvic acid and acetyl CoA, with CO_2, NADH, and $FADH_2$ being chief by-products.

Lactic Acid—by-product of anaerobic glycolysis.

Lipolysis—breakdown of triglycerides.

Metabolic Pathway—sequence of enzyme-mediated chemical reactions resulting in specific product(s).

Metabolic Power—rapidity with which a metabolic pathway produces ATP.

Metabolic Capacity—capacity of a metabolic pathway to produce quantities of ATP.

Metabolism—sum total of all the chemical reactions in the body.

Mitochondria—specialized cellular structures responsible for producing ATP during aerobic metabolism.

Oxygen Consumption—rate at which oxygen is utilized in the body (depicted as VO_2 and usually measured as liters/minutes or milliliters per kilogram of body mass per minute).

Phosphagen System—metabolic pathway using creatine phosphate as the substrate which donates a phosphate group to ADP in the anaerobic formation of ATP (used primarily during very intense exercise lasting a few seconds).

Phosphorylation—chemical process whereby a phosphate group is added to a molecule.

Potential Energy—energy stored in energy nutrients.

Resistance Exercise—form of exercise where muscles are contracting at large percentages of maximal voluntary contraction capability and results in a distinctly different hemodynamic and metabolic pattern of responses compared to endurance forms.

Stroke Volume—amount of blood pumped by the heart per beat.

CHAPTER 9: SPORT NUTRITION

Adiposity—the relative amount of body fat being carried by the individual.

Amine—nitrogen-containing compound which has gone through a slight chemical alteration.

Antioxidant—compounds which prevent the oxidation of substances in foods or in the body (includes vitamins A, C, E, and the mineral selenium).

Absorptive—ability to absorb; the body absorbs the majority of nutrients in the small intestine, the more absorptive a food is, the more the body absorbs that food.

Blood Glucose—blood sugar; glucose is a simple sugar and the breakdown product of carbohydrates.

Carbohydrate—class of energy nutrient including sugars, starches, and cellulose.

Cofactors—minerals and vitamins may act as cofactors as part of a reaction and are necessary for a reaction to move forward (they may be part of an enzyme).

Creatine Phosphate—high energy phosphate molecule which serves as a reservoir of phosphate units to resynthesis ATP from ADP.

Ergogenic Aids—ergogenic means "work enhancing"; thus, ergogenic aids are substances which would enhance exercise performance.

Diuretics—substances which result in water loss (increased urination).

Electrolytes—include sodium, chloride, and potassium and all are involved in fluid balance in the body, among other important functions.

Essential Amino Acids—the nine amino acids that must be obtained by the diet.

Fat—class of energy nutrient that contains twice as much energy as glucose. Its structure is very concentrated, with a higher ratio of hydrogen to carbon than carbohydrates contain.

Glycogen Stores—the storage form of carbohydrates found in liver and muscles.

Hypohydrated—low body water content.

Hyponatremia—below normal levels of sodium in the blood. Normal levels range from 135 to 145 milliequivalents per Liter (mEq/L).

Kilocalories (kcals)—the appropriate term used for "Calories" (Capital "C"). One kilocalorie = 1,000 calories (small "c"). However, calorie is commonly (and incorrectly) used for "kilocalorie."

Macronutrients—carbohydrates, fats, and proteins are considered macronutrients and are needed by the body in large quantities.

Major Minerals—essential mineral needed in the diet in amounts greater than 100 mg/day.

Micronutrients—vitamins and minerals are considered micronutrients and are needed by the body in small quantities.

Nonessential Amino Acid—the 11 amino acids which can be made in the body by the essential amino acids.

Picolinate—substance chelated (or combined) with such minerals as chromium because it is thought to enhance absorption of the mineral to which it has been chelated.

Quackery—a misrepresentation of the facts in order to deceive the consumer.

Sport Nutrition—principles of nutrition applied to individuals in sport and exercise.

Trace Minerals—essential mineral need in the diet in amounts less than 100 mg/day.

CHAPTER 10: PHYSICAL ACTIVITY EPIDEMIOLOGY

Biological Plausibility—the fact that your hypothesis and the relationship that you are proposing is in harmony with existing scientific information.

Clinical Trial—individuals free from the disease or condition are randomly assigned to receive either an intervention or no intervention (the control group). Subsequent follow-up of the groups over time would determine if the groups differ by the percent who eventually develop the disease.

Confounder—a variable whose effect is entangled with the effect of the risk factor of interest (e.g. physical activity). The variable must be related to the disease or health outcome of interest and be related to the risk factor.

Cross Sectional Studies—investigators collect information about the health outcome and the potential risk factor at the same time within the same group to determine if a relationship exists between these two variables.

Epidemiology—study of the distribution and determinants of health-related states or events in specified populations, and the application of this study to the control of health problems.

Experimental Study—investigators randomly assign varying levels of the risk factor of interest to individuals without the disease and then follows these individuals to compare the development of the disease in the future.

Incidence Rate—number of new cases of a disease in a specified time period divided by the population at risk of developing that disease over that given time period.

Mortality Rate—death rate.

Morbidity—any departure, subjective or objective, from state of physiological or psychological well-being.

Observational Study—investigator observes the occurrence of the disease or condition in individuals who differ by the risk factor of interest.

Physical Activity Epidemiology—involves the specific investigation of the relationship between physical activity (and/or exercise) and health and diseases within a population

Prevalence Rate—number of existing cases of the disease divided by the total population at a point in time or over a given time period.

Prospective Study—identifies and follows individuals initially free of the health outcome of interest and seeks to establish if initial or subsequent physical activity levels differentiate those who do and do not develop the disease.

Rate—number of cases or deaths divided by the population at risk in a given time period.

Risk Factors—biological, environmental, and behavioral variables (factors) which interact to cause disease in a population.

CHAPTER 11: APPLIED ANATOMY

Abduction—movement of a body part away from the midline of the body.

Adduction—movement of a body part toward the midline of the body.

Applied Anatomy—branch of anatomy that focuses on movement.

Anatomical Position—reference position for the body, consists of standing upright with the head facing forward, arms by the side of the trunk with the palms facing forward, and the legs together with the feet facing forward.

Anterior—toward the front of the body; situated in front or in the front part of an organism.

Distal—farthest from the center, from the medial line, or from the trunk; opposed to proximal; far or distant from the origin or point of attachment.

Sagittal Plane—a vertical plane that divides the body into left and right parts.

Frontal Plane—a vertical plane that divides the body into anterior and posterior parts.

Transverse Plane—a horizontal plane that divides the body into superior and inferior parts.

Agonist—the muscle or muscle group directly engaged in a movement through concentric development of tension.

Antagonist—the muscle or muscle group that are located on the opposite side of the joint from the agonist and oppose the action of the agonist.

Concentric—a muscle action that occurs when a muscle generates tension that produces a torque larger than the resistive torque at the joint, resulting in a shortening of the muscle and a change of the joint angle in the direction of the muscular force.

Eccentric—a muscle action that occurs when a muscle generates tension that produces a smaller torque than the resistive torque at the joint, resulting in a lengthening of the muscle and a change in the joint angle in the direction of the resistive force.

Isometric—a muscle action that occurs when a muscle generates tension that is equal to the resistance at the joint, resulting in no noticeable change in the joint angle.

CHAPTER 12: BIOMECHANICS

Biomechanics—application of mechanical principles to the study of biological systems.

Kinematics—branch of mechanics that describes motion without regard to the causative forces.

Kinetics—branch of mechanics that examines the forces that cause motion.

Force—the effect of one object or one body on another object or body.

Moment of force (Torque)—the rotational effect a force has about a fixed point.

Inertia—resistance to change in motion, measured by a person or object's mass.

Mechanopathology—the mechanics that cause an injury.

Pathomechanics—the mechanics that are the result of an injury.

CHAPTER 13: EXERCISE AND SPORT PSYCHOLOGY

Arousal—responsible for energizing an individual; ranges from deep sleep to extreme excitement

causal attribution—reason given for a particular outcome.

Exercise and Sport Psychology—applications of the principle of psychology to sport and exercise.

Extroversion-Introversion—personality dimension characterized by relative levels of being sociable and outgoing vs. being shy and inhibited.

Habit—most well-learned way of responding to a stimulus.

Motivation—energy thought to drive an individual; composed of direction, intensity, and persistence.

Self-Concept—core of personality containing our values, interests, beliefs, world-view, perceptions of self.

Self-Confidence—perception of ability.

Self-Efficacy—perception of ability to perform a specific task at a particular time; situation-specific self-confidence.

States—temporary thoughts or feelings easily changed.

Stressor—something which requires the need for adaptation by an individual.

Traits—more permanent ways of thinking or feeling; not easily changed.

CHAPTER 14: MOTOR BEHAVIOR

Capacity—amount of information that a memory store can hold.

Central Nervous System (CNS)—composed of the brain and spinal cord.

Challenge point—point at which the learner is being optimally challenged to enhance learning.

Chronometric Method—using reaction time to analyze a person's behavior between the presentation of a stimulus and their response.

Closed-loop—receiving feedback (i.e., sensory information) during the movement that helps us control the movement.

Contextual Interference—used to describe the interference that results from practicing a variety of tasks within the context of a single practice situation.

Duration—length of time that information can be held in that memory store.

Dynamical Systems Theory—views changes in motor patterns as occurring as a result of human behavior being inherently complex and dynamic and influenced by multiple internal and external factors.

Fading Knowledge of Results—method of providing KR whereby the frequency of the KR is faded or decreased throughout practice.

Fluid Intelligence—reasoning and abstract thought, such as mental rotation. Learning is considered a mechanism of fluid intelligence. Fluid intelligence is generally considered to reach a peak in the mid-30s.

Knowledge of Results (KR)—defined as post-response, augmented, error information. This means that KR is information given to the learner about the success of the response. This information is not something the learner would necessarily know by their self. Telling a pitcher he threw a strike would be KR.

Learning—defined as a relatively permanent change in behavior that results from practice or experience.

Longitudinal Method—study of motor development over time to see the impact of time on the subject.

Motor Behavior—application of psychology to movement, inclusive of control, development, learning.

Motor Control—concerned with understanding the mechanisms by which the neural and muscular system orchestrates the myriad of movements made by the organism and the manner in which these mechanisms are constrained.

Motor Development—concerned with understanding the change in movement orchestration that results more from system maturation than practice or experience.

Motor Learning—concerned with understanding the mechanisms of the relatively permanent change in behavior resulting from practice or experience that manifests itself in a more efficient orchestration of movements.

Neuron—a nerve cell that sends or receives messages throughout the CNS.

Open-loop—means that we do not receive feedback on-line (i.e., during the movement). Instead, we completely preplan the movement.

Primitive Reflexes—the reflexes associated with the infants basic needs such as nourishment and security.

Psychomotor Function—the ability to integrate cognition with motor abilities, such as communication and locomotion.

Reaction Time—time between stimulus onset and the initiation of a movement.

Regression—in the domain of motor development refers to a decrease in performance from peak and is generally associated with older adulthood.

Relative Task Difficulty—defined as the difficulty of the motor problem one must resolve to successfully complete a task relative to the performer completing the task.

Selective Attention—process whereby one actively chooses a single unit of information to pay attention to at a time.

Sensory (Afferent) Neurons—signals from the senses to the CNS.

Skills—learned movements consisting of the ability to bring about some end result with maximum certainty and minimum outlay of energy.

Summary Knowledge of Results—a method of providing KR that requires a subject to complete several trials of a simple motor task without receiving KR.

Task Difficulty—difficulty of the motor problem one must resolve to successfully complete a task.

CHAPTER 15: PHYSICAL AND OCCUPATIONAL THERAPY

Activities of Daily Living (ADL)—activities usually performed in the course of a normal day in a person's life, such as eating, dressing, bathing, grooming, and homemaking.

Ambulation—walking with or without aids, such as braces or crutches.

Assistive Device—any technology that enables a person with a disability to improve his or her functional level.

Functional Ability—level of skill to perform activities in a normal or accepted manner.

Geriatrics—branch of medicine dealing with the aging process and medical problems of aging.

Gerontology—study of aging.

Health Maintenance Organization—group healthcare agency that provides basic and supplemental health maintenance and treatment services to voluntary enrollees who prepay a fixed periodic fee without regard to the amount or kind of services received.

Individualized Treatment Plan—program designed to meet a client's treatment needs based on treatment goals and considering the client's unique background, psychological makeup, personal needs, and expectations.

Kinesthesis—muscle sense; the feel that accompanies a movement.

Mobility—ability to move from one location to another.

Modality—activity used as an intervention for treatment or rehabilitation purposes.

Occupational Therapy—purposeful mental and physical activities prescribed by medical doctors to enhance individuals' abilities to perform daily occupational roles. Clients include those with physical injuries or illnesses, developmental disorders, problems caused by aging, or social or emotional problems.

Physical Therapy—physical therapists are concerned with restoration of physical function and prevention of disability following disease, injury, or loss of body part. PT's apply therapeutic exercise and functional training procedures.

Rehabilitation—to restore or return the person to maximum functioning and optimal adjustment.

CHAPTER 16: CLINICAL EXERCISE PHYSIOLOGY

Angina Pectoris—heart pain that occurs when the blood supply to the heart muscle cannot meet the muscle's need for oxygen.

Asymptomatic—without symptoms.

Atherosclerosis—a progressive, degenerative disease that leads to a gradual blockage of arterial vessels, thereby reducing blood flow through them.

Beta Adrenergic Blocking Agents—medications which interfere with the transmission of nerve signals in the heart, thereby decreasing heart rate, blood pressure, cardiac muscle contractility, and oxygen demand.

Clinical Exercise Physiology—application of exercise physiology to treatment of patients, as in cardiac rehabilitation.

Contraindication—any condition, especially any condition of disease, which renders some particular line of treatment improper or undesirable.

Diabetic Ketoacidosis—a condition caused by a lack of insulin resulting in marked elevation of blood glucose and ketone bodies with a reduction of blood pH.

Diabetes Mellitus—a disease in which the body cannot produce insulin or cannot use insulin properly resulting in an elevation of blood glucose.

Diastole—the period of relaxation in the heart cycle alternating with periods of contraction.

Diastolic Blood Pressure—the point of lowest pressure in the arterial vascular system.

Double Product—a parameter used to monitor myocardial oxygen demands obtained by multiplying heart rate by systolic blood pressure.

Dyspnea—difficult or labored breathing.

Electrocardiogram—a record of the electrical activity of the heart.

Exercise Prescription—a plan for physical activity formulated to achieve specific outcomes of exercise training.

Exercise Protocol—method used for conducting an exercise test.

Hypoxemia—insufficient oxygenation of the blood.

Informed Consent—permission given by a client to be involved in a treatment procedure or research study.

Insulin Resistance—a condition in which the tissues of the body fail to respond normally to insulin.

Myocardial Infarction—damage to the heart muscle (myocardium) that results from severe or prolonged blockage of blood supply to the tissue.

Pharmacokinetics—study of the action of drugs with particular emphasis on time required for absorption, duration of action, distribution in the body, and method of excretion.

Rating of Perceived Exertion—rating of an individual's perception of exercise intensity.

Side Effect—drug's undesired action on the body.

Systolic Blood Pressure—the highest blood pressure in the arterial vascular system, occurring during contraction of the ventricles.

Type 1 Diabetes—form of diabetes caused when the immune system attacks the beta cells of the pancreas and the pancreas can no longer produce insulin.

Type 2 Diabetes—form of diabetes characterized by insulin resistance and a relative, rather than absolute, insulin deficiency.

CHAPTER 17: THERAPEUTIC RECREATION

Adapted Activities—altered activities which fit the needs, interests and capabilities of individuals; changes may be made in rules or equipment to accommodate the persons participating.

Case History—brief report on the client's background; often prepared by a social worker.

Case Management—problem-solving process through which appropriate healthcare services are provided to individuals and families.

Certified Therapeutic Recreation Specialist—certification by the National Council for Therapeutic Recreation Certification (NCTRC) for a healthcare practitioner to practice therapeutic recreation at the professional level. Certification requires the completion of the minimum of a bachelor's degree in therapeutic recreation and examination by NCTRC.

Efficacy—having the desired influence or outcome.

Family Therapy—treatment of more than one member of a family in the same session. The assumption is that a mental disorder in one member of a family may be manifestation of disorder in other members and may affect interrelationships and functioning.

Group Home—supervised living situation that helps persons to learn skills to prepare them for semi-independent or independent living.

Habilitation—encouragement and stimulation of the development and acquisition of skills and functions not previously attained.

Interdisciplinary Team—group of professionals with varied and specialized training who function together to provide clinical services for a client. Recreation therapists (or therapeutic recreation specialists) and occupational therapists are usually members of teams and, depending on type of setting, serve with professionals such as medical doctors, nurses, social workers, psychologists, speech therapists, and physical therapists.

Leisure Counseling—helping process in which the counselor attempts to assist the client to discover and change leisure attitudes or behaviors. Various verbal and nonverbal techniques are utilized in a counseling setting to help the client cope effectively with leisure problems and concerns, make decisions and develop plans for future leisure participation, become self-aware regarding perceptions toward leisure, and explore options for leisure.

Maladaptive Behavior—activity that is dysfunctional or counter-productive in coping effectively with stress.

Outcome Measure—instrument designed to gather information on the efficacy of a program; a means to determine if outcome goals and objectives have been reached.

Play Therapy—type of psychotherapy for children that utilizes play activities and toys.

Therapeutic Recreation—term sometimes used to encompass both recreation therapy and special recreation.

CHAPTER 18: ATHLETIC TRAINING

Closed Kinetic Chain—physical activity where the terminal end of a body segment is involved in functional forces.

Contusions—bruises usually caused by direct blows.

Emergency Care Plan—plan to be executed when a severe or catastrophic injury occurs.

Evaluation—assessment as to the nature and severity of an injury, information is transmitted to a physician who issues a diagnosis.

Functional Progression—stage of sport-specific activity an athlete is at during a rehabilitation program.

Health Care Administration—facility, financial, and personnel management including minimizing exposure to the legal system.

Inflammation—response of tissue to biological insult.

Injury History—what, when, where, why, and how an injury happened, including whether the part had been injured before and what the outcome was.

Injury Prevention—stopping an injury before it occurs.

Observation—visually inspecting an injury site, general body language, and facial expressions.

Overuse Injury—any of a number of injuries occurring as a result of repetitive microtrauma.

Palpation—placing hands on an injury site to feel for deformities, temperature changes, blood flow changes, and range of motion assessment.

Personnel Management—hiring and assignment of athletic trainers to job sites.

Primary Survey—part of an evaluation checking life-threatening situations.

Range of Motion—normal arc that a joint moves through.

Rehabilitation—restoring normal strength and function.

Repair—phase of rehabilitation dealing with scar tissue formation.

Secondary Survey—part of an evaluation assessing the nature and severity of an injury.

Sign—objective, quantifiable information about an athlete.

Sports Medicine—science applied to the individual in sport and exercise, with special attention to environment, psychological aspects, drugs, prevention and treatment of injuries, rehabilitation, and safety.

Symptom—subjective information obtained from an injured athlete.

Therapeutic Modalities—physical, thermal, and chemical agents used to modify the inflammatory response or speed the restoration of function after an athletic injury.

CHAPTER 19: SPORT PEDAGOGY

Adapted Physical Education—modified physical activity in educational settings for students with disabilities.

Assessment—collection and analysis of information to determine the status of the client.

Learning Domains—cognitive - mental skills (knowledge), affective - growth in feelings or emotional areas (attitude or self), psychomotor - manual or physical skills (skills)

Physical Education—discipline and/or profession that deals with education about physical activity and education through physical activity.

Sport Pedagogy—discipline concerned with understanding and optimizing the process of teaching movement skills.

CHAPTER 20: SPORT MANAGEMENT

Evaluation—a process whereby the worth of a product, service, experience, person, or concept is determined and established.

Experience Qualities—those aspects of the service or event that can be evaluated after the experience is over.

Intangibility—individuals cannot see, touch or inspect the service before they use it. Integrated marketing communications - suggests that all promotional information present a clear image with "one voice."

Legal Liability—the responsibilities and duties which exist among socially interacting people which are enforceable by law. As leisure, sport and fitness leaders, certain legal responsibilities and duties exist regarding actions involving clients and players. If these responsibilities are not fulfilled, then legal action may result.

Management—art and science of facilitating the effective and efficient achievement of organizational goals involving functions such as planning, organizing, leading, and controlling.

Marketing Strategy—contains five basic components - target market, product/service offering, promotion, pricing, and distribution.

Marketing Mix—the product/service, promotion, pricing, and distribution elements of the marketing strategy.

Mission Statement—manifestation of the philosophy of the organization, it tells us why the organization exists.

Organizational Triad—represents the three most essential areas of an organization: leadership, facilities/equipment, and programs.

Perceived Value—what one gives for what one gets.

Relationship marketing—focuses on making and keeping relationships with customers over the long term.

Risk Management—involves a systematic approach to minimizing the possibility of being successfully sued by players and clients for alleged torts such as negligence.

Secondary Services—those services which participants use while they are participating or using the primary service.

Service Quality—relates to how well the service meets or exceeds customers' expectations.

Servicescape—the ambient and design factors that make up the facility environment.

Sports Marketing—the development and management of the primary and secondary service offerings via promotion, pricing, and distribution aimed at satisfying viable target markets.

Target Market—consists of consumers who have similar characteristics and needs which can be best met by the coordinated efforts of the organization.

CHAPTER 21: RECREATION AND LEISURE

Leisure—Intrinsically motivated, self-determined experience allowing for a chosen level of mastery and competence that leads to feelings of self-efficacy, empowerment, excitement or enjoyment; having freedom to become.

Recreation—enjoyable, restorative activity in which individuals exercise choice and control; often associated with leisure time.

CHAPTER 22: HEALTH-FITNESS

Aerobic Physical Activity—activity in which the body's large muscles move in a rhythmic manner for a sustained period of time. Aerobic activity, also called endurance activity, improves cardiorespiratory fitness. Examples include walking, running, and swimming, and bicycling.

Agility—ability to quickly change body position or direction of the body.

Balance—performance-related component of physical fitness that involves the maintenance of the body's equilibrium while stationary or moving.

Baseline Activity—light-intensity activities of daily life, such as standing, walking slowly, and lifting light-weight objects. People who do only baseline activity are considered to be inactive.

Bone-Strengthening Activity—Physical activity primarily designed to increase the strength of specific sites in bones that make up the skeletal system. Bone strengthening activities produce an impact or tension force on the bones that promotes bone growth and strength. Running, jumping rope, and lifting weights are examples of bone-strengthening activities.

Cardiovascular Endurance—ability for the body to gather, deliver, and process oxygen.

Exercise—subcategory of physical activity that is planned, structured, repetitive, and purposive in the sense that the improvement or maintenance of one or more components of physical fitness is the objective. "Exercise" and "exercise training" frequently are used interchangeably and generally refer to physical activity performed during leisure time with the primary purpose of improving or maintaining physical fitness, physical performance, or health.

Flexibility—health- and performance-related component of physical fitness that is the range of motion possible at a joint. Flexibility is specific to each joint and depends on a number of specific variables, including but not limited to the tightness of specific ligaments and tendons. Flexibility exercises enhance the ability of a joint to move through its full range of motion.

Health—human condition with physical, social and psychological dimensions, each characterized on a continuum with positive and negative poles. Positive health is associated with a capacity to enjoy life and to withstand challenges; it is not merely the absence of disease. Negative health is associated with illness, and in the extreme, with premature death.

Health-Enhancing Physical Activity—activity that, when added to baseline activity, produces health benefits. Brisk walking, jumping rope, dancing, playing tennis or soccer, lifting weights, climbing on playground equipment at recess, and doing yoga are all examples of health-enhancing physical activity.

Lifestyle Activities—frequently used to encompass activities that a person carries out in the course of daily life and that can contribute to sizeable energy expenditure. Examples include taking the stairs instead of using the elevator, walking to do errands instead of driving, getting off a bus one stop early, or parking farther away than usual to walk to a destination.

Muscular Endurance—the ability of a muscle or group of muscles to sustain repeated contractions against a resistance for an extended period of time.

Muscular Strength—health component of physical fitness that is the ability of a muscle or muscle group to exert force.

Muscle-Strengthening Activity—physical activity including exercise that increases skeletal muscle strength, power, endurance, and mass.

Physical Activity—bodily movement produced by the contraction of skeletal muscle that increases energy expenditure above a basal level. In these Guidelines, physical activity generally refers to the subset of physical activity that enhances health.

Physical Fitness—ability to carry out daily tasks with vigor and alertness, without undue fatigue, and with ample energy to enjoy leisure-time pursuits and respond to emergencies. Physical fitness includes a number of components consisting of cardiorespiratory endurance (aerobic power), skeletal muscle endurance, skeletal muscle strength, skeletal muscle power, flexibility, balance, speed of movement, reaction time, and body composition.

Progression—The process of increasing the intensity, duration, frequency, or amount of activity or exercise as the body adapts to a given activity pattern.

Quality of Life—individual's perception of overall satisfaction with his or her life; perceptions include physical status and abilities, psychological well-being, social interactions, and economic conditions.

Speed—ability to minimize the time cycle of a repeated movement (running speed or how fast one can perform a repeated movement, such as a barbell movement, jump rope, etc).

CHAPTER 23: STRENGTH AND CONDITIONING COACHING

Body Part Training—bodybuilders (focus is on aesthetics over performance) view the body as individual parts and train one or two of those parts in isolation from the rest.

Bulgarian Method/Specificity Training—an extremely advanced periodization method using only competition movements and one or two other exercises to adapt and gain strength.

Circuit Training—performing back-to-back exercises (usually 2-4 different exercises) without rest intervals.

Concurrent Periodization—multiple physical skills are trained and improved, or at least maintained at the same time (most appropriate for intermediate lifters since strength training alone causes an increase in all physical abilities for a novice lifter).

Conjugate/Block Periodization—specific blocks of training (usually 2-6 weeks long) organized to focus on one specific physical skill or attribute while trying to maintain the others (most appropriate for advanced lifters and athletes.

Duration—time from the beginning of the workout to the end.

Deloading—planned period of training time (usually 1-2 weeks) during a periodization program where intensity, volume, or frequency is reduced to allow for the dissipation of accumulated fatigue.

Density—combination of volume and duration (amount of work in a set time).

Doubles—sets of two reps.

Failure—point in an exercise when the muscles are so fatigued they can't perform any more reps with strict form.

Forced Reps—reps that are performed past failure with the assistance of a spotter.

Full Body Training—Training the entire body in one session. CrossFit also utilizes full body training.

Frequency—how often – number of times a movement is trained in a week, how often a muscle group is trained a week, or how often a workout is performed in a week.

Intensity—how heavy a weight is in comparison to the one-rep max (the maximum amount of weight that can be lifted for a given exercise). The heavier the weight, the more intense the lift.

Linear Progression—one variable (usually intensity or weight) incrementally increased per workout to invoke the stress-recovery-adaptation response.

Loading—planned period of training time (usually 1-3 weeks) during a periodization program of increased intensity, volume, or frequency where the body is not allowed to fully recover. Fatigue is slowly allowed to build.

One Repetition Maximum—maximum amount of weight that can be lifted for a given exercise.

Over-Reaching—occurs when the stressor is such that it cannot be fully recovered from before the next session, and thus some fatigue accumulates.

Over-Training—occurs when over-reaching stressors occur with too much frequency or with such intensity that the body *cannot* recover and adapt, causing a break in the stress-recovery-adaptation cycle.

Periodization—planned programming, which includes a variation in volume, intensity, and/or frequency, and often involves loading and deloading for maximal strength and power benefit.

Personal Record—most weight ever lifted on a particular lift.

Plyometrics—type of exercise that involves a rapid eccentric contraction followed quickly by explosive concentric contraction. Used to increase power and speed. The most common plyometric exercises involve jumping movements.

Repetition—number of times a weight is lifted and lowered in one set of an exercise.

Set—group of repetitions.

Split Training—instead of doing lifts that train the entire body in a single workout, the focus is only on one major section or movement.

Stress-Recovery-Adaptation Cycle—based on the principle outlined in Hans Selye's "General Adaption Syndrome," stating that when the body is exposed to stress it will begin a biological process to deal with the stress, recover from it, and then adapt and compensate so that it is better prepared to handle it if exposed to the same stressors again.

Triples—sets of three reps.

Volume—number of total reps and sets in a given workout.

Western Periodization—the most popular form of programming for intermediate and early-advanced strength athletes, where programming moves from higher volume and lower intensity (12–16 weeks out from a competition), to high intensity and lower volume as the competition approaches.

CHAPTER 24: FUTURE KINESIOLOGY

Paradigm—a pattern, archetype or set of rules, especially as related to a set way of viewing or doing things within one's world view.

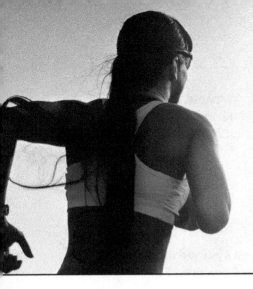

INDEX

CPSIA information can be obtained
at www.ICGtesting.com
Printed in the USA
FSHW011618150819
61057FS

9 781465 297686